Psychopharmacology Series 7

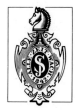

Clinical Pharmacology in Psychiatry

From Molecular Studies to Clinical Reality

Editors

S. G. Dahl L. F. Gram

With 76 Figures

Springer-Verlag Berlin Heidelberg New York
London Paris Tokyo Hong Kong

Prof. Dr. Svein G. Dahl

Professor of Pharmacology, Department of Pharmacology,
Institute of Medical Biology, University of Tromsø School of Medicine,
9001 Tromsø, Norway

Prof. Dr. Lars F. Gram

Professor of Clinical Pharmacology, Department of Clinical Pharmacology,
School of Medicine, Odense University, 5000 Odense C, Denmark

---

Vols. 1 and 2 of this series appeared under the titel "Psychopharmacology Supplementum"

ISBN 3-540-50770-1 Springer-Verlag Berlin Heidelberg New York
ISBN 0-387-50770-1 Springer-Verlag New York Berlin Heidelberg

Library of Congress Cataloging-in-Publication Data. Clinical pharmacology in psychiatrie: from molecular studies to clinical reality/editors, S.G.Dahl, L.F.Gram. p. cm. – (Psychopharmacology series; 7) Papers presented at the 5th International Meeting on Clinical Pharmacology in Psychiatry, held June 26–30, 1988 at the University of Tromsø, Norway. Includes index. ISBN 0-387-50770-1 (U.S.: alk. paper) 1. Psychopharmacology – Congresses. I. Dahl, S. G. (Svein G.), II. Gram, Lars F. III. International Meeting on Clinical Pharmacology in Psychiatry (5th: 1988: University of Tromsø) IV. Series. [DNLM: 1. Psychotropic Drugs – pharmacology – congresses. 2. Psychotropic Drugs – therapeutic use – congresses. W1 PS773J v. 7/QV 77 C6405 1988] RM300.C555 1989 615'.788–dc20 DNLM/DLC for Library of Congress.

© Springer-Verlag Berlin Heidelberg 1989
Printed in Germany

Typesetting, printing and bookbinding: Brühlsche Universitätsdruckerei, Giessen
2125/3130-543210 – Printed on acid-free paper

Preface

This volume collects the invited lectures and some selected contributions presented at the 5th International Meeting on Clinical Pharmacology in Psychiatry, which was held 26–30 June 1988 at the University of Tromsø, Norway. The 24 h of daylight at the northernmost university in the world allowed for long, pleasant and productive sessions. The title of the conference as well as a number of the topics covered represent a continuation of four previous conferences, the first held in Chicago in 1979 and organized by the late Earl Usdin and colleagues.

The earlier conferences have been documented in *Clinical Pharmacology in Psychiatry,* edited by E. Usdin (Elsevier, New York, 1981), *Clinical Pharmacology in Psychiatry. Neuroleptic and Antidepressant Research,* edited by E. Usdin, S. G. Dahl, L. F. Gram and O. Lingjærde (Macmillan Publishers Ltd., London, 1981), *Clinical Pharmacology in Psychiatry. Bridging the Experimental-Therapeutic Gap,* edited by L. F. Gram, E. Usdin, S. G. Dahl, P. Kragh-Sørensen, P. L. Morselli and F. Sjöqvist (Macmillan Publishers Ltd., London, 1983), and *Clinical Pharmacology in Psychiatry. Selectivity in Psychotropic Drug Action – Promises or Problems?* edited by S. G. Dahl, L. F. Gram, S. M. Paul and W. Z. Potter (Psychopharmacology Series 3, Springer, Heidelberg, 1987).

It seems to us that the key to the success of the IMCPP series, and the main reason for its continuation, lies in its interdisciplinary approach in discussing both clinical and basic research. The present volume contains a session on different strategies in the development of new psychotropic drugs, from molecular to clinical studies. The clinical advantages of the new generation of receptor-selective drugs in psychopharmacology was the main topic of the 4th International Meeting on Clinical Pharmacology in Psychiatry, and this theme is updated in one of the sessions presented in this volume. Clinical pharmacokinetics and the rationale for therapeutic plasma level monitoring of neuroleptic and antidepressant drugs have been important topics at this and all previous conferences. This volume extends the field with a session on pharmacogenetics and presents the first comprehensive analysis of the role of the sparteine-debrisoquine drug oxidation polymorphism in psychopharmacology, with clinical implications.

It is our hope that the scientific presentations in this volume may stimulate further research and development towards improved efficacy and safety of psychotropic drugs.

Tromsø, Odense, 1989   SVEIN G. DAHL · LARS F. GRAM

Acknowledgements

The 5th International Meeting on Clinical Pharmacology in Psychiatry would not have been possible without the generous financial support received from a number of institutions and pharmaceutical companies, which we gratefully acknowledge:

The University of Tromsø, The Norwegian Research Council for Science and the Humanities, Astra, Beecham, Ciba-Geigy, Delagrange, Delalande, Duphar, Eli Lilly, Essex, Fabre, Ferrosan Denmark, Ferrosan Sweden, I.C.I., I.R.I.S., Janssen, Lundbeck Foundation, Merrell Dow, Novo, Organon, Parke-Davis, Pfizer, Rhône-Poulenc, Roche, Roussel Uclaf, Sanofi, Schering, Upjohn.

The members of the organizing committee for the Fifth International Meeting on Clinical Pharmacology in Psychiatry were:

Svein G. Dahl, University of Tromsø, Norway.
Lars F. Gram, Odense University, Odense, Denmark.
Stuart A. Montgomery, St Mary's Hospital, London, UK.

The members of the Scientific Advisory Committee were:

Luc P. Balant, Université de Genève, Geneva, Switzerland.
Leif Bertilsson, Huddinge University Hospital, Huddinge, Sweden.
Herbert Y. Meltzer, Case Western Reserve University, Cleveland, Ohio, USA.
Steven M. Paul, National Institute of Mental Health, Maryland, USA.
William Z. Potter, National Institute of Mental Health, Maryland, USA.
Pierre Simon, Societé Sanofi Recherche, Paris, France.
Edouard Zarifian, Centre Psychiatrique Esquirol, Caen, France.

We would also like to thank Eldbjørg Heimstad and Gustav Wik, Tromsø, and the other staff members at the Department of Pharmacology, University of Tromsø and at Åsgård Psychiatric Hospital, who helped with the local arrangements during the conference.

Contents

Clinical Significance of Receptor-Selective Drugs

Pharmacogenetics in Psychopharmacology

Clinical Significance of Pharmacokinetic Variability

Dose-Finding Problems with Psychotropic Drugs

List of Contributors

You will find the addresses at the beginning of the respective contribution

Ågren, H.   40
Alfredsson, G.   303
Altamura, A.C.   263
Andersen, P.H.   3
Aravagiri, M.   269
Arnt, J.   109
Arrang, J.M.   10
Balant, L.P.   211, 228
Balant-Gorgia, A.E.   211, 228
Bareggi, S.R.   263
Baron, J.C.   20
Bech, P.   81
Benítez, J.   206
Bensimon, G.   296
Bertilsson, L.   52
Blin, J.   20
Boulenger, J.P.   20
Braestrup, C.   3
Brinkmann, R.   311
Brøsen, K.   172, 192
Caillard, V.   20
Cambon, H.   20
Cavallaro, R.   263
Charney, D.S.   94
Cobaleda, J.   206
Dahl, S.G.   60
Dahl-Puustinen, M.-L.   52
Dahlqvist, R.   201
Danjou, P.   296
Delgado, P.   94
Delini-Stula, A.   287
Dumont, E.   201
Edvardsen, Ø.   60
Farde, L.   32
Garbarg, M.   10
García, M.A.   206

Garver, D.L.   244
Gex-Fabry, M.   228
Goodman, W.   94
Gram, L.F.   172, 192
Grant, D.M.   141
Guengerich, F.P.   163
Haffner, F.   280
Hall, H.   123
Heimstad, E.   60
Heninger, G.R.   94
Hsiao, J.K.   40
Huret, J.D.   20
Hyttel, J.   109
Jatlow, P.I.   219
Jönsson, E.   303
Kalow, W.   148
Köhler, C.   123
Lacomblez, L.   296
Llerena, A.   206
Loc'h, C.   20
Magnusson, O.   123
Marder, S.R.   269
Mårtensson, E.   257
Martínez, C.   206
Martinot, J.L.   20
Mauri, M.   263
Maziere, B.   20
Mazure, C.   219
Meltzer, H.Y.   68
Meyer, U.A.   141
Montgomery, S.A.   105
Movin, G.   163
Nelson, J.C.   219
Nilsson, L.   32
Nordin, C.   52, 163
Nyberg, G.   257

Strategies in Psychotropic Drug Innovation

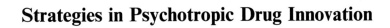

Receptor Subtypes and Endogenous Ligands: Rational Tools in the Search for Psychotropic Drugs?

C. Braestrup and P. H. Andersen [1]

1 Introduction

Relatively few new pharmacodynamic principles have been introduced in the late 1970s and early 1980s for the treatment of psychiatric disorders. This may reflect the type of experimental procedures used in the late 1960s and early 1970s, when animal models for psychiatric diseases were widely used for screening in the early discovery phases. These models, which were usually based on the performance of known efficacious psychotropic drugs, had a tendency to produce compounds which were similar to already known drugs. Today it seems that more rational approaches to the development of new CNS-active compounds have evolved in parallel with the explosive development in receptor research, and the results of these approaches are beginning to emerge.

In hindsight, it appears that most psychoactive drugs owe their therapeutic effects to an interaction with one or more brain receptors or receptor-like structures. Among the various receptor types depicted in Table 1, psychoac-

Table 1. Receptor types

Neurotransmitter receptors
Hormone receptors
Immune receptors
Drug receptors
Toxin receptors
Taste receptors
Uptake "receptors"

tive drugs are known to interact with neurotransmitter receptors, drug receptors and "uptake receptors". It is probable that new efficacious psychotropic drugs with fewer side effects can be developed from our current and future knowledge of brain receptors. In particular, it seems useful to pursue compounds with receptor subtype selectivity and those which mimic in one or another way the action of endogenously occurring neurotransmitters or brain modulators.

[1] Pharmaceuticals R&D, Novo-Nordisk A/S, 2880 Bagsværd, Denmark

Clinical Pharmacology in Psychiatry
Editors: S. G. Dahl and L. F. Gram
(Psychopharmacology Series 7)
© Springer-Verlag Berlin Heidelberg 1989

2 Receptor Subtypes

The concept of receptor subtypes is well known. Cholinergic receptors were divided into the nicotinic and muscarinic subtypes, named after the selective agonists used to identify their existence, and α- and β-receptors represent the early subclasses of adrenergic receptors. Since then, subclassification has continued, using either numbering systems (histamine H_3 for a recent example; Arrang et al. 1987) or naming systems (with quisqualate and nonquisqualate excitatory amino acid receptors as recent examples; Drejer and Honoré 1988).

The application of molecular biology has resulted in a new understanding of receptor classification and of receptor subtypes. Surprisingly, it appears that receptors seem to belong to relatively few major families which are the products of gene superfamilies. Receptors which were previously classified in quite distinct groups, such as γ-aminobutyric acid (GABA) and nicotinic receptors, belong to one single family and must be regarded, in principle, as subclasses of the same ancient receptor. Nicotinic and GABAergic receptors belong to an ion channel gating receptor family to which glycine receptors also belong. Cloning has revealed that nicotinic receptors, GABA receptors and glycine receptors are homologous proteins having certain highly conserved regions; they clearly seem to originate from a common ancestor gene (Barnard et al. 1987).

Receptors which are coupled to G proteins and adenylate cyclase represent another superfamily; receptors within this category span from α- and β-adrenergic receptors to the light receptor rhodopsin (Lefkowitz and Caron 1988).

Subclasses for each of the receptor types in a superfamily easily emerge from further mutations, and we must foresee the discovery of many additional receptor subclasses which will be identified by cloning and sequencing of their genes, and which might constitute new specific targets for drugs. Examples are available today; the CNS nicotinic receptor seems to exist in several genetic forms, the pharmacology of which is still unknown (Boulter et al. 1987). Genetically defined receptor subtypes will be available for pharmacological screening and investigation after expression of the receptor on the surface of appropriate cell systems.

Before receptor subtypes were defined genetically, subclassification was based primarily on data obtained from binding or functional studies (e.g. the muscarinic receptor; Hulme et al. 1976; Birdsall et al. 1978). Further, before the definite genetic evidence for the existence of such muscarinic receptor subtypes was available (Bonner et al. 1987), compounds selective for the proposed subtypes were developed (e.g. pirenzepine and McN A-343; Hammer and Giachetti 1982; Hammer et al. 1980). Several other neurotransmitter receptors have been proposed to exist in one or more subtypes, e.g. the α_1-receptor (Morrow and Creese 1986), the α_2-receptor (Kaposci et al. 1987) and recently the dopamine D_1 receptor (Andersen and Braestrup 1986). Since none of these three receptor classes has yet been cloned, no genetic evidence is available to support the presence of a distinct genetic variety.

Table 2. Pharmacological charateristics of [^{3}H]SCH 23390 binding and dopamine-stimulated adenylate cylase in rat striatum

Compound	Dopamine-stimulated adenylate cyclase (K_i, nM)	[^{3}H]SCH 23390 binding (K_i, nM)	(Rank)
SCH 23390	39.9	0.14	(1)
cis-Flupentixol	40.0	0.32	(2)
(+)-Butaclamol	81.8	0.95	(3)
Fluphenazine	212	4.5	(4)
Chlorpromazine	463	25	(5)
Bulbocapnine	865	270	(6)
trans-Flupentixol	1200	474	(7)
Spiroperidol	1720	360	(8)
(−)-Butaclamol	> 5000	> 9000	(9)
NB 106-094	> 5000	> 5000	(9)
Dibenzepin	> 5000	> 5000	(9)
l-Sulpiride	> 5000	> 15000	
Clopazine	32.5	55	
Fluperlapine	26.6	85	
Clothiapine	33.9	8	

K_i values obtained from [^{3}H]SCH 23390 binding were calculated from $K_i = IC_{50}/(1 + L/K_D)$, where IC_{50} is the drug concentration that inhibits specifically bound [^{3}H]SCH 23390 by 50%, L is the concentration of [^{3}H]SCH 23390 (0.2 nM), and K_i is the dissociation constant of [^{3}H]SCH 23390 (0.14 nM). K_i values are means from at least three independent experiments using three to eight different inhibitor concentrations. K_i values for inhibition of dopamine-stimulated adenylate cyclase were obtained by Schild analyses using three different antagonist concentrations and five different concentrations of dopamine (10, 30, 60, 100, 200 nM). Values are means from two to eight independent experiments (Andersen et al. 1985; Andersen and Braestrup 1986).

With respect to psychiatric diseases, and in particular to one of the major psychoses, schizophrenia, dopamine is thought to play a major role. The dopamine D_1 receptor subtype was originally defined as a receptor associated with the enzyme adenylate cyclase in a stimulatory way (Kebabian and Calne 1979). No selective compounds for the dopamine D_1 receptor were available, however, before the introduction of SCH 23390 (Hyttel 1983). Radiolabelling of this compound produced a ligand highly specific for the dopamine D_1 receptor (Billard et al. 1984; Schulz et al. 1984). In a later study, where both binding to and a functional measurement of the dopamine D_1 receptor was investigated under identical biochemical conditions, an unexpected discrepancy was observed. The absolute K_i values obtained for inhibition of [^{3}H]SCH 23390 binding and dopamine-stimulated adenylate cyclase for a variety of typical neuroleptics were not identical, although the rank order of potencies was similar (see Table 2; Andersen et al. 1985).

In a follow-up study it was further shown that whereas typical neuroleptics exhibited much higher affinity for the D_1 receptor labelled with [^{3}H]SCH 23390 than for inhibition of the dopamine-stimulated adenylate cyclase, atypical neuroleptics of the clozapine type showed the opposite characteristic, i.e.

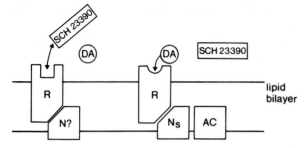

Fig. 1. Diagrammatic representation of an extended two-state model for the two subtypes of states of the dopamine D_1 subtype, illustrating the adenylate cyclase coupled and uncoupled receptors. Included is the guanosine triphosphate (GTP) sensitive protein (*N?*) to explain data with dopamine inhibition of [^{3}H]SCH 23390 binding. *DA*, Dopamine; *R*, D_1 receptor; *Ns* and *N?*, GTP regulatory protein; *AC*, adenylate cyclase catalytic unit

highest affinity for inhibition of the adenylate cyclase (Andersen and Braestrup 1986). These data indicated the existence of subtypes or of different coupling states of the dopamine D_1 receptor. A model was suggested postulating the existence of two states of the D_1 receptor, one coupled to the adenylate cyclase and the other uncoupled (Fig. 1; Andersen and Braestrup 1986). This model was later corroborated in radiation inactivation experiments (Andersen and Nielsen 1987). Several lines of evidence have since accumulated in support of the existence of subtypes of the dopamine D_1 receptor subtype. In some of these studies, selective dopamine D_1 agonists exhibiting various efficacies were used. Waddington et al. (1988) rated the dopamine D_1 mediated behaviour grooming in rodents and showed that both partial and full efficacy agonists induced behavioural changes to the same extent. This observation was confirmed in a study by Arnt et al. (1988) using selective dopamine D_1 receptor depletion with EEDQ (*N*-ethoxycarbonyl-2-ethoxy-1,2-dihydroquinoline), thereby excluding the spare-receptor explanation. Furthermore, data from electrophysiological studies have supported a subdivision of the dopamine D_1 receptor. Thus, a variety of dopamine D_1 agonists stimulate dopamine D_1 mediated changes in cell firing irrespective of their efficacy in stimulating the adenylate cyclase (White et al. 1987). Also, lipophilic cyclic adenosine monophosphate (cAMP) derivatives or blockers of cAMP degradation had no effect on the dopamine D_1 stimulation (Johansen and White 1988), as would be expected if all the receptors were coupled to adenylate cyclase. Finally, the action of concurrent dopamine D_1 and D_2 receptor stimulation is additive or synergistic and not opposite (White 1987), as observed in biochemical studies (Kelly and Nahorski 1987).

All these behavioural, biochemical, and electrophysiological data are best interpreted by the presence of dopamine D_1 receptor subtypes; one subtype is linked to the adenylate cyclase whereas the other is not linked to this enzyme.

Table 3. Occupation of receptors in vivo by neuroleptic compounds

Compound	Administration	ED_{50} (mg/kg)			
		D_1	D_2	5-HT_2	Muscarinic
SCH 23390	sc, 0.5 h	0.017	5.6	1	> 30
cis-Flupentixol	ip, 2 h	0.3	0.1	0.4	> 10
Clozapine	sc, 1 h	10.2	1	0.7	3
Fluperlapine	sc, 1 h	0.8	9.6	2.8	> 10
dl-Sulpiride	ip, 2 h	90	25	35	>100
Molindone	ip, 2 h	51	0.6	43	59

ED_{50} is the dose which occupies by 50% the receptor population available for each specific ligand. D_1 receptor, [^{3}H]SCH 23390; D_2, [^{3}H]spiroperidol; 5-HT_2, [^{3}H]ketanserin; muscarinic, [^{3}H]QNB. (Values from Andersen et al. 1986, and unpublished).

In the development of new neuroleptics, the two most important goals seem to be improvement of therapeutic efficacy and reduction in the incidence of side effects such as extrapyramidal effects and tardive dyskinesias.

Clozapine – the prototype atypical neuroleptic – is efficacious, with effects against both the negative and the positive symptoms of schizophrenia and is virtually without extrapyramidal side effects. Surprisingly, clozapine and the closely related analogue fluperlapine show an appreciable affinity for the dopamine D_1 receptor (Table 2). In addition to the dopamine D_1 receptor, clozapine also affects several other receptors (see Hyttel et al., this volume). The high in vitro affinity of clozapine and fluperlapine for the dopamine D_1 receptor is also reflected in in vivo studies (Table 3); clozapine and fluperlapine act on [^{3}H]SCH 23390 labelled receptors in the low mg/kg range. Fluperlapine even showed preference for D_1 receptors, as compared to the other receptors measured (Table 3).

The unexpectedly high dopamine D_1 activity found for clozapine and fluperlapine becomes even more pronounced when the adenylate cyclase coupled dopamine D_1 receptor is considered. While all other neuroleptics were most active on the [^{3}H]SCH 23390 labelled dopamine D_1 receptor, clozapine and fluperlapine showed preference for the adenylate cyclase coupled dopamine D_1 receptor. This unique feature may explain why early proposals of a dopamine receptor involvement in the mechanism of action of clozapine seemed evasive in biochemical experiments. Having the adenylate cyclase linked dopamine D_1 sub-subtype as a target for the atypical neuroleptic, clozapine opens a screening possibility which may lead to new classes of atypical neuroleptics with a clozapine-like profile.

3 Conclusion

The preceding section describes how the detailed investigation of subtypes, or potential subtypes, of the dopamine D_1 receptor may lead to new strategies for screening putatively useful new psychotropic drugs. Another useful approach has been the search for endogenous ligands for drug receptors which may represent a source of new leads, with new mechanisms of action and new spectra of activity.

Recently, Barbaccia et al. (1988) reviewed this approach for the GABA/benzodiazepine receptor chloride channel complex by highlighting β-carbolines, diazepam binding inhibitor (DBI) and other peptides as leads for developing new psychotropic drugs. It should be recognized in this respect, however, that the discovery of new drug receptors may not guarantee the existence of an endogenous ligand to form new drug leads. Our current understanding is that drug receptors may exist which do not have natural modulators, i.e. drug receptors may simply be random regions of macro-molecules which happen to bind certain drugs.

With exact determination of the three-dimensional structure of proteins, the identification of new "drug binding regions" should be possible. Future drug development combining molecular biology with knowledge of the three-dimensional protein structure may result in a new generation of highly specific drugs.

References

Andersen PH, Braestrup C (1986) Evidence for different states of the dopamine D1 receptor: clozapine and fluperlapine may preferentially label an adenylate cyclase-coupled state of the D1 receptor. J Neurochem 47:1822–1831

Andersen PH, Nielsen M (1987) Irradiation inactivation studies of the dopamine D_1 receptor and dopamine-stimulated adenylate cyclase in rat striatum. Neurosci Lett 83:167–172

Andersen PH, Grønvald FC, Jansen JAa (1985) A comparison between dopamine-stimulated adenylate cyclase and ^{3}H-SCH 23390 binding in rat striatum. Life Sci 37:1977–1983

Andersen PH, Nielsen EB, Grønvald FC, Braestrup C (1986) Some atypical neuroleptics inhibit [^{3}H]SCH 23390 binding in vivo. Eur J Pharmacol 120:143–144

Arnt J, Hyttel J, Meier E (1988) Inactivation of dopamine D-1 or D-2 receptors differentially inhibits stereotypes induced dopamine agonists in rats. Eur J Pharmacol (in press)

Arrang JM, Garbarg M, Lancelot JC, Lecomte JM, Pollard H, Robba M, Schunack W, Schartz JC (1987) Highly potent and selective ligands for histamine H3-receptors. Nature 327:117–123

Barbaccia ML, Costa E, Guidotti A (1988) Endogenous ligands for high-affinity recognition sites of psychotropic drugs. Annu Rev Pharmacol Toxicol 28:451–476

Barnard EA, Darlison MG, Seeburg P (1987) Molecular biology of the $GABA_A$ receptor: the receptor/channel superfamily. Trends Neurosci 10:502–509

Billard W, Ruperto V, Crosby G, Iorio LC, Barnett A (1984) Characterization of the binding of ^{3}H-SCH 23390, a selective D1 receptor antagonist ligand, in rat striatum. Life Sci 35:1885–1893

Birdsall NJM, Burgen ASV, Hulme EC (1978) The binding of agonists to brain muscarinic receptors. Mol Pharmacol 14:723–736

Bonner TI, Buckley NJ, Young AC, Brann MR (1987) Identification of a family of muscarinic acetylcholine receptor genes. Science 237:527–532

Boulter J, Connolly J, Deneris E, Goldman D, Heinemann S, Patrick J (1987) Functional expression of two neuronal nicotinic acetylcholine receptors from cDNA clones identifies a gene family. Proc Natl Acad Sci USA 84:7763–7767

Casey PJ, Gilman AG (1988) G protein involvement in recepter-effector coupling. Biol Chem 263:2577–2580

Drejer J, Honoré T (1988) Excitatory amino acid receptors. In: Elling K (ed) Glutamine and glutamate in mammals, vol 2. CRC, Boca Raton, pp 89–109

Hammer R, Giachetti A (1982) Muscarinic receptor subtypes M1 and M2: biochemical and functional characterization. Life Sci 31:2991–2998

Hammer R, Berrie CP, Birdsall NJ, Burgen AS, Hulme EC (1980) Pirenzepine distinguishes between different subclasses of muscarinic receptors. Nature 283:90–92

Hulme EC, Burgen ASV, Birdsall NJM (1976) Interactions of agonists and antagonists with the muscarinic receptor. In: Worcel M, Vassort G (eds) Smooth muscle pharmacology and physiology. Inserm, Paris, pp 49–70

Hyttel J (1983) SCH 23390 – the first selective dopamine D1 antagonist. Eur J Pharmacol 91:153–154

Johansen PA, White FJ (1988) D1/D2 dopamine receptor interactions in the nucleus accumbens: the role of cAMP in electrophysiological responses. Soc Neurosci Abstr 14(2):931

Kapocsi J, Somogyi GT, Ludvig N, Sefozo P, Harsin LG Jr, Woods RJ, Vizi ES (1987) Neurochemical evidence for two types of presynaptic alpha$_2$-adrenoceptors. Neurochem Res 12:141–147

Kebabian JW, Calne DB (1979) Multiple receptors for dopamine. Nature 277:93–96

Kelly E, Nahorski SR (1987) Endogenous dopamine functionally activates D-1 and D-2 receptors in striatum. J Neurochem 49:115–120

Lefkowitz RJ, Caron MG (1988) Adrenergic receptors as models for the study of receptors coupled to guanine nucleotide regulatory proteins. J Biol Chem 263:4993–4996

Morrow AL, Creese I (1986) Characterization of α_1-adrenergic receptor subtypes in rat brain: a reevaluation of [^{3}H]WB4104 and [^{3}H]prazosin binding. Mol Pharmacol 29:321–330

Nielsen EB, Randrup K, Andersen PH (1989) Amphetamine discrimination: effects of dopamine receptor agonists. Eur J Pharmacol 160:253–262

Schulz DW, Wyrick SD, Mailman RB (1984) ^{3}H-SCH 23390 has the characteristics of a dopamine receptor ligand in the rat central nervous system. Eur J Pharmacol 106:211–212

Wachtel SR, Galloway MP, White FJ (1988) D1 dopamine receptor stimulation enables the postsynaptic but not autoreceptor effects of D2 dopamine agonists. Soc Neurosci Abstr 14(2):1077

Waddington JL, O'Boyle KM, Murray AM (1988) Stimulation of dopamine-sensitive adenylate cyclase and induction of grooming behaviour by new selective D-1 agonists. Neurochem Int [Suppl 1] 13:F326

White FJ (1987) D-1 dopamine receptor stimulation enables the inhibition of nucleus accumbens neurons by a D-2 receptor agonist. Eur J Pharmacol 135:101

White FJ, Wachtel SR, Johansen PA, Einhorn LC (1987) Electrophysiological studies of the rat mesoaccumbens dopamine system: focus on dopamine receptor subtypes, interactions, and the effects of cocaine. In: Chiodo LA, Freeman AS (eds) Neurophysiology of dopaminergic systems – current status and clinical perspectives. Lakeshore, Grosse Pointe, pp 317–365

Histamine H$_3$ Receptors in the Brain: Potent and Selective Ligands

J. C. SCHWARTZ, J. M. ARRANG, M. GARBARG, and H. POLLARD [1]

1 Introduction

Histamine is a recently admitted neurotransmitter in the brain, and few drugs are available which selectively modify histaminergic neurotransmission for either research or, possibly, therapeutic purposes.

Most histaminergic neurons are located in the tuberomamillary nucleus, a group of a few hundred magnicellular neurons in the ventral part of the posterior hypothalamus. Their axons constitute long ascending pathways projecting mainly in an ipsilateral fashion, to the entire CNS. Hence the general disposition of the histamine neuronal system, with a few compact cell groups and a widespread distribution of long axons, resembles that of catecholaminergic and serotoninergic systems. These similarities extend to receptor-mediated cellular events and to functional roles. Although the latter are still incompletely understood, it appears that histaminergic neurons may control arousal, energy metabolism, cerebral circulation, cardiovascular reflexes, pituitary hormone release and body temperature. Some histaminergic neurons also store γ-aminobutyric acid, the gastrointestinal peptide galanin, or, possibly, adenosine, but the functional significance of these co-localizations is still unknown. In addition, the CNS contains a small number of histamine-rich mast cells. These connective tissue cells seem closely associated with vascular elements in the CNS. As in peripheral tissues, they may be involved in immune and inflammatory processes, but this remains to be established (reviewed in Schwartz et al. 1986).

2 Post-Synaptic Histamine Receptors

Until recently two subclasses of receptors were believed to mediate the actions of histamine on target cells. They can be distinguished by their pharmacology and by the intracellular responses which they mediate (Hill 1987).

[1] Unité de Neurobiologie et Pharmacologie (U. 109) de l'Inserm, Centre Paul Broca, 2ter rue d'Alésia, 75014 Paris, France

Clinical Pharmacology in Psychiatry
Editors: S. G. Dahl and L. F. Gram
(Psychopharmacology Series 7)
© Springer-Verlag Berlin Heidelberg 1989

2.1 H$_1$ Receptors

H$_1$ receptors are pharmacologically defined by their blockade by many "classical" antihistamines, the prototype of which is mepyramine (pyrilamine; Table 1).

H$_1$ receptors visualized by autoradiography are widely and heterogeneously distributed in the CNS (Bouthenet et al. 1988), but their distribution, which differs among animal species, does not match exactly that of histaminergic axons. From their decrease following ablation of neurons by kainate, a

Table 1. Pharmacology of the three subclasses of histamine receptors

		Receptor subclasses		
		H$_1$	H$_2$	H$_3$
	Agonists (relative potencies)			
Histamine		100	100	100
2-Thiazolylethylamine		26	2.2	<0.01
Impromidine		<0.01	4800	<0.01
(R)α-Methylhistamine		0.5	1	1500
	Antagonists (K$_i$ values, nM)			
Mepyramine		0.4	–	>3000
Cimetidine		450000	800	33000
Thioperamide		>100000	>10000	4

neurotoxin, they appear to be at least partly located on neuronal membranes, where they may act as post-synaptic receptors. H_1 receptors also seem to be present on glial cells and cerebral microvessels (Gross 1985), on which they may mediate smooth-muscle contraction or permeability changes, or both, elicited by histamine.

H_1-receptor stimulation triggers various responses in neural tissues such as cyclic guanosine monophosphate formation, glycogenolysis, or augmentation of cyclic adenosine monophosphate (cyclic AMP) accumulation, which all have in common a requirement for intact cells and the presence of Ca^{2+} in the external medium. It is therefore likely that Ca^{2+} mobilization is a universal consequence of H_1-receptor activation.

An early cellular event associated with activation of many receptors mediating Ca^{2+} mobilization is the hydrolysis of inositol phospholipids with generation of the two second messengers: diacylglycerol, a protein kinase C activator, and inositol phosphates which mobilize Ca^{2+} from intracellular stores. That H_1 receptors belong to this category was first suggested by the observation that their stimulation accelerates the incorporation of inorganic ^{32}P into cerebral phospholipids in vivo. More recently, activation of the phosphatidylinositol cycle by stimulation of H_1 receptors in brain slices was demonstrated by monitoring accumulation of [^3H]inositol phosphate in the presence of Li^+, an inositol phosphatase inhibitor (Carswell et al. 1985).

Although H_1 receptors are not directly coupled to adenylate cyclase, their activation in brain slices results in an increased accumulation of cyclic AMP when cyclase-coupled receptors, e.g. histamine H_2 receptors, adenosine A_2 receptors, or β-adrenoreceptors, are simultaneously activated. Both types of intracellular second messengers generated by the phosphatidylinositol cycle, diacylglycerol and inositol phosphates, seem to be involved in this potentiating effect (Garbarg and Schwartz 1988).

From a physiological point of view, stimulation of cerebral H_1 receptors powerfully triggers the release of vasopressin and, possibly, of adrenocorticotropin.

Finally, most H_1-receptor antagonists easily crossing the blood-brain barrier cause sedation or drowsiness ("mental clouding"), presumably attributable to impairment of the arousal function of histaminergic neurons (Schwartz 1977). This common side effect of "classical" antihistamines used in allergy has led to the recent development of several compounds, such as mequitazine, terfenadine, and astemizole, which do not easily cross the blood-brain barrier and are, therefore, largely devoid of sedative side effects.

2.2 H_2 Receptors

Impromidine, a partial but highly potent and rather selective agonist, and a series of antagonists, the prototype of which is cimetidine, define the H_2 receptor pharmacologically (Table 1). These two compounds, as well as other selective agonists (e.g. dimaprit) or antagonists (e.g. ranitidine, tiotidine, and famotidine) are hydrophilic molecules which do not easily cross the blood-brain barrier.

As in other tissues, H_2 receptors in the brain are coupled with adenylate cyclase, and their stimulation in guinea-pig hippocampal membranes increases the activity of the enzyme by about threefold. By contrast, histamine stimulates cyclic AMP accumulation in hippocampal slices by 10- to 20-fold, but in this preparation, the response involves both H_1 and H_2 receptors. Another difference between the H_2-receptor mediated cyclic AMP response in cell-free and whole-cell preparations is that, in the former, a number of compounds, e.g. several tricyclic antidepressants, display anomalously high antagonist activity. This is not the case in whole-cell preparation, a difference which is still poorly understood, but which casts some doubts on the hypothesis that H_2-receptor blockade in brain represents the common mechanism of antidepressant action of tricyclic compounds (Nowak et al. 1983).

Lesion and subcellular fraction studies suggest that H_2 receptors are located on neurons, and that some synaptic actions of histamine are mediated by cyclic AMP. The cyclic nucleotide could well act in the target neuron by decreasing a Ca^{2+}-activated K^+ conductance, presumably via protein phosphorylation reactions. In turn, this conductance effect results in a disinhibition of target neurons, which thereby become more sensitive to a variety of excitatory signals such as those mediated by the neurotransmitter glutamate (Haas 1984). Because histamine also has a slight hyperpolarizing effect, also mediated by H_2 receptors, stimulation of the latter results in an enhancement of signal-to-noise ratio in targets cells: their responses to stimuli near action potential threshold are inhibited whereas responses to larger stimuli are enhanced. Other neurotransmitters which, like histamine, are released by highly divergent neurons projecting to the whole cerebral cortex (e.g. noradrenaline or acetylcholine) seem to act through similar mechanisms (when α_1-adrenoreceptors and M_1 muscarinic receptors are involved). All these neurotransmitters, by sharing this essentially modulatory mechanism, may have a "waking" effect, increasing the awareness to a variety of specific stimuli.

In agreement with this idea, the activity of histaminergic neurons, like that of noradrenergic neurons, is increased during arousal and almost abolished during slow-wave sleep (Vanni-Mercier et al. 1984).

Finally, H_2 receptors in the hypothalamus mediate hypothermia and, possibly, the release of the pituitary hormone prolactin.

3 The Presynaptic H_3 Receptor: Definition and Design of Potent and Selective Ligands

The third histamine receptor was only recently discovered and differs from the two others both by its pharmacology (hence its designation as H_3) and by its localization (Arrang et al. 1983, 1985, 1987a, b). It is exquisitely sensitive to histamine and, even more, to the chiral agonist $(R)\alpha$-methylhistamine, which is active at nanomolar concentrations whereas the S isomer is approximately 100-fold less potent. A potent and highly selective antagonist, thioperamide, has also recently been rationally designed (Arrang et al. 1987b). Whereas H_1-receptor antagonists are ineffective, some H_2-receptor agonists (e.g. impromidine) or antagonists (e.g. burimamide) are reasonably potent H_3-receptor antagonists. This last feature suggests that some actions of histamine previously categorized as being mediated by H_2 receptors might, in fact, be attributable to H_3-receptor activation.

Histamine inhibits its own depolarization-induced release via stimulation of H_3 receptors in slices of various brain regions as well as in isolated nerve endings, indicating that they are autoreceptors involved in a local feedback regulation of histamine neurons. It should be underlined that this action is only observed when endogenous stores are labelled with the precursor ^{3}H-labelled amino acid and not with preformed [^{3}H]histamine, presumably because the latter is not selectively taken up into histaminergic axons. In addition, activation of H_3 receptors inhibits the depolarization-induced stimulation of [^{3}H]histamine synthesis (Arrang et al. 1987a).

4 Radioligand Assay and Visualization of H_3 Receptors

The high apparent affinity of $(R)\alpha$-methylhistamine in functional studies suggested that the drug might constitute, when radiolabelled, a suitable probe for H_3-receptor assay and visualization.

Indeed, [^{3}H]$(R)\alpha$-methylhistamine was found to bind in a reversible and saturable manner to cerebral cortex membranes with a K_D of 0.5 nM derived from either saturation kinetics or dissociation/association rates and a maximal number of sites representing 30 ± 3 fmol/mg protein (Table 2; Arrang et al., in preparation). In comparison, H_1 and H_2 receptors appear significantly more abundant.

Sites labelled with [^{3}H]$(R)\alpha$-methylhistamine were pharmacologically identified as H_3 receptors by competition studies with a variety of compounds whose potencies relative to histamine (for agonists) or K_i (for antagonists) were in good agreement with corresponding values derived from functional stu-

Table 2. [^{3}H] (R) α-Methylhistamine binding to H_3 receptors of membranes from rat cerebral cortex

Parameter	Value
Rate of association	0.146 min^{-1} nM^{-1}
Rate of dissociation	0.045 min^{-1}
Dissociation constant (kinetic)	0.31 nM
Dissociation constant (at equilibrium)	0.43 nM
Capacity (B_{max})	30 ± 3 fmol/mg protein
Capacity in the presence of 0.1 mMGppNHp	12 ± 5 fmol/mg protein (-60%)

dies (Table 1). Nevertheless, it can be noticed that K_i values of histamine and agonists in binding studies were generally five to ten times lower than their corresponding EC$_{50}$ values in functional studies. This difference might correspond to differences in the ionic composition of media used in binding and functional studies or to the selective labelling of H$_3$ receptors in a discrete conformational state with high affinity for agonists. The latter hypothesis is consistent with the effect of a non-hydrolysable analogue of the nucleotide guanosine triphosphate which markedly decreases the binding of the agonist (Table 2).

In autoradiographic studies performed with the same ligand (Fig. 1), H$_3$ receptors were found fairly widespread in rat brain, as previously shown in release studies. Telencephalic areas such as the cerebral cortex (particularly in its most rostral part), striatum, hippocampus (molecular layer of the dentate gyrus), lateral septum, bed nucleus of the stria terminalis, and olfactory nuclei, to which diffuse projections of the ascending histaminergic neurons have been evidenced, showed the highest grain densities. In contrast, the cerebellum (all layers), brainstem or mesencephalon (except a few areas, such as the substantia nigra), which contain a lower density of projections, showed fainter labelling. In posterior hypothalamus a thin band of dense labelling was observed in the perimamillary area, which is known to contain most histamine perikarya, suggesting the presence of H$_3$ receptors on the latter. However, in the remainder of hypothalamus, in which levels of L-histidine decarboxylase and histamine are much higher than in telencephalon, a relatively low labelling was

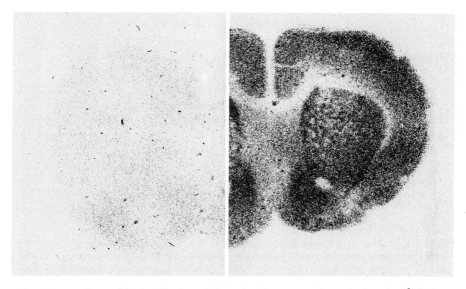

Fig. 1. Autoradiographic visualization of histamine H$_3$ receptors in rat brain using [^{3}H](R)α-methylhistamine as a probe. *Left,* non-specific binding (in the presence of thioperamide); *right,* total binding

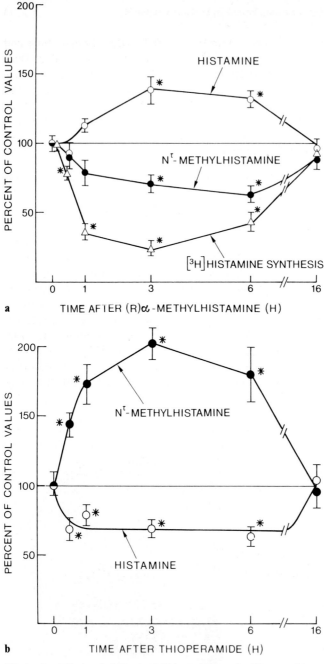

Fig. 2a, b. Effect of $(R)\alpha$-methylhistamine and thioperamide on histamine and N^τ-methylhistamine levels and on [^{3}H]histamine synthesis in rat cerebral cortex. Animals received an oral dose of 10 mg/kg $(R)\alpha$-methylhistamine (**a**) or 5 mg/kg thioperamide (**b**). Histamine levels were measured by a radio-enzymatic assay in a crude P_2 synaptosomal fraction. N^τ-Methylhistamine was measured with a novel radio-immunoassay. [^{3}H]Histamine synthesis was measured 10 min after intravenous administration of [^{3}H]L-histidine; [^{3}H]histamine was isolated by ion-exchange chromatography

observed. This may indicate that H_3 receptors are not restricted to histaminergic neurons, a hypothesis recently confirmed by lesion studies (Pollard et al., in preparation).

5 Histamine H_3 Receptors Control Cerebral Histamine Turnover In Vivo

With the recent design of brain-penetrating ligands selectively interacting with H_3 receptors, it has become feasible to test the role of these receptors in the control of histamine turnover in rat brain in vivo.

Whereas the activity of some monoaminergic neurons, e.g. the dopaminergic neurons, seems at least partly controlled via neuronal feedback loops involving post-synaptic receptors, the activity of others, such as the noradrenergic neurons, seems to be controlled mainly if not solely via autoreceptors.

In the case of histamine the administration of a combination of mepyramine, a H_1-receptor antagonist, and zolantidine, a H_2-receptor antagonist which, like the former, easily crosses the blood-brain barrier, failed to affect [³H]histamine synthesis in the cerebral cortex. In contrast, the administration of $(R)\alpha$-methylhistamine significantly decreased histamine turnover, as shown on a series of indexes: (a) the rate of [³H]histidine, its precursor amino acid; (b) the rate of endogenous histamine depletion after administration of a suicide inhibitor of L-histidine decarboxylase; (c) the steady-state level of tele-methylhistamine, a major histamine metabolite (Fig. 2a).

These actions were not only antagonized by thioperamide but this agent, when administered alone in rather low dosage, also elicited a marked elevation of turnover, indicated on the same indexes (Fig. 2b).

These observations indicate that these agents may constitute useful tools for behavioural investigations on the role of histaminergic neuronal systems in the brain.

6 Histamine H_3 Receptors Control Histamine Release in Human Brain

It is very likely that histamine plays a neurotransmitter role in the human brain as in the brain of other species. Its regional distribution and that of L-histidine decarboxylase, its specific synthetizing enzyme, seem to be roughly parallel to those of these markers in rodent brain. Also H_1 receptors could be characterized in membranes from human brain, and their blockade is likely to account for the sedative effects of many classical H_1 antihistamines (see Schwartz et al. 1986). However, no information is available concerning histamine release in the human brain.

We have recently studied this problem using samples of fresh human cerebral cortex obtained during surgical removal of deep tumors (Arrang et al.

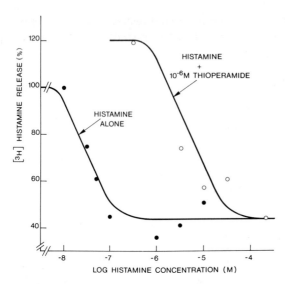

Fig. 3. Evidence for histamine H_3 receptors in human brain. Slices of human cerebral cortex were prepared from fresh tissue samples raised during neurosurgery and preincubated in the presence of [^{3}H]histidine. Neo-synthetized [^{3}H]histamine was released by 30-mM K$^+$ in the absence (100% release) or the presence of exogenous histamine added in increasing concentration. The maximal inhibition elicited by exogenous histamine was about 60% and occurred with an EC_{50} of 35 nM, which was shifted to 2200 nM in the presence of 1-μM thioperamide, leading to a K_i of 16 nM for the latter

1988). Slices were prepared and labelled with [^{3}H]histidine according a procedure essentially similar to that used with rat brain tissues (Arrang et al. 1983). [^{3}H]Histamine was released upon depolarization elicited by 30-mM K$^+$, and this release was progressively inhibited, by up to 60%, in the presence of exogenous histamine with an EC_{50} of 35 ± 5 nM (Fig. 3). The concentration-response curve to the amine was rightward shifted in the presence of thioperamide, leading to a K_i value of the compound of around 10 nM.

These observations identify H_3 receptors as mediating the autoinhibition of histamine release in human brain and suggest that their pharmacology is similar to that of corresponding receptors in rodents.

References

Arrang JM, Garbarg M, Schwartz JC (1983) Autoinhibition of brain histamine release mediated by a novel class (H_3) of histamine receptor. Nature 302:832–837

Arrang JM, Garbarg M, Schwartz JC (1985) Autoregulation of histamine release in brain by presynaptic receptors. Neuroscience 15:553–562

Arrang JM, Garbarg M, Schwartz JC (1987a) Autoinhibition of histamine synthesis mediated by presynaptic H_3-receptors. Neuroscience 23:149–157

Arrang JM, Garbarg M, Lancelot JC et al. (1987b) Highly potent and selective ligands for histamine H_3-receptors. Nature 327:117–123

Arrang JM, Devaux B, Chodkiewicz JP, Schwartz JC (1988) H_3-receptors control histamine release in human brain. J Neurochem 51:105–108

Bouthenet ML, Ruat M, Salès N, Garbarg M, Schwartz JC (1988) A detailed mapping of histamine H_1-receptors in guinea-pig central nervous system established by autoradiography with ^{125}I-iodobolpyramine. Neuroscience 26:553–600

Carswell H, Daum PR, Young JM (1985) Histamine H_1-agonist stimulated breakdown of inositol phospholipids. In: Ganellin CR, Schwartz JC (eds) Frontiers in histamine research. Pergamon, London, pp 27–38

Garbarg M, Schwartz JC (1988) Synergism between histamine H$_1$- and H$_2$-receptors in the cAMP response in guinea pig brain slices: effects of phorbol esters and calcium. Mol Pharmacol 33:38–43

Gross PM (1985) Multiple actions of histamine on cerebral blood vessels. In: Ganellin CR, Schwartz JC (eds) Frontiers in histamine research. Pergamon, London, pp 341–349

Haas HL (1984) Histamine potentiates neuronal excitation by blocking a calcium-dependent potassium conductance. Agents Actions 14:534–537

Hill SJ (1987) Histamine receptors in the mammalian central nervous system: biochemical studies. Prog Med Chem 24:29–84

Nowak JZ, Arrang JM, Schwartz JC, Garbarg M (1983) Interaction between mianserin, an antidepressant drug, and central H$_1$- and H$_2$-histamine-receptors: in vitro and in vivo studies and radioreceptor assay. Neuropharmacology 22:259–266

Schwartz JC (1977) Histaminergic mechanisms in brain. Annu Rev Pharmacol Toxicol 17:325–339

Schwartz JC, Garbarg M, Pollard H (1986) Histaminergic transmission in the brain. In: Mountcastle VB, Bloom FE, Geiger SR (eds) The nervous system, vol 4: Intrinsic regulatory systems of the brain. American Physiological Society, Philadelphia, pp 257–316 (Handbook of physiology, Sect 1)

Vanni-Mercier G, Sakai K, Jouvet M (1984) Neurones spécifiques de l'éveil dans l'hypothalamus postérieur du chat. CR Acad Sci [III] 298:195–200

Targets for Neurotransmitter Receptor Research Using PET Scan: The Neuroleptic Binding Site *

J. C. Baron [1,2], J. L. Martinot [1], H. Cambon [1], J. P. Boulenger [2],
M. F. Poirier [3], V. Caillard [2], J. Blin [1], J. D. Huret [1],
C. Loc'h [1], and B. Maziere [1]

1 Introduction

Using positron emission tomography (PET) and high-affinity positron-emitting labelled radioligands administered in trace amounts, it is possible to investigate in vivo in humans a variety of brain neuroreceptors (Baron 1987). With this method one obtains a series of transaxial tomographic brain images that quantitatively represent the specifically bound radioligand an ("in vivo receptor autoradiography"). Various approaches and models have been and are still being developed in order to measure, in a quantitative or semi-quantitative way, the regional density and affinity of the neuroreceptor under study (Baron 1987).

Presently available applications in clinical PET research in the field of neurotransmitter receptors include studies of the dopamine D_2 receptor using spiperone derivatives (Wagner et al. 1983; Mazière et al. 1985; Hägglund et al. 1987; Perlmutter et al. 1987; Arnett et al. 1985) or raclopride (Farde et al. 1986), the dopamine D_1 receptor using SCH 23390 (Farde et al. 1987b), the serotonin S_2 receptor using setoperone (Blin et al. 1988) or methylbromo-LSD (Wong et al. 1987), the μ-opiate receptor using carfentanil (Frost et al. 1985) and the central-type benzodiazepine receptor using flumazenil (Samson et al. 1985; Persson et al. 1987; Shinotoh et al. 1986; Pappata et al. 1988).

In vivo studies of dopamine D_2 receptors in the corpus striatum using PET have mainly been pathophysiological investigations in ageing and extrapyramidal disorders (Wong et al. 1984; Baron et al. 1986; Hägglund et al. 1987; Perlmutter et al. 1987) and in drug-naive schizophrenics (Wong et al. 1986; Farde et al. 1987). More recently, however, preliminary studies have used PET to evaluate the rate of occupancy of striatal dopamine D_2 receptors by orally given neuroleptics. For example, Farde et al. (1986, 1988) reported that a wide range of typical and atypical neuroleptics administered in doses titrated for antipsychotic efficacy induced a narrow range of dopamine D_2 receptor occupancy (65%–84%). This was taken as evidence for a dopamine D_2 receptor related mechanism of action of antipsychotic drugs. Farde et al. (1988) also reported that for up to 54 h following withdrawal of haloperidol or

---
* J. L. M. and J. D. H. are supported financially by the Fondation de France
[1] Service Hospitalier Frédéric Joliot, CEA, Département de Biologie, 91406 Orsay, France
[2] Centre Psychiatrique Esquirol and INSERM, Unit 320, 14000 Caen, France
[3] Service de Thérapeutique et de Santé Mentale, Hôpital Sainte-Anne, 75014 Paris, France

sulpiride, there was a rapid fall in serum drug level without significant changes in D_2 receptor occupancy, suggesting a curvilinear relationship between specific binding of the drug in striatum and free drug concentration in the brain. In six patients on chronic neuroleptic treatment, Cambon et al. (1987) demonstrated a curvilinear relationship between daily drug dosage and occupancy rate, suggesting that the latter can be confidently predicted from knowledge of the former. They also showed that, following drug withdrawal in eight patients, return to normal levels of available sites occurred within 3–12 days. This indicated that neuroleptics are rapidly cleared from their central binding sites after withdrawal, and that the prolonged remission of psychotic symptoms after drug withdrawal is not due to persistent dopamine D_2 receptor occupation but to a more protracted pharmacological effect.

We have expanded this study and present here the updated results.

2 Patients

Ten patients were studied while on chronic treatment with phenothiazine or butyrophenone neuroleptics for over 1 month; one patient (case 10) had been treated for 11 days only (Table 1). A wide range of doses was ensured by selecting patients with a variety of neurological or psychiatric indications for neuroleptics. Other drugs such as anticholinergics, benzodiazepines, or antidepressants were not withdrawn. The daily dose of neuroleptic was expressed in terms of chlorpromazine equivalents, based on standard equipotence tables and, when unavailable for a given drug, on the in vitro K_i for [^{3}H]haloperidol

Table 1. Studies on neuroleptic treatment

Patient no.	Age	Sex	Clinical Diagnosis	Neuroleptic treatment	Dose (mg/kg per day)	Chlorpromazine-equivalent dose (μmol/kg per day)
1	62	M	Alzheimer's disease	Haloperidol	0.010	1.4
2	82	M	Senile dementia	Haloperidol	0.017	2.4
3	21	M	Schizophrenic disorder	Haloperidol	0.031	4.4
4	79	F	Senile dementia	Alimemazine	0.741	6.5
5	50	M	Syphilitic dementia	Haloperidol, levomepromazine	0.042 0.174	13.9
6	27	M	Schizophrenia	Haloperidol	0.538	75.7
7	21	M	Schizophrenic disorder	Haloperidol, levomepromazine	0.254 1.271	94.3
8	28	M	Schizophrenia	Thioproperazine	1.111	222.0
9	43	F	Schizophrenia	Thioproperazine	1.429	285.4
10	65	F	Korsakov's psychosis	Propericiazine	0.167	13.8
11	83	F	Schizophrenic disorder	Haloperidol, alimemazine	0.039 1.11	15.2

Table 2. Studies after neuroleptic withdrawal

Patient no.	Age	Sex	Clinical diagnosis	Neuroleptic treatment	Dose (mg/kg per day)	Days stopped
1	68	F	Chronic hallucinatory psychosis	Haloperidol	0.205	1
2 [a]	50	M	Syphilitic dementia	Haloperidol, levomepromazine	0.042 0.174	3
3 [a]	21	M	Schizophrenic disorder	Haloperidol, levomepromazine	0.254 1.271	3
4 [a]	43	F	Schizophrenia	Thioproperazine	1.429	3
5	25	M	Schizophrenic disorder	Pipotiazine, chlorpromazine	0.145 2.899	3
6 [a]	28	M	Schizophrenia	Thioproperazine	1.111	3
7	72	F	Post-stroke agitation	Haloperidol	0.027	7
8 [a]	21	M	Schizophrenic disorder	Haloperidol	0.031	7
9	28	M	Post-traumatic depression	Levomepromazine	0.291	8
10 [a]	27	M	Schizophrenia	Haloperidol	0.538	8
11	33	M	Alcoholism	Propericiazine	0.526	10
12	60	M	Vertigo	Thiethylperazine	0.375	12
13	35	M	Schizophrenia	Pipotiazine	0.143	90
14	24	M	Schizophrenia	Pimozide	0.026	15
15	33	M	Schizophrenia	Haloperidol	0.107	40
16 [a]	83	F	Schizophrenic disorder	Haloperidol, alimemazine	0.039 1.11	3
17	54	M	Schizophrenia	Alimemazine, clotiapine	0.58 1.15	2.5

[a] Patients also studied during neuroleptic treatment.

Table 3. Depot neuroleptics

Patient no.	Age	Sex	Clinical diagnosis	Drug	Dose/month	Duration of treatment	Days after last injection
1	58	M	Schizophrenia	Haloperidol, decanoate	50 mg	2 years	34 3
2	26	M	Schizophrenia	Haloperidol, decanoate	250 mg	2 years	3 19
3	27	M	Schizophrenia	Haloperidol, decanoate	150 mg	>6 months	120
4	28	M	Schizophrenia	Haloperidol, decanoate	200 mg	8 months	26
5	54	M	Schizophrenia	Pipotiazine, palmitate	100 mg	>2 years	1 20
6	34	M	Schizophrenia	Fluphenazine, decanoate	200 mg	1 year	31

binding and the published correlation between K_i and daily dose (Leysen 1984; Creese et al. 1976).

Seventeen patients were studied after a drug-withdrawal period of 1–90 days. Seven of these patients had been previously studied while on drug (Table 2). Finally, six patients on chronic treatment with depot neuroleptics were also studied. Three of these were studied twice at varying intervals, the delay between the PET study and the last intramuscular injection ranging from 1 to 120 days (Table 3). Except for four patients, each patient had a determination of plasma prolactin concentration (ng/ml) in the morning of the PET study.

3 Methods

The method has been described in detail elsewhere (Baron et al. 1986; Cambon et al. 1987). In brief it consists of injecting intravenously trace amounts (ca. 1–3 µg) of [^{76}Br]bromospiperone and imaging seven slices of the brain for 10 min starting 5 min after injection and for 30 min starting 4.5 h after injection. From the last series of scans, the mean striatum/cerebellum (S/C) ratio of radioactive concentration was calculated by means of a validated computer-controlled method of regions-of-interest (ROI) delineation. Repeated PET studies after withdrawal of neuroleptics allowed delineation of the striatal area during the first, full-occupation study by means of dedicated copy-translation ROI software. In patients in whom no washout study was available, determination of the striatal ROI was presumably less reliable.

In the applied conditions of negligible radioligand concentrations in brain tissue and quasi-equilibrium imaging, "cold" neuroleptics reduce the binding of [^{76}Br]bromospiperone to a density of available binding sites, B'_{max}, lower than the total receptor population B_{max}. The ratio of available binding sites, A, is therefore equal to B'_{max}/B_{max}. It may be assumed that the free (F) and non-specifically bound (NS) ligand concentrations are constant, as shown by the lack of effects of neuroleptic treatment on the cerebellar tracer concentration at 4.5 h, which represents F + NS (Cambon et al. 1987). Therefore, B_{max} = (B/F) (K_d + F) and B'_{max} = (B'/F) (K_d + F), where B and B' are the concentrations of specifically bound tracer in striatum in the normal and neuroleptic-treated conditions, respectively. It follows that A = B'/B. As B and B' are equal to the striatal (S) minus the cerebellar (C) radioligand concentration (assuming similar non-specific binding in these two structures), it follows that A = (S' − C)/(S − C). Dividing each term by C leads to A = (S'/C − 1)/(S/C − 1) (Eq. 1). The basal value for S/C could not be measured before therapy was initiated, therefore the theoretical age-adjusted value was taken instead, using the significant ($p < 0.05$) linear relationship found with the same method in our laboratory in 28 control subjects ranging in age from 18 to 76 years: S/C = 2.222 − 0.006 age (years).

4 Results

The observed A as a function of the daily dose in chlorpromazine equivalents followed a typical S-shaped dose-dependent saturation curve (Fig. 1). The curve shows little variability of A for similar dosages among different patients. The value found in the patient treated for only 11 days was not remarkably different from the values in other patients.

Following withdrawal, there was a sharp increase in the observed value of A, which indicated a return to the 100% level within 6–12 days, with four exceptions. In three cases, values of A were already normal or above-normal 1–3 days after withdrawal (patients 1, 5 and 17, Table 2), while in patient 16 the value was almost unchanged from pre-withdrawal value at 3 days (Fig. 2). Of the two patients studied long after drug withdrawal, patient 15 had a very high value (150%) after 40 days, while patient 13 had a close to normal value (86%) after 90 days.

All patients on depot neuroleptics showed a significant receptor occupation (A range: 20%–50%), which exhibited either no change over time or a slight trend for increased occupation around 20 days (Fig. 3). The only subject studied after interruption of treatment showed a close to normal A value (83%) 4 months after the last injection.

The prolactin plasma levels were linearly correlated with the corresponding chlorpromazine-equivalent dosage ($r=0.70$, $n=9$, $p<0.05$), but the distribution of values was large, and the predictive value of the two variables upon each other was low. During treatment with depot neuroleptics the prolactin plasma levels were very variable from subject to subject (4–39 ng/ml), despite more consistent receptor occupation (50%–80%). After drug withdra-

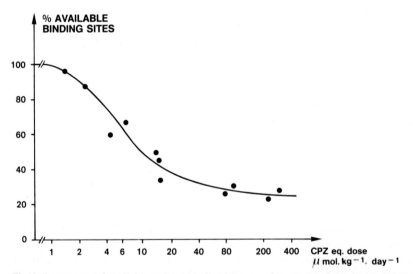

Fig. 1. Percentage of available striatal binding sites as a function of daily dosage of oral neuroleptics, expressed as chlorpromazine (*CPZ*) equivalents (μmol/kg per day) in 11 patients

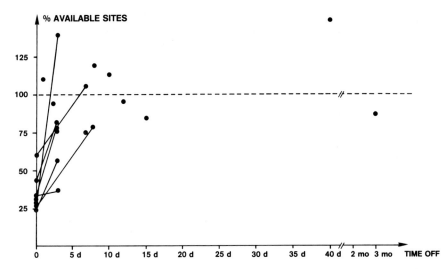

Fig. 2. Percentage of available striatal binding sites over time since withdrawal of neuroleptics. Seventeen PET studies after drug withdrawal are represented here, as well as seven performed during treatment. Lines join pre- and post-withdrawal data in the same subject

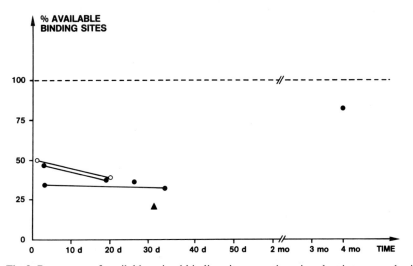

Fig. 3. Percentage of available striatal binding sites over time since last intramuscular injection of depot neuroleptics (see Table 3). *Lines* join data obtained at two different occasions in the same subject. ● Haloperidol decanoate; ○ pipotiazine palmitate; ▲ fluphenazine decanoate

wal, the prolactin plasma concentrations showed a rapid decline towards normal values, all values except one being within the normal range (<18 ng/ml) within 3 days of withdrawal. Patient 16 showed almost no change in receptor occupancy 3 days after withdrawal. After drug withdrawal there was a curvilinear relationship between the percentage decline in prolactin plasma levels

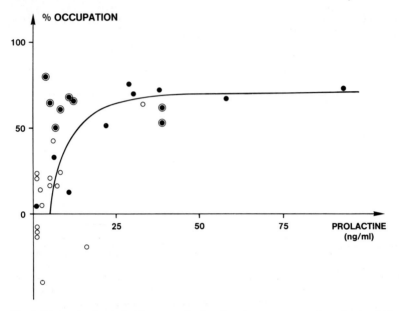

Fig. 4. Plasma prolactin level versus calculated percentage occupation of striatal binding sites in studies of patients receiving oral neuroleptic treatment ($n=9$), after withdrawal of such treatment ($n=15$), or receiving depot neuroleptics ($n=8$). The curvilinear relationship indicated was determined visually, not taking into consideration the latter category of studies. ● On treatment; o off treatment; ☉ depot neuroleptics

and the increase in receptor availability ($n=5$). Similarly, there was a curvilinear relationship between the prolactin plasma level and the receptor occupation (Fig. 4) during or following oral treatment. Therefore the prolactin values did not accurately predict either low or high receptor occupancy rates. For patients on depot neuroleptics, no correlation at all was apparent (Fig. 4).

5 Discussion

The results of the present study confirm our preliminary findings (Cambon et al. 1987) in a larger number of subjects. New information regarding depot neuroleptics and correlations with prolactin levels were also obtained.

Despite a relatively high non-specific binding of bromospiperone, which results in a comparatively low S/C ratio, our method is particularly reliable because the amount of labelled drug administered is consistently very low, and because the S/C ratio is measured between 4.5 and 5 h after injection, when "quasi-equilibrium" is achieved and dependence on accessibility rate and blood flow is negligible (Baron et al. 1986; Maziére et al. 1985). The latter point is probably the reason for the remarkable stability of C, the cerebellar relative tracer uptake, in ageing, degenerative brain disease and under neuroleptic medication (Baron et al. 1986; Cambon et al. 1987). Under these conditions, and assuming a stable K_d, the S/C ratio is a reliable representation of the density of available binding sites in striatum, as shown by its ability to detect in vivo the loss of dopamine D_2 receptors that occurs during ageing and in progressive supranuclear palsy (Baron et al. 1986).

The calculation of A, the percentage of available sites, using Eq. (1) relies on a number of assumptions:

1. *Stable value for C* among normals, treated, and untreated patients, which was verified earlier (Cambon et al. 1987).
2. *Similar non-specific binding* of [^{76}Br]bromospiperone in striatum and cerebellum. Data from rat studies (Laduron et al. 1978; Barone et al. 1985) and from one normal human brain in our laboratory (unpublished) suggest a ca. 25% higher NS in striatum. The overestimation of A resulting from this error is only a few percent at low occupancy and up to 25% for the highest occupancy found here, indicating that full receptor occupation was almost reached in our most heavily treated subjects (Fig. 1). On the other hand, this error underestimates abnormally with A values, up to 16% in patient 15, whose uncorrected A value 40 days after drug withdrawal was 150%.
3. *A "normal" baseline S/C ratio,* i.e. no effect of either the underlying psychopathology or the neuroleptic treatment on the dopamine D_2 receptors in the striatum. At variance with the report of Wong et al. (1986), both Farde et al. (1987a) and we (Martinot et al. 1989) found no significant change in striatal dopamine D_2 receptors in whole samples of drug-naive schizophrenics. Although up-regulation of the dopamine D_2 receptors has been well described in rats chronically treated with neuroleptics (Jenner and Marsden 1983), no definitive evidence for this effect has yet been reported in humans. However, following drug withdrawal the A value was above 140% in two of our patients, possibly reflecting receptor up-regulation (Fig. 2). If a 50% increase in dopamine D_2 receptor density is assumed during treatment, then the calculated A values are consistently overestimated by only a few percent at high occupation rates but by up to 33% at an uncorrected A value of 100%. This would suggest a somewhat slower rate of neuroleptic washout than indicated in Fig. 2. PET studies of patients withdrawn from neuroleptics for 15–40 days would be needed to address this issue.

The dose-dependent occupation of striatal dopamine D_2 receptors shown in Fig. 1 suggests that a reliable estimation of the rate of receptor blockade can be inferred from the oral daily dose of neuroleptics. Since the chlorpromazine-equivalent dose was calculated from clinically determined equipotence tables, our finding would support the hypothesis that the antipsychotic action of neuroleptic drugs is related to their dopamine D_2 receptor blocking effect. The lack of complete receptor occupation, as discussed above, is presumably an artefact of the method, which could easily be corrected. The data shown in Fig. 2 indicate that a dose of about 6 µmol/kg per day (ca. 2 mg/kg per day) is needed to achieve a 50% receptor occupation, while full occupation would be reached for doses of about 80 µmol/kg per day (ca. 28 mg/kg per day). Beyond this dose range no further benefit concerning antipsychotic effect, but unwanted side effects, may be anticipated. Also, our data, showing no therapeutic window, suggest that patients who do not respond to large doses of neuroleptics are nevertheless likely to have achieved full occupancy of their dopamine D_2 receptors, pointing to a dopamine-unrelated psychosis.

The reliability of our method to estimate dopamine D_2 receptor occupation despite the well-known variability in pharmacokinetics and bioavailability of neuroleptics, is striking. It suggests that the poor correlation observed between therapeutic effects and plasma concentration of neuroleptics (Midha et al. 1987; Ortiz and Gershon 1987) is due to the variable occurrence of pharmacologically active metabolites. In support of this hypothesis, the radioreceptor assay of antidopamine potency in serum has provided better correlations both between drug dosage and serum level and between the latter and clinical effects (Krska et al. 1986; Midha et al. 1987). We found our PET method much more sensitive in the evaluation of receptor occupancy than the plasma prolactin level (Fig. 4). This is in accordance with recent reviews indicating a wide inter-subject variability in this peripheral marker, presumably because of inter-subject differences in both response and long-term tolerance to dopamine receptor blockade (Meltzer et al. 1983; Davis et al. 1984; Gunnet and Moore 1988).

Treatment with depot neuroleptics resulted in a 50%-80% occupancy rate of dopamine D_2 receptors (Fig. 3), indicating that the regimens were consistently efficient despite the variety of drugs and doses used. The fact that this range of occupancy was maintained throughout the whole monthly interval demonstrates a genuinely stable delivery of neuroleptics to the pharmacological targets in the central nervous system by this route, consistent with pharmacokinetic data (Jørgensen 1986). The latter, however, indicate a progressive drop in plasma level concentrations which probably is too small to have significant influence on elevated occupancy rates. The fact that there was a complete lack of correlation between prolactin levels and receptor occupation in depot-treated patients (Fig. 4) would indicate a particularly efficient tolerance effect in the endocrine response when the plasma drug level is not subject to nyctohemeral variations, as has been shown in rats for dopamine upregulation (Kashihara et al. 1986).

After interruption of chronic oral neuroleptic treatment, there was a rapid return towards normal receptor occupation (Fig. 2), which paralleled and was curvilinearly related to the fall in prolactin levels. Although difficult to ascertain because of possibly increased receptor density as an effect of treatment itself (see above discussion), the actual time necessary for complete elimination of neuroleptic drugs from striatum lies between 5 and 15 days at most, although it could be shorter in some cases and slower in others (Fig. 2). This is perhaps a function of the pharmaceutical used or of individual factors such as age (the only patient with essentially no change in occupation after 3 days of withdrawal was 83 years old) or associated medication (Dahl and Hals 1987). Farde et al. (1988) reported no fall in D_2 receptor occupation following withdrawal of sulpiride or haloperidol, but the interval was 27–54 h, and only two patients were studied. Previous belief that receptor occupation would last for weeks or even months following oral neuroleptic withdrawal was based not only on the slow rate of relapse of psychotic symptoms (Davis and Andriukaitis 1986) but also on the duration of both extrapyramidal side effects in patients and behavioural disturbances in rats (Hershon et al. 1972; Campbell et al. 1985; Marsden et al. 1975). From our data, it must be inferred that these pharmacological effects are not due to sustained dopamine receptor blockade. This has implications not only for the long-term antipsychotic action of neuroleptics, which may involve more durable changes either in the dopaminergic transmission, or in a step beyond drug-receptor interaction, but also for some of their side effects as well as for the pathophysiology of psychosis.

Our results are consistent with the reported 96% fall in serum neuroleptic activity 2 weeks after withdrawal (Bagdy et al. 1985) and with the rapid fall in prolactin level observed after drug interruption (Meltzer et al. 1983; Gunnet and Moore 1988). Although phenothiazines accumulate to some extent in rat brain after repeated systemic administration, their rate of elimination from brain is not affected, with a $t_{1/2}$ remaining around 6 h for chlorpromazine (Mahju and Maickel 1969). After chronic dosage with tritium-labelled chlorpromazine or prochlorperazine to monkeys, recovery of radioactivity from excretion was complete in 10–20 days (Forrest et al. 1974). Finally, in vivo [^{3}H]spiperone studies in rats have shown a return to normal or above-normal radioactivity levels in the striatum within days of neuroleptic withdrawal (Saelens et al. 1980; Ferrero et al. 1983; Owen et al. 1983).

In two of our patients, a significant up-regulation of the D_2 receptors, unmasked by neuroleptic washout, was observed (Fig. 2), as early as 3 days postwithdrawal in one patient. The time course and clinical correlates, if any, of this effect require further investigation.

References

Arnett CD, Fowler JS, Wolf AP, Shiue CY, McPherson DW (1985) ^{18}F-N-methylspiroperidol: the radioligand of choice for PET studies of the dopamine receptor in human brain. Life Sci 36:1359–1366

Bagdy G, Perenyi A, Frecska E, Revai K, Pappa Z, Fekete MIK, Arato M (1985) Decrease in dopamine, its metabolites, and noradrenaline in cerebrospinal fluid of schizophrenic patients after withdrawal of long-term neuroleptic treatment. Psychopharmacology (Berlin) 85:62–64

Baron JC (1987) In vivo study of central receptors in man using PET. In: Tucek S (ed) Synaptic transmitters and receptors. Academia, Prague, pp 80–88

Baron JC, Mazière B, Loc'h C, Cambon H, Sgouropoulos P, Bonnet AM, Agid Y (1986) Loss of striatal ^{76}Br-bromospiperone binding sites demonstrated by positron tomography in progressive supranuclear palsy. J Cereb Blood Flow Metab 6:131–136

Barone D, Luzzani F, Assandri A, Galliani G, Mennini T, Garattini S (1985) In vivo stereospecific ^{3}H-spiperone binding in rat brain: characteristics, regional distribution, kinetics and pharmacological properties. Eur J Pharmacol 116:63–74

Blin J, Pappata S, Kiyosawa M, Crouzel C, Baron JC (1988) ^{18}F-setoperone: a new high affinity ligand for in vivo study of the serotonin-2 receptors in baboon brain. Eur J Pharmacol 147:73–82

Cambon H, Baron JC, Boulenger JP, Loc'h C, Zarifian E, Mazière B (1987) In vivo assay for neuroleptic receptor binding in the striatum: positron tomography in humans. Br J Psychiatry 151:824–830

Campbell A, Baldessarini RJ, Teicher MH, Kula NS (1985) Prolonged antidopaminergic actions of single doses of butyrophenones in the rat. Psychopharmacology (Berlin) 87:161–166

Creese I, Burt DR, Snyder SH (1976) Dopamine receptors and average clinical doses. Science 194:546

Dahl SG, Hals PA (1987) Pharmacokinetic and pharmacodynamic factors causing variability in response to neuroleptic drugs. In: Dahl SG, Gram LF, Paul SM, Potter WZ (eds) Clinical pharmacology in psychiatry. Springer, Berlin Heidelberg New York, pp 266–274

Davis JM, Andriukaitis S (1986) The natural course of schizophrenia and effective maintenance drug treatment. J Clin Psychopharmacol 6:25–105

Davis JM, Vogel C, Gibbons R, Parkovic I, Zhang M (1984) Pharmacoendocrinology of schizophrenia. In: Brown GM et al. (eds) Neuroendocrinology and psychiatric disorder. Raven, New York, pp 29–53

Farde L, Hall H, Ehrin E, Sedvall G (1986) Quantitative analysis of D$_2$ dopamine receptor binding in the living human brain by PET. Science 231:258–261

Farde L, Wiesel FA, Hall H, et al. (1987a) No D$_2$ receptor increase in PET study of schizophrenia. Arch Gen Psychiatry 44:671

Farde L, Halldin C, Stone-Elander S, Sedvall G (1987b) PET analysis of human dopamine receptor subtypes using ^{11}C-SCH 23390 and ^{11}C-raclopride. Psychopharmacology (Berlin) 92:278–284

Farde L, Wiesel FA, Halldin C, Sedvall G (1988) Central D$_2$-dopamine receptor occupancy in schizophrenic patients treated with antipsychotic drugs. Arch Gen Psychiatry 45:71–76

Ferrero P, Vaccarino F, Guidotti A, Costa E, di Chiro G (1983) In vivo modulation of brain dopamine recognition sites: a possible model for emission computed tomography studies. Neuropharmacology 22:791–795

Forrest IS, Fox J, Green DE, Melikian AP, Serra MT (1974) Total excretion of ^{3}H-chlorpromazine in chronically dosed animals: balance sheet. In: Forrest IS, Carz CJ, Usdin E (eds) The phenotiazines and structurally related drugs. Raven, New York, pp 347–356

Frost JJ, Wagner HN, Dannals RF, et al. (1985) Imaging opiate receptors in the human brain by positron tomography. J Comput Assist Tomogr 9:231–236

Gunnet JW, Moore KE (1988) Neuroleptics and neuroendocrine function. Annu Rev Pharmacol Toxicol 28:347–366

Hägglund J, Aquilonius SM, Eckernas SA, Hartrig P, Lundquist H, Gullberg P, Langstrom B (1987) Dopamine receptor properties in Parkinson's disease and Huntington's chorea evaluated by positron emission tomography using ^{11}C-N-methyl-spiperone. Acta Neurol Scand 75:87–94

Hershon HI, Kennedy PF, McGuire RJ (1972) Persistence of extra-pyramidal disorders and psychiatric relapse after withdrawal of long-term phenothiazine therapy. Br J Psychiatry 120:41–50

Jenner P, Marsden CD (1983) Neuroleptics and tardive dyskinesia. In: Coyle JT, Enna SJ (eds) Neuroleptics neurochemical, behavioral and clinical perspectives. Raven, New York, pp 223–253

Jørgensen A (1986) Metabolism and pharmacokinetics of antipsychotic drugs. Prog Drug Metab 9:111–174

Kashihara K, Sato M, Fujiwara Y, Harada T, Ogawa T, Otsuki S (1986) Effects of intermittent and continuous haloperidol administration on the dopaminergic system in the rat brain. Biol Psychiatry 21:650–656

Krska J, Sampath G, Shah A, Sori SD (1986) Radio-receptor assay of serum neuroleptic levels in psychiatric patients. Br J Psychiatry 148:187–193

Laduron PM, Janssen PFM, Leysen JE (1978) Characterization of specific in vivo binding of neuroleptic drugs in rat brain. Life Sci 23:581–586

Leysen JE (1984) Receptors for neuroleptic drugs. In: Burrows GD, Werry JS (eds) Advances in human psychopharmacology, vol 3. JAI, Greenvich, pp 315–356

Mahju MA, Maickel RP (1969) Accumulation of phenothiazine tranquillizers in rat brain and plasma after repeated dosage. Biochem Pharmacol 18:2701–2710

Marsden CD, Tarsy D, Baldessarini RJ (1975) Spontaneous and drug-induced movement disorders in psychotic patients. In: Benson DF, Blumer D (eds) Psychiatric aspects of neurologic disease. Grune and Stratton, New York, pp 219–265

Martinot JL, Peron-Magnan P, Huret JD, Mazoyer B, Baron JC, Boulenger JP, Mazière B, et al. (1989) Striatal D_2 dopaminergic receptors assessed in vivo by positron emission tomography and ^{76}Br-bromospiperone in untreated schizophrenics. Amer J Psychiat (in press)

Mazière B, Loc'h C, Baron JC, Sgouropoulos P, Duquesnoy N, d'Antona R, Cambon II (1985) In vivo quantitative imaging of dopamine receptors in human brain using positron emission tomography and ^{76}Br-bromospiperone. Eur J Pharmacol 114:267–272

Meltzer HY, Kane JM, Kolakowska T (1983) Plasma levels of neuroleptics, prolactin levels and clinical response. In: Coyle JT, Enna SJ (eds) Neuroleptics: neurochemical, behavioral and clinical perspectives. Raven, New York, pp 255–279

Midha KK, Hawes EM, Hubbard JW, Korchinski ED, McKay G (1987) The search for correlations between neuroleptic plasma levels and clinical outcome: a critical review. In: Meltzer HY (ed) Psychopharmacology: the third generation of progress. Raven, New York, pp 1341–1351

Ortiz A, Gershon S (1987) Plasma levels of neuroleptics in clinical treatment of acute psychotic states. ISI Atlas of Science (pharmacology) 1:60–62

Owen F, Poulter M, Mashal RD, Crow TJ, Veall N, Zanelli GD (1983) ^{77}Br-p-bromospiperone: a ligand for in vivo labelling of dopamine receptors. Life Sci 33:765–768

Pappata S, Samson Y, Chavoix C, et al. (1988) Regional specific binding of ^{11}C-Ro15 1788 to central type benzodiazepine receptors in human brain: quantitative evaluation by PET. J Cereb Blood Flow Metab 8:304–313

Perlmutter JS, Kilbourn MR, Raichle ME, Welch MT (1987) PET demonstration of upregulation of radioligand-receptor binding in human MPTP-induced parkinsonism. J Cereb Blood Flow Metab [Suppl 1] 7:371

Persson A, Stone-Elander S, Pauli S, Sedvall G (1987) Saturation analysis of benzodiazepine receptor binding in the brain of healthy human subjects using ^{11}C-RO 15 1788 and PET. J Cereb Blood Flow Metab [Suppl 1] 7:344

Saelens JK, Simke JP, Neale SE, Weeks BJ, Selwyn M (1980) Effects of haloperidol and d-amphetamine on in vivo ^{3}H-spiroperidol binding in the rat forebrain. Arch Int. Pharmacodyn Ther 246:98–107

Samson Y, Hantraye P, Baron JC, Soussaline F, Comar D, Mazière M (1985) Kinetics and displacement of ^{11}C-RO 15-1788, a benzodiazepine antagonist, studied in human brain in vivo by positron tomography. Eur J Pharmacol 110:147–250

Shinotoh H, Yamasaki T, Inoue U, et al. (1986) Visualization of specific binding of benzodiazepine in human brain. J Nucl Med 77:1593–1599

Wagner HN Jr, Burns HD, Dannals RF, Wong DF, Langstrom B, Duelfer T, Frost JJ, et al. (1983) Imaging dopamine receptors in the human brain by positron tomography. Science 221:1264–1266

Wong DF, Wagner HN Jr, Dannals RF, Links JM, Frost JJ, Ravert HT, Wilson AA, et al. (1984) Effects of age on dopamine and serotonin receptors measured by positron tomography in the living human brain. Science 226:1393–1396

Wong DF, Wagner HN, Tune LE, et al. (1986) Positron emission tomography reveals elevated D_2. Dopamine receptors in drug-naive schizophrenics. Science 234:1558–1563

Wong DF, Lever JR, Hartig PR, et al. (1987) Localization of serotonin $5HT_2$ receptors in living human brain by PET using $N1$-^{11}C-methyl-2-Br-LSD. Synapse 1:393–398

The Potential of Positron-Emission Tomography for Pharmacokinetic and Pharmacodynamic Studies of Neuroleptics *

L. Farde [1], F.-A. Wiesel [1], L. Nilsson [2], and G. Sedvall [2]

1 Introduction

The antipsychotic effect of neuroleptic drugs is well established (Delay and Deniker 1957; Klein and Davis 1962). The individual response to treatment with neuroleptic drugs is, however, highly variable. Some patients do not respond to treatment, and in some patients severe side effects are recorded. For such reasons there is a need for useful methods to examine the mechanism of antipsychotic drug action in patients and for measures to guide the determination of proper dosage. During the past 20 years techniques have been available for the measurement of drug concentrations in body fluids. Despite a large number of studies on the relationships between serum drug concentrations and antipsychotic effect, no consistent relationships have been generally confirmed (Dahl 1986).

It is widely accepted that the therapeutic effect of neuroleptic drugs is related to their ability to antagonize the action of the neurotransmitter dopamine (Carlsson and Lindqvist 1963; Creese et al. 1976; Seeman et al. 1976). This hypothesis is supported by the demonstration of a linear relationship between drug affinity for central dopamine D_2 receptors in animals and antipsychotic potency in man, while no such relationship has been demonstrated for any other central receptor (Peroutka and Snyder 1980). Previously it had not been possible to test this hypothesis in man. The development of positron emission tomography (PET) has now made it feasible to study radioligand binding to receptors in the living human brain (Wagner et al. 1983; Sedvall et al. 1986). After intravenous injection of a ligand labelled with a positron-emitting isotope, the PET camera system measures regional brain radioactivity over time. Measurements of radioactivity and ligand metabolism in arterial blood and plasma during the PET experiment provides additional information for the interpretation of regional brain activity in terms of quantitative receptor characteristics.

* This research was supported by the National Institute of Mental Health (MH 41205-01), the Swedish Medical Research Council, the Bank of Sweden Tercentenary Fund, and the Karolinska Institute.
[1] Department of Psychiatry and Psychology, Karolinska Institute and Hospital, 104 01 Stockholm, Sweden
[2] Astra Alab AB, 151 85 Södertälje, Sweden

Clinical Pharmacology in Psychiatry
Editors: S. G. Dahl and L. F. Gram
(Psychopharmacology Series 7)
© Springer-Verlag Berlin Heidelberg 1989

Each radiolabelled ligand has a unique set of characteristics that determines its usefulness for PET studies (Sedvall et al. 1986). Not only receptor characteristics such as specificity, affinity and the relative degree of non-specific binding are of importance but also ligand metabolism, distribution volume and lipophilicity. Although only a few compounds are suitable as radioligands for receptor studies with PET, the receptor binding of a great number of drugs can be characterized in vivo, since the receptor binding can be examined indirectly by studying the interaction of those unlabelled drugs with a selective labelled compound.

Raclopride is a highly selective dopamine D_2 receptor antagonist. Equilibrium is rapidly established after ligand injection, allowing the determination of receptor density (B_{max}) and affinity (K_d) by a saturation procedure. By varying the specific activity in a series of experiments, B_{max} and K_d have been calculated from saturation curves and Scatchard plots (Farde et al. 1986 b). Initial studies with clinical doses of raclopride in schizophrenic patients indicate that the receptor population examined with PET is a population by which antipsychotic effect may be mediated (Farde et al. 1988 c).

In the present paper, the application of PET will be discussed in relation to the examination of four issues: (a) The relationship between drug concentration in plasma and drug concentration in brain; (b) identification of the receptor population by which the antipsychotic effect of neuroleptics is mediated; (c) the relationship between the drug concentration in brain and the degree of central dopamine D_2 receptor occupancy; and (d) the relationship between central dopamine D_2 receptor occupancy and antipsychotic effect or side effects.

2 Methods

Patients recruited for the studies satisfied DSM-IIIR criteria for schizophrenic disorder. Patients on antipsychotic drug treatment had been treated for at least 1 month. The reference group of 15 drug-naive schizophrenics has been described elsewhere (Farde et al. 1987).

The synthesis of [^{11}C]-raclopride in PET experiments has been described in detail elsewhere (Farde et al. 1988 b). In brief, [^{11}C]raclopride was prepared by alkylation of the corresponding desmethyl analogue using [^{11}C]methyliodide. In each experiment 100 MBq [^{11}C]raclopride was injected intravenously (specific activity, 110–800 Ci/mmol). Brain radioactivity was followed with a PC384B PET system (Scanditronix, Sweden) by sequential scans for 51 min. Regional radioactivity was measured for each sequential scan, corrected for ^{11}C decay, and plotted against time. Radioactivity in venous blood was measured using a well counter. Specific binding in the putamen (B) was defined as the difference between radioactivity in the putamen, a region with a high density of dopamine D_2 receptors and the cerebellum, a region with a negligible density of dopamine D_2 receptors.

Radioactivity in cerebellum was used as an estimate of the free radioligand concentration in the brain (F). The concept of dopamine D_2 receptor occupancy was defined as the percentage reduction in the ratio B/F in relation to the mean value in 15 drug-naive schizophrenic patients (mean, 3.55; SD, 0.63).

The level of protein binding in plasma was also determined in PET experiments on eight drug-naive schizophrenic patients. A blood sample was drawn before the experiment, and the plasma was frozen for an in vitro determination of the protein binding of raclopride. Protein binding was determined by ultrafiltration. Plasma blanks from each subject were used, and raclopride was added, giving plasma concentrations of 2 μM. The samples were kept at 37 °C, and the pH was adjusted to 7.4 prior to ultrafiltration. The compounds were extracted from the ultrafiltrate to an organic phase at alkaline pH. After evaporation of the organic phase and redissolution in buffer, the concentration of raclopride was determined by reversed-phase liquid chromatography.

3 Relationship Between Drug Concentration in Plasma and Drug Concentration in Brain

After the intravenous injection of [^{11}C]raclopride in eight patients with schizophrenia, radioligand concentration was measured in brain with PET and in plasma with a well counter. The concentration values 12 min after ligand injection were chosen for analysis; at this time point a constant ratio has been established between radioligand in brain and in plasma, and more than 90% of radioactivity in blood represents unchanged [^{11}C]raclopride (Farde et al. 1987). The patients had similar radioligand concentrations in plasma but a nearly three-fold variation in the brain concentration of radioligand (Fig. 1, inset). Plasma protein binding varied from 92% to 97%. A correlation was

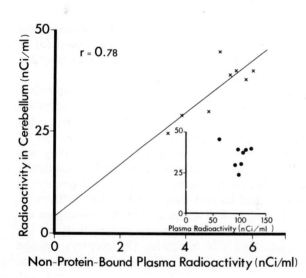

Fig. 1. Relationship between radioactivity in a brain region (white matter) and the not protein-bound (free) radioactivity in plasma after the injection of [^{11}C]raclopride in eight patients with schizophrenia. *Inset*, relationship between radioactivity in brain and the total radioactivity in plasma. Radioactivity concentrations were obtained 12 min after ligand injection

shown ($r=0.78$) between free (not protein-bound) radioligand concentration in plasma and ligand concentration in brain (Fig. 1). This correlation indicates that the brain concentration of drugs reflects the free concentration and not the total concentration in plasma.

Several neuroleptics have a high and sometimes concentration-dependent degree of protein binding in plasma (Jörgensen 1986). In future studies on the relationship of plasma levels to antipsychotic effect, efforts must be made to correct for individual variation in plasma protein binding.

4 Identification of Target Receptors for the Antipsychotic Drug Action

In each of the patients treated with one of 11 chemically distinct antipsychotic drugs, there was a marked reduction of radioactivity in the putamen when

Table 1. Dopamine D_2 receptor occupancy in patients treated with psychoactive drugs

	Dose (mg)	Receptor occupancy (%)
Phenothiazines		
Chlorpromazine	100 b.i.d.	80
Thioridazine	100 t.i.d.	75
Trifluoperazine	5 b.i.d.	80
Perphenazine	4 b.i.d.	79
Perphenazine	30 b.i.d.	88 [a]
Thioxanthenes		
Flupenthiol	5 b.i.d.	74
Buthyrophenones		
Haloperidol	6 b.i.d.	86 [a]
Haloperidol	3 b.i.d.	85 [a]
Haloperidol	3 b.i.d.	89 [a]
Haloperidol	2 b.i.d.	81 [a]
Melperone	100 t.i.d.	70
Diphenylbutyls		
Pimozide	4 b.i.d.	77 [a]
Dibenzodiazepines		
Clozapine	300 b.i.d.	65
Substituted benzamides		
Sulpiride	400 b.i.d.	82
Sulpiride	400 b.i.d.	73
Sulpiride	400 b.i.d.	68
Raclopride	4 b.i.d.	72
Raclopride	3 b.i.d.	65

[a] Extrapyramidal effects were recorded in connection with the PET experiment.

compared to the mean value previously obtained in the drug-naive schizophrenic patients (Table 1). The dopamine D_2 receptor occupancy calculated for the different antipsychotic drug treatments varied between 65% and 89%.

The dopamine D_2 receptor is the only central receptor to which all classes of antipsychotic drugs have affinity in vitro (Peroutka and Snyder 1980). Our finding that clinical doses of all the 11 chemically distinct antipsychotic drugs induce a 65%–87% occupancy of the central dopamine D_2 receptors represents strong support for the hypothesis that the mechanism of action of antipsychotic drugs is indeed related to a substantial degree of dopamine D_2 receptor occupancy.

5 Relationship Between Drug Concentration in Brain and Central Dopamine D_2 Receptor Occupancy

The theoretically expected curvilinear relationship between neuroleptic drug concentration in plasma and dopamine D_2 receptor occupancy (Fig. 2) has been confirmed either by repeated PET scans at different plasma concentrations in the same individual (Farde et al. 1986b, 1988a), by one PET scan in each patient of a group treated with different doses of various neuroleptics (Cambon et al. 1987) or by one PET experiment in each patient of a group treated with different doses of haloperidol (Smith et al. 1988).

The findings are illustrated by an experiment in a patient treated with sulpiride (600 mg b.i.d.). Receptor occupancy and serum drug concentrations were followed for 27 h after withdrawal (Farde et al. 1988). PET experiments were performed 3, 6 and 27 h after the last dose. The dopamine D_2 receptor occupancy remained above 65% for 27 h, in spite of a several-fold reduction in the serum concentration. In a patient withdrawn from haloperidol (6 mg b.i.d.) receptor occupancy and serum drug concentrations were followed for 54 h. Three PET experiments were performed 6, 30 and 53 h after the last dose. A reduction of only a small percentage in dopamine D_2 receptor oc-

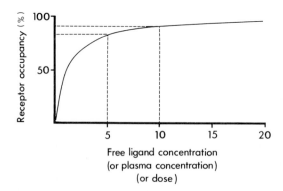

Fig. 2. Theoretical hyperbolic relationship between free radioligand concentration and the degree of receptor occupancy. During antipsychotic drug treatment a part of the hyperbola is reached that approaches a horizontal asymptote. *Dotted lines* show that a major increase in free ligand concentration at the asymptotic part of the hyperbola causes only a minor increase in dopamine D_2 receptor occupancy

cupancy was observed, in spite of a several-fold reduction of the haloperidol serum concentration (Fig. 2).

In a patient treated with sulpiride (800 mg b.i.d.) the dose was reduced stepwise from 1600 to 1200, 800, 400 and 0 mg daily. A period ranging from 9 days to 3 weeks elapsed between each dose reduction. The reduction in dopamine D_2 receptor occupancy in relation to dose followed a curve with a hyperbolic (curvilinear) shape while the curve of reduced serum concentration of sulpiride had a linear shape.

Clinical doses of neuroleptics are high enough to give a receptor occupancy that approaches the horizontal part of the binding hyperbola (Fig. 2). An increased or reduced dose at this part of the hyperbola produces only a small alteration in receptor occupancy at the already nearly saturated dopamine D_2 receptors. In several studies, similar antipsychotic effects have been reported on widely different doses and concentration levels of neuroleptic drugs in schizophrenic patients (Wode-Helgodt et al. 1978; Baldessarini and Davis 1980; Marder et al. 1984; Wiesel et al., this volume). This marked variation of doses and concentrations producing similar effects may be expected if the horizontal part of the hyperbola is approached during treatment with antipsychotic drugs.

6 Relationship of Central Dopamine D_2 Receptor Occupancy to Antipsychotic Effect and Side Effects

By relating dopamine D_2 receptor occupancy to antipsychotic effect it may be possible to define a "threshold occupancy" for the effect. The detailed relationships between the degree of dopamine D_2 receptor occupancy and drug effects have, so far, not been studied. However, it is of interest that all the patients in our study with a receptor occupancy above 65% responded well to the treatment. Six patients had observable extrapyramidal side effects (Table 1). One of these patients had akathisia when treated with 6 mg haloperidol b.i.d. His dopamine D_2 receptor occupancy was then 86%. He was subsequently treated with 4 mg b.i.d., with a maintained antipsychotic effect but no extrapyramidal side effects. At that time his receptor occupancy was 84%. The observable extrapyramidal side effects were recorded only in patients with a comparatively high dopamine D_2 receptor occupancy (Table 1). On the basis of these initial results we suggest that a threshold occupancy also may exist for the extrapyramidal side effects.

Acknowledgement. The assistance of the members of the Stockholm PET group involved in the PET experiments is gratefully acknowledged.

References

Baldessarini RJ, Davis JM (1980) What is the best maintenance dose of neuroleptics in schizophrenia? Psychiatry Res 3:115–122

Cambon H, Baron JC, Boulenger JP, Loch C, Zarifian E, Mazière B (1987) In vivo assay for neuroleptic receptor binding in the striatum. Positron tomography in humans. Br J Psychiatry 151:824–830

Carlsson A, Lindqvist M (1963) Effect of chlorpromazine or haloperidol on formation of 3-methoxytyramine and normetanephrine in mouse brain. Acta Pharmacol Toxicol (Copenh) 20:140–144

Creese I, Burt DR, Snyder SH (1976) Dopamine receptor binding, clinical and pharmacological potencies of antischizophrenic drugs. Science 192:481–483

Dahl SG (1986) Plasma level monitoring of antipsychotic drugs' clinical utility. Clin Pharmacokinet 11:36–61

Deniker P (1978) Impact of neuroleptic chemotherapies on schizophrenic psychosis. Am J Psychiatry 135:923–927

Farde L, Wiesel F-A, Ehrin E, Hall H, Sedvall G (1986a) Quantitative PET-scan determination of dopamine-D₂ receptor binding in schizophrenic patients treated with distinct classes of antipsychotic drugs. In: Shagass C, et al. (eds) World Congress of Biological Psychiatry, 8–13 September 1985. Elsevier, New York, pp 363–365 (Developments in psychiatry, vol 7)

Farde L, Hall H, Ehrin E, Sedvall G (1986b) Quantitative analysis of dopamine-D₂ receptor binding in the living human brain by positron emission tomography. Science 231:258–261

Farde L, Wiesel F-A, Hall H, Halldin C, Stone-Elander S, Sedvall G (1987) No D₂ receptor increase in PET study of schizophrenia. Arch Gen Psychiatry 44:671

Farde L, Wiesel F-A, Halldin H, Sedvall G (1988a) Central D₂-dopamine receptor occupancy in schizophrenic patients treated with antipsychotic drugs. Arch Gen Psychiatry 45:71–76

Farde L, Pauli S, Hall H, Eriksson L, Halldin C, Högberg T, Nilsson, Sjögren I (1988b) Stereoselective binding of ¹¹C-raclopride in living human brain – a search for extrastriatal central D2-dopamine receptors by PET. Psychopharmacology (Berlin) 94:471–478

Farde L, Wiesel F-A, Jansson P, Uppfeldt G, Wahlén A, Sedvall G (1988c) An open label trial of raclopride in acute schizophrenia. Confirmation of D₂-dopamine receptor occupancy by PET. Psychopharmacology (Berlin) 94:1–7

Jörgensen A (1986) Metabolism and pharmacokinetics of antipsychotic drugs. In: Bridges JW, Chasseaud LF (eds) Progress in drug metabolism, vol 9. Taylor and Francis, London, pp 111–174

Klein D, Davis J (1962) Diagnosis and drug treatment of psychiatric disorders. Williams and Williams, Baltimore

Marder SR, van Putten T, Mintz J, et al. (1984) Costs and benefits of two doses of fluphenazine. Arch Gen Psychiatry 41:1025–1029

Peroutka SJ, Snyder SH (1980) Relationship of neuroleptic drug effects at brain dopamine, serotonin, adrenergic and histamine receptors to clinical potency. Am J Psychiatry 137:1518–1522

Sedvall G, Farde L, Persson A, Wiesel F-A (1986) Imaging of neurotransmitter receptors in the living human brain. Arch Gen Psychiatry 43:995–1005

Seeman P, Lee T, Chau-Wong M, Wong K (1976) Antipsychotic drug doses and neuroleptic/dopamine receptors. Nature 261:717–719

Smith M, Wolf AD, Brodie JD, Arnett CD, Barouche F, Shine C-Y, Fowler JS, Russell JAG, MacGregor RR, Wolkin A, Angrist B, Rotrosen J, Peselow E (1988) Serial [¹⁸F]N-Methylspiroperidol PET studies to measure changes in antipsychotic drug D-2 receptor occupancy in schizophrenic patients. Biol Psychiatry 23:653–663

Wagner HN, Burns HD, Dannals RF, Wong DF, Långström B, Duelfer T, Frost JJ, et al. (1983) Imaging dopamine receptors in the human brain by positron tomography. Science 221:1264–1266

Wode-Helgodt B, Borg S, Fyrö B, Sedvall G (1978) Clinical effects and drug concentrations in plasma and cerebrospinal fluid in psychotic patients treated with fixed doses of chlorpromazine. Acta Psychiatr Scand 58:149–173

Neurotransmitter Interactions as a Target of Drug Action

W. Z. Potter [1], J. K. Hsiao [1], and H. Ågren [2]

The characterization of neuroleptics and antidepressants as dopamine antagonists and monoamine uptake or monoamine oxidase (MAO) inhibitors led to various strategies for measuring these biochemical parameters in humans. Not until the late 1970s, however, were relevant analytical methods sufficiently developed to permit widespread clinical investigations. We will briefly review the results emerging from application of these methods in clinical studies designed to ascertain whether drugs alter or correct the postulated abnormalities in particular neurotransmitters. We will then focus on relationships between neurotransmitters as additional targets of drug action and consider the possibility that such actions may ultimately prove more important than effects on any single neurotransmitter.

1 Drug Effects on Neurotransmitters in Man

Until recently, there have been no methods to study directly pharmacologic effects on neurotransmitters; positron-emission tomography (PET) may be the first. Psychopharmacologists therefore relied on indirect measures of neurotransmitter turnover, first in animals and then in humans. A useful definition of turnover as a rate term is: the amount moving in (or out) of a fixed pool at steady state per unit time. It should be immediately apparent that the only compartments in which one can directly measure a total amount produced are those from which no elimination occurs; for all practical purposes in clinical studies this means urine. For instance, we have found that the total excretion in urine of norepinephrine plus its metabolites, normetanephrine, 3-methoxy-4-hydroxyphenylglycol (MHPG), and vanillylmandelic acid (VMA), under steadystate conditions is reduced in patients following 3–4 weeks of treatment with at least four biochemically different classes of antidepressants (Table 1). At the same time we demonstrated that changes in the relative proportion of, for instance, normetanephrine, which is formed by extraneuronal O-methylation of norepinephrine, compared to changes in that of MHPG and VMA, much of which is formed via intraneuronal deamination, were characteristic of a drug's primary effects.

[1] Section on Clinical Pharmacology, Laboratory of Clinical Science, National Institute of Mental Health, 9000 Rockville Pike, Bethesda, MD 20892, USA
[2] Department of Psychiatry, University Hospital, 751 85 Uppsala, Sweden

Clinical Pharmacology in Psychiatry
Editors: S. G. Dahl and L. F. Gram
(Psychopharmacology Series 7)
© Springer-Verlag Berlin Heidelberg 1989

Table 1. Differential effects on NE metabolic pathways of antidepressants that similarly reduce total NE turnover in patients and/or volunteers following 3–4 weeks of treatment

Drug	First-degree acute action	Fractional excretion (% change with treatment)[a]	
		Normetanephrine	MHPG + VMA
Desipramine	NE uptake inhibition	+ 36%	NS
Zimelidine	5-HT uptake inhibition	NS	NS
Clorgyline	MAO inhibition	+ 574%	− 35%
Bupropion	DA + ?NE uptake inhibition	NS	NS

[a] Calculated as [(fraction posttreatment − fraction pretreatment)/fraction pretreatment] × 100 from data in Linnoila et al. (1982a, b), Rudorfer et al. (1984), Golden et al. (1988), where fractional excretion is the amount of NM or of MHPG + VMA divided by the sum of NE + NM + MHPG + VMA in urine. NE, Norepinephrine; NM, normetanephrine; DA, dopamine; 5-HT, serotonin; MAO, monoamine oxidase.

Hence, as is shown in Table 1, an MAO inhibitor dramatically increased the proportion of normetanephrine, and a norepinephrine uptake inhibitor modestly increased it, whereas an uptake inhibitor of serotonin (5-hydroxytryptamine, 5-HT) and a probable dopamine uptake inhibitor do not affect the relative proportion of normetanephrine excreted. The inherent limitation of such urinary studies is that they primarily reflect output from peripheral tissues although, as reviewed by Maas (1984), in the case of the noradrenergic system this may be functionally linked to the CNS.

An alternative approach to studying neurotransmitter turnover in humans has been to measure the steady-state concentrations of the major metabolites of norepinephrine, dopamine, and serotonin – MHPG, homovanillic acid (HVA), and 5-hydroxyindoleacetic acid (5-HIAA), respectively – in lumbar cerebrospinal fluid (CSF). A comprehensive summary on the first decade of aplication of CSF studies in humans is available elsewhere (Wood 1980). The first studies utilizing definitive gas chromatography/mass spectrometry techniques for HVA and 5-HIAA were carried out in Sweden and demonstrated reductions of 5-HIAA after the antidepressant nortriptyline (Åsberg et al. 1973) and elevations of HVA after antipsychotics (Sedvall et al. 1974). Subsequent studies from the same groups showed that both classes of drugs also affected other neurotransmitter metabolites, with the tricyclics and antipsychotics reducing both MHPG and 5-HIAA but differentially affecting HVA (Träskman et al. 1979; Wode-Helgodt et al. 1977).

Of particular interest are results from studies designed to demonstrate selective effects on MHPG and 5-HIAA after specific uptake inhibitors of norepinephrine or serotonin. It has emerged that even the selective norepinephrine uptake inhibitor desipramine reduces 5-HIAA in the CSF (Potter et al. 1985), and the selective serotonin uptake inhibitors zimelidine and citalopram reduce MHPG (Bertilsson et al. 1980; Potter et al. 1985; Bjerkenstedt et al. 1985). As summarized in Table 2, it appears instead that

Table 2. Effects of antidepressants on monoamine metabolites in cerebrospinal fluid (CSF)

Drug	% Change			Study
	5-HIAA	MHPG	HVA	
Imipramine	−35	−39	+ 7	Bowden et al. (1985)
Desipramine	−37	−49	−19	Potter et al. (1985)
Amitriptyline	−36	−41	− 3	Bowden et al. (1985)
Nortriptyline	−25	−36	(not done)	Åsberg et al. (1973)
				Bertilsson et al. (1974)
Clomipramine	−48	−33	+14	Träskman et al. (1979)
Zimelidine	−39	−20	+ 8	Potter et al. (1985)
Citalopram	−29	−11	+15	Bjerkenstedt et al. (1985)

5-HIAA, 5-hydroxyindoleacetic acid; MHPG, 3-methoxy-4-hydroxyphenylglycol; HVA, homovanillic acid.

potent serotonin uptake inhibitors can be distinguished by their tendency to increase HVA. It is important to consider possible interpretations for the common tendency of classic tricyclics and selective serotonin uptake inhibitors to reduce both 5-HIAA and MHPG while having different effects on HVA. This phenomenon has been noted by Åsberg et al. (1977) and Bjerkenstedt et al. (1985). They observed a high correlation between drug-induced changes in HVA and 5-HIAA and interpreted this to suggest a functional linkage between the dopaminergic and serotonergic systems.

2 Correlations: Theoretical Correlations

A sufficiently high correlation between two or more variables indicates that their values are determined by the same controlling process, or that they directly interact, or a combination of the two. In human studies we are usually limited in terms of the experiments that we perform to administration of safe drugs in order to explore the meaning of correlations. For example, the commonly observed high correlation between 5-HIAA and HVA in CSF, which reaches a value of $r = 0.90$ in some studies (reviewed in Ågren et al. 1986), could theoretically be a result of their common clearance site, an active acid transport pump which can be blocked by probenecid. Indeed, probenecid administration increases the concentrations of both 5-HIAA and HVA roughly proportionately such that the increases are highly correlated (Goodwin et al. 1973). On the other hand, since under basal steady-state conditions the acid transport pump is not saturated, and since 5-HIAA can be increased by administration of a precursor, *l*-tryptophan, or decreased by a synthesis inhibitor, parachlorophenylalanine (Goodwin et al. 1973), the bulk of the variance of 5-HIAA in CSF cannot be accounted for by changes in clearance. Obviously, the validity of this argument depends on the specificity of action of the pharmacologic agents utilized. It also raises another interesting point: If 5-

HIAA is selectively altered, then how is the correlation with HVA maintained? In other words, if one rules out a common controlling factor such as the same clearance mechanism, what determines the correlation? Under such conditions, the correlation presumably reflects some other interaction.

We have directly studied various correlation matrices of monoamine metabolites and determined whether they can be systematically altered. As we will show below, once one has an acceptable method for managing the statistics, this open-ended approach to correlations of variables that we usually consider separately provides a very interesting target of drug action, i.e., increasing or decreasing correlations. At the very least this allows us to conclude whether a drug alters a relationship between two or more variables. Moreover, it can provide data consistent with notions that interactions between neurotransmitters, which are certainly part of the cascade of determinants of monoamine metabolites, are involved in the response to drugs.

There are new methods for structural analysis which have been developed by mathematicians/statisticians working largely with social scientists (for review see Bentler 1980). Elsewhere we have presented an application of one such method, linear structural relationships (LISREL) from Jöreskog and Sörbom (1984), to analysis of the correlation between HVA and 5-HIAA using age, height, and weight as exogenous variables (Ågren et al. 1986). This analysis yielded a unidirectional, significant LISREL correlation coefficient such that 5-HIAA "determines" HVA but not vice versa. Such a result could be taken as support for a mechanistic interpretation, based on animal studies which show projections from the raphe (serotonin cell bodies) to the substantia nigra (dopamine cell bodies; Fuxe 1965) and that electrical stimulation of the raphe alters firing of dopamine neurons in the substantia nigra (Dray et al. 1976).

In this instance, deriving information of possible mechanistic relevance from observed correlations depended on the concomitant measure of exogenous physiologic variables such as age, height, and weight. A drug known to have a biochemical effect on one or another of the variables under consideration (e.g., 5-HIAA or HVA) could function as an exogenous variable if there was a reasonable correlation between drug concentration and biochemical change. Such data, however, are very hard to come by, and the observed correlations are not robust (e.g., Muscettola et al. 1978). Much more work remains to be done, therefore, before deciding on the value of such structural analyses to extract mechanistic information from the effects of drugs on correlations. Could we gain more information from studying ratios of variables than looking at their correlations?

3 Ratios: Theoretical Considerations

Ratios involve a numerator and denominator and hence necessarily say something about the relationship of two terms. Take, for instance, the ratio of 5-HIAA and HVA concentrations in CSF. If one uses a standard two-dimensional plot with 5-HIAA on the ordinate and HVA on the abscissa (Fig. 1), it is immediately apparent that the point of intersection can be mathematically described as a distance from the origin, r, which is the hypotenuse of a right triangle with an angle of elevation, α, which is the arc tangent of HVA/5-HIAA. The ratio, and hence the angle α, can remain constant over an infinite range of values of 5-HIAA and HVA, i.e., the hypotenuse can vary infinitely for a fixed angle (Fig. 1). Conversely, the ratio and angle can change between $0°$ and $90°$ without affecting the length of the hypotenuse, as would be described by a quarter circle. Clearly, if the HVA/5-HIAA ratio (angle) does not change, the length of the hypotenuse (radius) will vary directly with the value of either HVA or 5-HIAA. Therefore, it is the ratio or angle which contains additional information beyond the value of a single parameter. The application of polar coordinates to drug effects on ratios between monoamine metabolites has been described elsewhere (Ågren et al. 1988) and will be summarized below.

Here we wish to address the question of whether the ratios provide information on any relationship between two measures. It can be easily appreciated from inspection of Fig. 1 that, simply by holding one measure fixed (e.g., 5-HIAA) and varying the other (HVA), the ratio will be altered. In pharmacologic terms, this means that any drug which selectively affects one variable will produce changes in the ratio. This adds no separate information under these circumstances – or does it? In this instance, it depends on whether an underlying model can be specified from prior and independent data. This is where the structural analysis of correlational data added to the much more critical neuroanatomical and physiological data from animals may be useful.

Specifically, we can mathematically describe the determinants of HVA in terms of 5-HIAA based on a model whereby 5-HIAA "determines" HVA. In

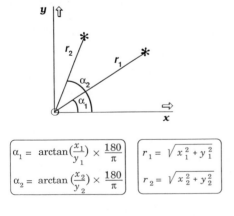

$$\alpha_1 = \arctan\left(\frac{x_1}{y_1}\right) \times \frac{180}{\pi}$$

$$\alpha_2 = \arctan\left(\frac{x_2}{y_2}\right) \times \frac{180}{\pi}$$

$$r_1 = \sqrt{x_1^2 + y_1^2}$$

$$r_2 = \sqrt{x_2^2 + y_2^2}$$

Fig. 1. General description of polar coordinates whereby the angle, α, formed by a line from the origin to point of intersection of x and y, is equivalent to the arc tangent of the ratio and can be expressed in degrees after multiplying by $180/\pi$, as shown. The distance from the origin to the intersect is the hypotenuse of a right triangle and therefore can be calculated from values of x and y as shown. See text for specific application to neurotransmitter measures

brief, one can introduce the term R to summarize any and all processes relating serotonin turnover and release to dopamine turnover. Under conditions during which the fractional conversions of serotonin and dopamine to 5-HIAA and HVA are constant, and the clearances of 5-HIAA and HVA from CSF are stable, the ratio of HVA to 5-HIAA can be expressed as:

$$\frac{[HVA]}{[5\text{-}HIAA]} = \frac{DA_I}{5\text{-}HT} + R$$

where DA_I refers to the rate of formation of dopamine independent of serotonin and 5HT refers to the rate of formation of serotonin. The details of the derivation of this expression are provided in the "Appendix."

It immediately follows from the equation that the ratio of metabolites directly reflects the ratio of dopamine and serotonin turnover as R approaches zero, i.e., when there is little or no effect of serotonin on dopamine turnover. The more interesting situation is when the R term is large (as suggested by the high correlation coefficient of HVA to 5-HIAA in most CSF studies); then the value of the ratio is substantially influenced by the degree of linkage between serotonin and dopamine as well as their actual rates of synthesis. Hence a change in the ratio, even if it appears to be accounted for by "selective" alterations in the numerator or denominator may include a change in the R function. For example, even if 5HT uptake inhibitors specifically reduced 5-HIAA, the observed increase in the HVA/5-HIAA ratio might reflect the combination of a decrease in 5HT turnover and an altered contribution of serotonin to dopamine turnover. Indeed, if there *is* a basal functional link, then a decrease of serotonin turnover without a change in that of dopamine (i.e., no change in HVA) would indicate that there is an alteration in the relationship.

There is another potential methodologic benefit to be gained from using the ratio of substances such as HVA and 5-HIAA which may share some common extraneous sources of variance. When one is comparing values before and after treatment, there are numerous methodologic problems such as (hopefully) small variations in acid transport over time which may effect both variables to the same extent; a ratio cancels out the noise (see "Appendix") and clearer data may result.

4 Correlations: Application to Analysis of Drug Effects

To our knowledge, no one has yet prospectively looked at drug effects on the intercorrelations between all monoamine metabolites. One study that we have done provides an example of what to look for. Briefly, we compared the correlation matrices of CSF monoamine concentrations from patients who respond ($n=23$) or failed to respond ($n=17$) to a variety of antidepressant treatments. Responders had correlations between monoamine metabolites

Table 3. Cerebrospinal fluid metabolite product-moment correlations

Metabolite	Correlation			
	Nonresponders		Responders	
	5-HIAA	MHPG	5-HIAA	MHPG
Pretreatment				
HVA	0.22	0.20	0.74[a]	0.54[b]
5-HIAA		0.37		0.44[c]
Posttreatment				
HVA	0.48[d]	0.39	0.69[a]	0.58[b]
5-HIAA		−0.08		0.42[d]
Change with treatment				
HVA	0.23	−0.18	0.63[c]	0.69[b]
5-HIAA		−0.10		0.38[d]

Data taken from Hsiao et al. (1987).
[a] $p < 0.001$. [b] $p < 0.01$. [c] $p < 0.05$. [d] $p < 0.10$.

similar to those observed in healthy volunteers (Sedvall et al. 1980) whereas nonresponders revealed no significant correlations (Table 3). The correlation of $r = 0.22$ between 5-HIAA and HVA is far below that reported in any previously studied population (Ågren et al. 1986), and the correlation matrices for the change with treatment were significantly different from one another ($p < .01$). The details of this analysis have been presented elsewhere (Hsiao et al. 1987). The interesting trend (which did not quite reach statistical significance in our retrospective study) was for the treatment to "normalize" the correlation of HVA vs with 5-HIAA. Prospective studies are under way to determine whether a single drug can systematically alter monoamine correlations.

5 Ratios: Application to Analysis of Drug Effects

At least one major psychotropic drug, chlorpromazine, systematically affects the CSF ratios of monoamine metabolites. In particular, the HVA/5-HIAA ratio is affected in a dose-dependent manner, at least in men (Wode-Helgodt et al. 1977). Subsequently, in an attempt to distinguish better between three treatments which all reduced 5-HIAA in the CSF (Potter et al. 1985), we compared the HVA/5-HIAA ratio after desipramine, an norepinephrine uptake inhibitor, zimelidine, a 5HT uptake inhibitor, and clorgyline, an MAO type A inhibitor (Risby et al. 1987). HVA in CSF was reduced by clorgyline but was not consistently altered by zimelidine or desipramine. The HVA/5-HIAA ratio (Table 4) was dramatically and significantly increased by zimelidine, was reduced by clorgyline, and was unchanged by desipramine. This analysis has been extended to other drugs with the finding that the HVA/5-HIAA ratio in CSF (Risby et al. 1987) or HVA–5-HIAA angle (Ågren et al. 1988) is con-

Table 4. Cerebrospinal fluid HVA, 5-HIAA, and the HVA/5-HIAA ratio before and after chronic treatment with antidepressants

Drug	HVA (nmol/l)		5-HIAA (nmol/l)		Ratio (HVA/5-HIAA)	
	Before	After	Before	After	Before	After
Zimelidine	160 ± 9	196 ± 30	109 ± 9	72 ± 9[a]	1.51 ± 0.08	2.68 ± 0.14[a]
Clorgyline	172 ± 23	117 ± 15[a]	107 ± 14	84 ± 8[b]	1.68 ± 0.22	1.40 ± 0.16[c]
Desipramine	183 ± 22	168 ± 24	108 ± 10	86 ± 8[b]	1.68 ± 0.08	1.88 ± 0.16

Data taken from Risby et al. (1987).
Significance of differences between pre- and posttreatment values calculated using paired t test.
[a] $p < 0.002$. [b] $p < 0.02$. [c] $p < 0.005$.

sistently increased by serotonin uptake inhibitors, unchanged by norepinephrine uptake inhibitors and is reduced by MAO inhibitors. Simply in terms of clarifying the action of certain classes of psychotropic drugs in vivo in humans, the ratio therefore provides a useful pharmacodynamic measure.

Some additional variations on this theme should be mentioned. Either the ratios or the polar coordinates of HVA, 5-HIAA, and MHPG can be simultaneously plotted using three dimensions, as presented in a poster presentation at this conference (Ågren et al.). Put simply, if we plot the points describing the change in HVA, 5-HIAA, and MHPG after various treatments (see Fig. 1 in Hsiao et al. 1987, for an example of such a plot), the values for 5HT uptake inhibitors cluster in one area of three-dimensional space, while those for norepinephrine uptake and MAO inhibitors each again cluster in distinctly different areas. It is perhaps not surprising that the more variables we consider, the better we can discriminate the effects of drugs. What is impressive is that the effects of drugs with clear preclinical biochemical specificity do produce unique *combinations* of effects on monoamine metabolites in CSF of patients following chronic administration. Nonetheless the broad target therapeutic effect, alleviation of depression, is nonspecific. In the future, it will be of interest to compare specific drug effects on possible measures of neurotransmitter interaction versus specific components of the clinical response (e.g., sleep and mood).

6 Future Directions

The possible application of correlation matrices, ratios, or polar coordinates as indirect indices of neurotransmitter interaction has been presented above. What is necessary is to assess in any available experimental model whether changes in measures of relative levels of neurotransmitter can be explained in terms of demonstrable neurotransmitter interaction. For instance, Scheinin (1986) has looked at the effects of a possible psychotropic drug, the α_2 antagonist idazoxan, on MHPG and HVA in the CSF in rats. He found dose-dependent increases of both monoamine metabolites, increases that were highly correlated ($r=0.95$), and concluded not that this provided evidence of noradrenergic/dopaminergic interaction, but that the acute idazoxan-induced change in HVA reflected HVA released from noradrenergic neurons (Scheinin 1986). Moreover, one of the earlier models for the modulation of dopamine by norepinephrine (Antelmen and Caggiula 1977) has been challenged by recent behavioral studies suggesting that interactions occur as a consequence of parallel activation producing complex end-organ responses without involving an effect of one neurotransmitter on the other (Cole and Robbins 1987). Other investigators, however, have been able convincingly to demonstrate modulation of dopamine and serotonin release from the nucleus accumbens through α_2 adrenergic receptors (Nurse et al. 1985; Benkirane et al. 1985). The actual role of such possible interactions in determining the steady-state balance between neurotransmitter metabolites therefore remains very much an open question.

Appendix. Making the assumption that there is a unidirectional influence of 5-HT on dopamine turnover, a model for interpreting the HVA/5-HIAA ratio can be constructed.

Terms are defined as follows:

[HVA]	= concentration of HVA in CSF (mol/ml)
f_1	= proportion of dopamine metabolized to HVA
DA_1	= rate of formation of dopamine independent of serotonin influence (mol/min)
DA_s	= rate of formation of dopamine dependent on serotonin influence (mol/min)
Cl_1	= clearance of HVA from CSF (ml/min)
R	= function relating dopamine turnover to serotonin turnover and release
[5-HIAA]	= concentration of 5-HIAA in CSF (mol/ml)
f_2	= proportion of serotonin metabolized to 5-HIAA
5HT	= rate of formation of serotonin (mol/min)
Cl_2	= clearance of 5-HIAA from CSF (ml/min)

Only three terms require special comment. The first is DA_s which allows for a certain proportion of dopamine synthesis to be under serotonergic control. DA_1 is the synthesis rate of dopamine dependent on all other influences. The R term is intentionally left vague since the linkage between the turnover of serotonin and its release at sites where it could act on dopamine or norepinephrine neurons to stimulate the synthesis and/or turnover of dopamine remains to be established. For instance, under certain situations it has been shown that the turnover of serotonin as reflected in 5-HIAA concentrations has no discernible link to serotonergic function (Commissiong 1985). Thus, we must allow for complex relationships between serotonin turnover and any target function, alteration of dopamine turnover being the one under consideration here.

With these definitions in mind, the following equations can be derived: first, relating the concentration of HVA to the synthesis rate of dopamine,

$$[HVA] = \frac{f_1(DA_1 + DA_s)\,mol/min}{Cl_1\,ml/min} = mol/ml$$

second, relating the concentration of 5-HIAA to the synthesis rate of serotonin

$$[5\text{-}HIAA] = \frac{f_2(5\text{-}HT)}{Cl_2}$$

third, relating dopamine synthesis which is dependent on some connection with serotonin synthesis,

$$DA_s = R\,(5\text{-}HT)$$

the ratio of HVA/5-HIAA then becomes,

$$\frac{[HVA]}{[5\text{-}HIAA]} = \frac{f_1}{f_2}\frac{Cl_2}{Cl_1}\frac{DA_1 + R\,(5\text{-}HT)}{(5\text{-}HT)}$$

Under conditions in which the fractional conversion rates of the parent amines to their metabolites (f_1 and f_2) are similar or covary, the term f_1/f_2 will be close to unity or a constant. Likewise, the clearance rates of 5-HIAA and HVA from the CSF (Cl_2 and Cl_1) may be very similar or covary across individuals, in which case Cl_2/Cl_1 will be close to unity or another constant. If these conditions hold, then leaving out the constant terms yields:

$$\frac{[HVA]}{[5\text{-}HIAA]} = \frac{(DA_1)}{(5\text{-}HT)} + R\,.$$

References

Ågren H, Mefford I, Rudorfer M, Linnoila M, Potter W (1986) Interacting neurotransmitter systems. A non-experimental approach to the 5-HIAA-HVA correlation in human CSF. J Psychiatr Res 20:175–193

Ågren H, Nordin C, Potter WZ (1988) Antidepressant drug action and CSF monoamine metabolites: new evidence for selective profiles on monoaminergic interactions. In: Belmaker RH, Sandler M, Dahlstrom A (eds) Progress in catecholamine research, Part C: Clinical aspects, Alan R. Liss, Inc, New York, in press

Antelman SM, Caggiula AR (1977) Norepinephrine-dopamine interactions and behaviour. Science 195:646–653

Åsberg M, Bertilsson L, Tuck O, Cronholm R, Sjöqvist F (1973) Indoleaminic metabolites in the cerebrospinal fluid of depressed patients before and during treatment with nortriptyline. Clin Pharmacol Ther 14:277–286

Åsberg M, Ringberger VA, Sjöqvist F, Thoren P, Träskman L, Tuck JR (1977) Monoamine metabolites in cerebrospinal fluid and serotonin uptake inhibition during treatment with chlorimipramine. Clin Pharmacol Ther 21:201–207

Benkirane S, Arbilla S, Langer SZ (1985) Supersensitivity of alpha$_2$-adrenoceptors modulating [^{3}H]5-HT release after noradrenergic denervation with DSP4. Eur J Pharmacol 119:131–133

Bentler PM (1980) Multivariate analysis with latent variables – causal modeling. Annu Rev Psychol 31:419–456

Bertilsson L, Åsberg M, Thoren P (1974) Differential effect of chlorimipramine and nortriptyline on cerebrospinal fluid metabolites of serotonin and noradrenaline in depression. Eur J Clin Pharmacol 7:365–368

Bertilsson L, Tuck JR, Siwers B (1980) Biochemical effects of zimelidine in man. Eur J Clin Pharmacol 18:483–487

Bjerkenstedt L, Edman G, Flyckt L, Hagenfeldt L, Sedvall G, Wiesel FA (1985) Clinical and biochemical effects of citalopram, a selective 5-HT reuptake inhibitor – a dose-response study in depressed patients. Psychopharmacology (Berlin) 87:253–259

Bowden CL, Koslow SH, Hanin I, Maas JW, Davis JM, Robins E (1985) Effects of amitriptyline and imipramine on brain amine neurotransmitter metabolites in cerebrospinal fluid. Clin Pharmacol Ther 37:316–324

Cole BJ, Robbins TW (1987) Amphetamine impairs the discriminative performance of rats with dorsal noradrenergic bundle lesions on a 5-choice serial reaction time task: new evidence for central dopaminergic-noradrenergic interactions. Psychopharmacology (Berlin) 91:458–466

Commissiong JW (1985) Monoamine metabolites: their relationship and lack of relationship to monoaminergic neuronal activity. Biochem Pharmacol 34:1127–1131

Dray AL, Gonye TJ, Oakley NR, Tanner T (1976) Evidence for the existence of a raphe projection to the substantia nigra in rat. Brain Res 113:45–57

Esler M, Jackman G, Leonard P, Skews H, Bobik A, Korner P (1981) Effect of norepinephrine uptake blockers on norepinephrine kinetics. Clin Pharmacol Ther 29:12–20

Fuxe K (1965) Evidence for the existence of monoamine neurons in the central nervous system. Acta Physiol Scand [Suppl 247] 65:37–85

Golden RN, Rudorfer MV, Sherer MA, Linnoila M, Potter WZ (1988) Bupropion in depression. I. Biochemical effects and clinical response. Arch Gen Psychiatry 45:139–143

Goodwin FK, Post RM, Dunner DL, Gordon EK (1973) Cerebrospinal fluid amine metabolites in affective illness: the probenecid technique. Am J Psychiatry 130:73–79

Hsiä JK, Ågren H, Rudorfer MV, Linnoila M, Potter WZ (1987) Monoamine metabolite interactions and the prediction of antidepressant response. Arch Gen Psychiatry 44:1078–1083

Jöreskog KG, Sörbom D (1984) LISREL VI. Analysis of structural relationships by the method of maximum likelihood. User's guide, 3rd edn. Department of Statistics at Uppsala University, Scientific Software, Mooresville

Linnoila M, Karoum F, Calil HM, Kopin IJ, Potter WZ (1982a) Alteration of norepinephrine metabolism with desipramine and zimelidine in depressed patients. Arch Gen Psychiatry 39:1025–1028

Linnoila M, Karoum F, Potter WZ (1982b) Effect of low dose clorgyline on 24-hour urinary monoamine secretion in rapidly cycling bipolar affective disorder patients. Arch Gen Psychiatry 39:513–516

Maas JW (1984) Relationships between central nervous system noradrenergic function and plasma and urinary concentrations of norepinephrine metabolites. In: Usdin E, Åsberg M, Bertilsson L, Sjöqvist F (eds) Frontiers in biochemical and pharmacological research in depression. Raven, New York, pp 45–55

Muscettola G, Goodwin FK, Potter WZ, Claeys MM, Markey SP (1978) Imipramine and desimipramine in plasma and spinal fluid: relationship to clinical response and serotonin metabolism. Arch Gen Psychiatry 35:621–625

Nurse B, Russell VA, Taljaard JJF (1985) Effect of chronic desipramine treatment on adrenoceptor modulation of [³H]dopamine release from rat nucleus accumbens slices. Brain Res 334:235–242

Potter WZ, Scheinin M, Golden RN, Rudorfer MV, Cowdry RW, Calil HM, Ross RJ, Linnoila M (1985) Selective antidepressants lack specificity on norepinephrine and serotonin metabolites in cerebrospinal fluid. Arch Gen Psychiatry 42:1171–1177

Risby ED, Hsiao JK, Sunderland T, Ågren H, Rudorfer MV, Potter WZ (1987) The effects of antidepressants on the HVA/5-HIAA ratio. Clin Pharmacol Ther 42:547–554

Rudorfer MV, Scheinin M, Karoum F, Ross RJ, Potter WZ, Linnoila M (1984) Reduction of norepinephrine turnover by serotonergic drugs in man. Biol Psychiatry 19:179–193

Scheinin H (1986) Enhanced noradrenergic neuronal activity increases homovanillic acid levels in cerebrospinal fluid. J Neurochem 47:665–667

Sedvall G, Fyrö B, Nybäck H, Wiesel F-A, Wode-Helgodt B (1974) Mass fragmentometric determination of homovanillic acid in lumbar cerebrospinal fluid of schizophrenic patients during treatment with antipsychotic drugs. J Psychiatr Res 11:75–80

Sedvall G, Fyrö B, Gullberg B, Nybäck H, Wiesel F-A, Wode-Helgodt B (1980) Relationships in healthy volunteers between concentrations of monoamine metabolites in cerebrospinal fluid and family history of psychiatric morbidity. Br J Psychiatry 136:366–374

Träskman L, Åsberg M, Bertilsson L, Cronholm B, Mellstrom B, Neckers IM, Sjöqvist F, Thoren P, Tybring G (1979) Plasma levels of chlorimipramine and its desmethyl-metabolite during treatment of depression. Clin Pharmacol Ther 26:600–610

Wode-Helgodt B, Fyrö B, Gullberg B, Sedvall G (1977) Effect of chlorpromazine treatment on monoamine metabolite levels in cerebrospinal fluid of psychotic patients. Acta Psychiatr Scand 56:129–142

Wood JH (ed) (1980) Neurobiology of cerebrospinal fluid. Plenum Press, New York

E-10-Hydroxynortriptyline: Effects and Disposition of a Potential Novel Antidepressant *

L. Bertilsson, M.-L. Dahl-Puustinen, and C. Nordin [1]

1 Metabolism of Nortriptyline

Nortriptyline is one of the most studied antidepressants, and a therapeutic plasma concentration interval has been established (Sjöqvist et al. 1980). When similar doses of nortriptyline are given, the plasma levels vary extensively among individual patients (Sjöqvist, this volume). This is due to the great variation in the liver cytochrome P-450 enzyme, which hydroxylates nortriptyline. In several studies both in vivo and in vitro, we have shown that E-10-hydroxylation of nortriptyline covaries with the debrisoquin hydroxylation phenotype (see Sjöqvist, this volume).

The major metabolite of nortriptyline in man is E-10-hydroxynortriptyline (E-10-OH-NT; Fig. 1). The Z isomer accounts for only 10%–20% of the amount of 10-OH-NT formed in vivo (Bertilsson and Alexanderson 1972; Mellström et al. 1981) and in human liver microsomes (Mellström et al. 1983).

2 Noradrenaline Uptake Inhibition of E-10-Hydroxynortriptyline and the Concentration of this Active Metabolite in Plasma and CSF

Results from early biochemical studies (Borgå et al. 1970) indicated that nortriptyline per se accounted for the noradrenaline uptake inhibition seen during treatment with the drug. In 1979, we showed that E- and Z-10-OH-NT were equipotent in inhibiting the uptake of noradrenaline into neurons from rat brain in vitro (Bertilsson et al. 1979). In this system the major isomer (E form) had a mean activity that was 57% that of nortriptyline. In the same study we found that in 87 patients treated with nortriptyline or amitriptyline, the mean ratio between the plasma levels of 10-OH-NT (sum of E and Z isomers) and nortriptyline was 1.4 ± 0.9 (range, 0.3–5.0).

We could later show that in 25 patients treated with nortriptyline, the mean cerebrospinal fluid (CSF) concentration of 10-OH-NT (67 nmol/l) was

* These studies have been supported by the Swedish Medical Research Council (3902 and 8270) and the Karolinska Institute
[1] Departments of Clinical Pharmacology and Psychiatry, Karolinska Institute, Huddinge Hospital, 141 86 Huddinge, Sweden

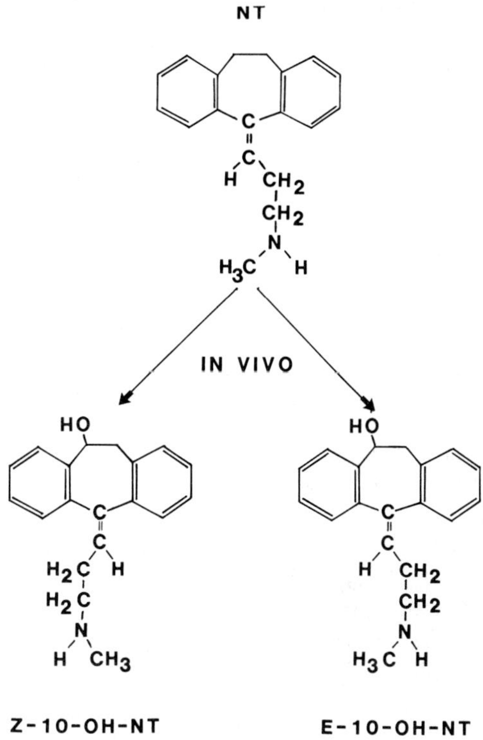

NT

Fig. 1. Formation of Z- and E-10-hydroxynortriptyline from nortriptyline

Z-10-OH-NT

E-10-OH-NT

higher than that of nortriptyline (39 nmol/l; Nordin et al. 1985; Fig. 2). These studies show that E-10-OH-NT passes the blood-brain barrier and probably contributes to increased transmission in central noradrenaline neurons. A clinical study on the treatment of depression with nortriptyline indicated that the therapeutic effect was related not only to the plasma concentration of nortriptyline but also to that of 10-OH-NT (Nordin et al. 1987b). This study and that of Malmgren et al. (1987) show that the serotonergic effect seen during nortriptyline treatment is due to the parent drug itself and not to hydroxy metabolites.

3 Anticholinergic Effect of E-10-Hydroxynortriptyline

The affinity of nortriptyline and its hydroxy metabolites to rat brain muscarinic receptors was determined by receptor-binding techniques (Wägner et al. 1984). E-10-OH-NT had only 1/18 the affinity of nortriptyline for such receptors, suggesting fewer anticholinergic side effects of the metabolite than of nortriptyline itself. This was supported by a case report (Bertilsson et al. 1985). A depressed patient had extremely rapid hydroxylation of both debrisoquin and nortriptyline and had been treated for a long period of time

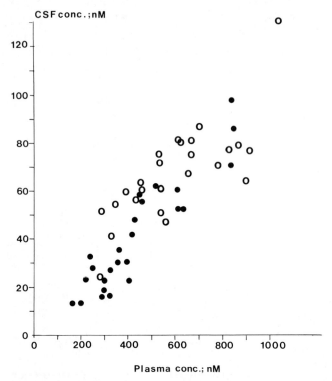

Fig. 2. Relationship between CSF and plasma concentrations of NT (●) and 10-OH-NT (○) (sum of unconjugated E and Z isomers) in 25 patients treated with nortriptyline. (From Nordin et al. 1985). ● NT r = 0.92, p < 0.001; ○ 10-OH-NT unconj. r = 0.77, p < 0.001

with high doses of nortriptyline to obtain "therapeutic plasma concentrations". On a 300-mg daily dose of nortriptyline, she had plasma concentrations of nortriptyline and 10-OH-NT that were 350 and 2730 nmol/l, respectively. Even at this extremely high plasma level of 10-OH-NT, she experienced no side effects.

In a later study we confirmed that E-10-OH-NT has less anticholinergic effect than nortriptyline (Nordin et al. 1987a). In a double-blind crossover

Table 1. Changes from baseline in saliva flow after single oral doses of placebo, E-10-OH−NT (75 mg hydrogen maleate) and nortriptyline (50 mg) in eight healthy subjects. (From Nordin et al. 1987a)

Compound	% Change (mean ± SD)	Significance (paired t test)
Placebo	−12.5±20.8 ⎫ NS	⎫
E-10-OH-NT	−22.1± 9.6 ⎭	⎬ p < 0.01
Nortriptyline	−37.8±17.1 ⎫ p < 0.05	⎭

study equimolar single oral doses of nortriptyline and *E*-10-OH-NT (and placebo) were given randomly to eight healthy volunteers. Nortriptyline significantly decreased saliva flow compared with both placebo ($p < 0.01$) and *E*-10-OH-NT ($p < 0.05$; Table 1). By contrast, there was no difference between *E*-10-OH-NT and placebo.

4 Disposition of the Enantiomers of *E*-10-Hydroxynortriptyline In Vivo and In Vitro

Increasing single oral doses (from 10 to 100 mg) of racemic *E*-10-OH-NT were given as the hydrogen maleate to nine healthy subjects (Bertilsson et al. 1986). The absorption was complete, as shown by the high urinary recovery ($86.1 \pm 9.9\%$) of the given dose. A mean of 51% of the administered dose was excreted as conjugate, and 24% was recovered as unchanged compound. The mean plasma half-life of *E*-10-OH-NT was 8.0 h.

We have developed an HPLC method for analysis of the glucuronides of the two enantiomers of *E*-10-OH-NT (Dumont et al. 1987). As these two glucuronides are diastereo-isomers, they could be separated on a regular C_{18} reversed-phase column. The unconjugated enantiomers of *E*-10-OH-NT were separated on an α_1-acid glycoprotein HPLC column and quantified by mass fragmentography (Perry et al. 1989). These methods have been used to quantitate the enantiomers of *E*-10-OH-NT and their glucuronides.

In a subsequent study, 75 mg racemic *E*-10-OH-NT was given orally as a single dose to ten healthy subjects (Dahl-Puustinen et al. 1989b). The disposition of the two enantiomers was quite different. The plasma concentration of $(-)$-*E*-10-OH-NT was two to five times higher than that of the $(+)$ enantiomer. A higher proportion of the given dose of $(+)$-*E*-10-OH-NT than that of the $(-)$ enantiomer was recovered in urine as glucuronide conjugate, while more $(-)$-*E*-10-OH-NT was recovered unchanged in the urine (Table 2). The plasma clearance of non-protein-bound enantiomer by the formation of glucuronide was higher for $(+)$-*E*-10-OH-NT (1.77 ± 0.60 l/kg

Table 2. Recovery in urine (% of dose) of unconjugated and glucuronidated enantiomers of *E*-10-OH-NT after an oral dose of 75 mg racemic *E*-10-OH-NT hydrogen maleate to 10 healthy subjects (mean $\pm$ SD)

E-10-OH-NT	Enantiomers		Significance
	+	−	
Unconjugated	14.4 ± 5.1	35.8 ± 10.0	$p < 0.0001$
Glucuronide	64.4 ± 12.1	35.3 ± 9.7	$p < 0.0001$
Total	78.8 ± 13.6	71.1 ± 10.3	$p < 0.05$

per hour) than for the $(-)$ form $(0.45 \pm 0.15; p < 0.0001)$. This shows that the glucuronidation of the $(+)$ enantiomer is more efficient than that of $(-)$-E-10-OH-NT.

We studied the glucuronidation of racemic E-10-OH-NT in the liver microsomal fraction in vitro (Dumont et al. 1987). The rat liver catalysed the formation of both glucuronides, while only $(+)$-E-10-OH-NT was glucuronidated in liver microsomes from 13 humans. We were surprised that the $(-)$-E-10-OH-NT glucuronide was not formed in human liver microsomes, since this compound is excreted in urine from subjects given the racemate (Table 2). In a subsequent study (Dahl-Puustinen et al. 1989a) it was shown that $(-)$ but not $(+)$-E-10-OH-NT was glucuronidated in homogenate of human intestinal mucosa. These studies show that there is an organ-specific glucuronidation of the enantiomers of E-10-OH-NT, i.e. $(+)$-E-10-OH-NT is glucuronidated with a high capacity in the liver, while the $(-)$ enantiomer is glucuronidated in the intestine with less capacity.

5 Initial Trial of E-10-Hydroxynortriptyline in Depressed Patients

Increasing daily doses (from 3×25 mg to 3×75 mg, given at 8 a.m., 2 and 10 p.m.) of racemic E-10-OH-NT have been given to the first patient in a clinical trial (Fig. 3). A 32-year-old man with recurrent major depression was given this compound for 18 days (Fig. 3), and then for another 5 days as an outpatient at a dose of 3×50 mg. Trough plasma levels of E-10-OH-NT (sum of the two enantiomers) before the morning dose were proportional to the dose. At the highest dose, plasma levels of 400 and 375 nmol/l were recorded. These levels are close to the levels usually measured during treatment of depression with nortriptyline (Nordin et al. 1987b; Fig. 2). The patient's condition ameliorated, and his score on the Montgomery-Åsberg Depression Rating Scale (Montgomery and Åsberg 1979) decreased from 34 before treatment to 16 after 18 days (Fig. 3). During the following 5 days as an outpatient the patient continued to improve. The patient was thereafter switched to nortriptyline with good results. During treatment with E-10-OH-NT no side effects were experienced by the patient. Of course, an open trial in one patient can not tell us very much about the antidepressant effect of the drug, but the results show dose-independent kinetics during maintenance therapy with E-10-OH-NT and, as expected, no side effects of this compound. Continued studies will evaluate the antidepressant effect.

6 A Comparison Between the Properties of E-10-Hydroxynortriptyline and Nortriptyline

In Table 3 certain properties of E-10-OH-NT and nortriptyline are compared in a schematic way. One major advantage of E-10-OH-NT is the slight inter-individual variation in the disposition, and it seems likely that similar doses of this compound may be given to different patients. If E-10-OH-NT can be

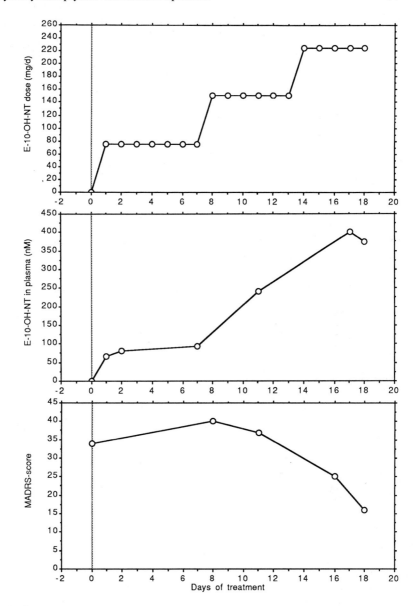

Fig. 3. The first patient treated with racemic *E*-10-OH-NT for 18 days as an inpatient. *Top*, time course of the dose; *middle*, plasma concentration (sum of the unconjugated enantiomers of *E*-10-OH-NT); *bottom*, Montgomery-Åsberg Depression Rating scale (*MADRS*) score

Table 3. Comparison between the properties of nortriptyline and those of E-10-OH-NT

	Nortriptyline	E-10-OH-NT
Disposition	Mainly E-10-hydroxylation	Glucuronidation and renal excretion (see Table 1)
Variation in disposition between individuals	Pronounced	Slight
Inhibition of noradrenaline uptake	+ + +	+ +
Inhibition of serotonin uptake	+	−
Anticholinergic effect	+ +	−
Antidepressant effect	Yes	To be evaluated

shown to have an antidepressant effect, its lack of anticholinergic effect could make it a valuable drug, especially in the elderly, who are sensitive to such side effects. As E-10-OH-NT is a specific inhibitor of noradrenaline uptake, it may also be used as a tool to evaluate the importance of changed noradrenaline transmission for the aetiology of depression.

Acknowledgements. We thank Jan Lundvall and Jolanta Widén for excellent assistance.

References

Bertilsson L, Alexanderson B (1972) Stereospecific hydroxylation of nortriptyline in man in relation to interindividual differences in its steady-state plasma level. Eur J Clin Pharmacol 4:201–205

Bertilsson L, Mellström B, Sjöqvist F (1979) Pronounced inhibition of noradrenaline uptake by 10-hydroxy metabolites of nortriptyline. Life Sci 25:1285–1292

Bertilsson L, Åberg-Wistedt A, Gustafsson LL, Nordin C (1985) Extremely rapid hydroxylation of debrisoquine – a case report with implication for treatment with nortriptyline and other tricyclic antidepressants. Ther Drug Monit 7:478–480

Bertilsson L, Nordin C, Otani K, Resul B, Scheinin M, Siwers B, Sjöqvist F (1986) Disposition of single oral doses of E-10-hydroxynortriptyline in healthy subjects with some observations on pharmacodynamic effects. Clin Pharmacol Ther 40:261–267

Borgå O, Hamberger B, Malmfors T, Sjöqvist F (1970) The role of plasma protein binding in the inhibitory effect of nortriptyline on the neuronal uptake of norepinephrine. Clin Pharmacol Ther 11:581–588

Dahl-Puustinen M-L, Dumont E, Bertilsson L (1989a) Glucuronidation of E-10-hydroxynortriptyline in human liver, kidney and intestine – organ-specific differences in enantioselectivity. Drug Metab Dispos (in press)

Dahl-Puustinen M-L, Perry TL Jr, Dumont E, von Bahr C, Nordin C, Bertilsson L (1989b) Stereoselective disposition of racemic E-10-hydroxynortriptyline in human beings. Clin Pharmacol Ther (in press)

Dumont E, von Bahr C, Perry TL Jr, Bertilsson L (1987) Glucuronidation of the enantiomers of E-10-hydroxynortriptyline in human and rat liver microsomes. Pharmacol Toxicol 61:335–341

Malmgren R, Åberg-Wistedt A, Bertilsson L (1987) Serotonin uptake inhibition during treatment of depression with nortriptyline caused by parent drug and not by 10-hydroxymetabolites. Psychopharmacology (Berlin) 92:169–172

Mellström B, Bertilsson L, Säwe J, Schulz HU, Sjöqvist F (1981) E- and Z-hydroxylation of nortriptyline in man – relationship to polymorphic hydroxylation of debrisoquine. Clin Pharmacol Ther 30:189–193

Mellström B, Bertilsson L, Birgersson C, Göransson M, von Bahr C (1983) E- and Z-10-hydroxylation of nortriptyline by human liver microsomes – methods and characterization. Drug Metab Dispos 11:115–119

Montgomery SA, Åsberg M (1979) A new depression scale designed to be sensitive to change. Br J Psychiatry 134:382–389

Nordin C, Bertilsson L, Siwers B (1985) CSF and plasma levels of nortriptyline and its 10-hydroxy metabolites. Br J Clin Pharmacol 20:411–413

Nordin C, Bertilsson L, Otani K, Widmark A (1987a) Little anticholinergic effect of E-10-hydroxynortriptyline compared with nortriptyline in healthy subjects. Clin Pharmacol Ther 41:97–102

Nordin C, Bertilsson L, Siwers B (1987b) Clinical and biochemical effects during treatment of depression with nortriptyline – the role of 10-hydroxynortriptyline. Clin Pharmacol Ther 42:10–19

Perry TL Jr, Drayer DE, Widén J, Bertilsson L (1989) Analysis of the enantiomers of E-10-hydroxynortriptyline in plasma and urine using chiral alpha-1-acid glycoprotein HPLC and mass fragmentography. J Chromatogr (to be published)

Sjöqvist F, Bertilsson L, Åsberg M (1980) Monitoring tricyclic antidepressants. Ther Drug Monit 2:85–93

Wägner A, Ekqvist B, Bertilsson L, Sjöqvist F (1984) Weak binding of 10-hydroxymetabolites of nortriptyline to rat brain muscarinic acetylcholine receptors. Life Sci 35:1379–1383

Molecular Graphics of Antidepressant Drugs and Metabolites *

S. G. Dahl, Ø. Edvardsen, and E. Heimstad [1]

1 Three-Dimensional Molecular Graphics

Along with the rapid advance in molecular biology, methods and concepts have evolved which have provided new insight into the three-dimensional molecular structures of macromolecules and into the mechanisms of their interaction with various types of ligands.

Many research laboratories involved in drug design have recently acquired computer graphics equipment with software designed for three-dimensional molecular modelling. This has become feasible through recent developments in computer technology which have provided commercial workstations with rapidly increasing power at decreasing prices. As reviewed by Langridge (1988), the first static line drawings of molecular structures on the screen of a computer were made by Bushing in 1961, and the first interactive two-dimensional computer graphics program was described in 1963. The first interactive three-dimensional graphics hardware was built in 1964 and was applied to proteins and nucleic acids. In the same period, the use of a pen plotter in the ORTEP program package (Johnson 1971) became a standard, which since has been widely used for illustration of three-dimensional molecular structures determined by X-ray crystallography. The ORTEP technique was previously used in our laboratories to produce drawings of solid-state molecular structures of phenothiazine drugs and their metabolites (Dahl et al. 1983, 1986).

Modern workstations offer high-quality raster or vector colour graphics, perspective, depth cueing, three-dimensional clipping and real-time translation and rotation. Combined with other computational methods, these techniques have enormous potential for increasing our insight into the spatial arrangements of atoms in molecules, the charge distribution over molecules, and the dynamics of molecular interactions. Such methods may provide important information about the molecular mechanisms of action of drugs and other biologically active compounds.

* This work was supported by grants from Troms Fylkeskommune and the Norwegian Research Council for Science and the Humanities
[1] Institute of Medical Biology, University of Tromsø, P.O. Box 977, 9001 Tromsø, Norway

Clinical Pharmacology in Psychiatry
Editors: S. G. Dahl and L. F. Gram
(Psychopharmacology Series 7)
© Springer-Verlag Berlin Heidelberg 1989

2 Molecular Structures in Crystals and Solution

X-ray diffraction techniques have been and still are the most widely used experimental methods for determination of three-dimensional molecular structures. Many computational methods used in molecular modelling are based on atomic coordinates from crystal structures. Up to now the number of three-dimensional protein structures which have been solved at atomic resolution have been less than 20 per year. Ongoing research in several laboratories is aimed at the cloning, purification and crystallization of neurotransmitter receptors, but no three-dimensional crystal structure of a neurotransmitter receptor, solved at atomic resolution, has yet been reported.

As a result of recently developed techniques for fast amino acid sequencing in proteins, a large number of such sequences are currently being reported each year. Among these have been human nicotinic (Noda et al. 1983; Shibahara et al. 1985) and muscarinic acetylcholine receptors (Bonner et al. 1987) and β_2-adrenergic receptors (Kobilka et al. 1987). These authors proposed that the α carbon chain of the β_2-receptor passes through the cell membrane seven times, which points out the difficulties encountered in obtaining a crystal of such a receptor protein in its functional state. Several research groups are trying to develop methods to predict tertiary peptide and protein structures from amino acid sequences based on artificial intelligence (Eccles and Saldanha 1988) and other approaches. However, problems in this extremely difficult task remain unsolved. Predictions of three-dimensional protein structures may be based on substitution of chemical groups in known structures of analogous proteins (Stewart et al. 1987), but this method has its obvious limitation in the lack of such analogous structures.

Recent studies from our laboratories on the structures of antipsychotic drugs and their metabolites (Dahl et al. 1987) have demonstrated that significant information about the structures and dynamics of psychotropic drug molecules may be gained by molecular modelling techniques. Although no definite three-dimensional models of neurotransmitter receptor molecules are available yet, these studies have demonstrated that molecular modelling of drug molecules may provide increased insight into how the drug interacts with receptor molecules.

3 Structures of Tricyclic Antidepressants

We have used the program package, Assisted Model Building with Energy Refinement (AMBER; Weiner et al. 1984, 1986), to calculate molecular structures by molecular mechanics methods. The Molecular Interactive Display And Simulation programs (MIDAS; Jarvis et al. 1986) were used for molecular graphics on an Evans and Sutherland PS390 computer graphics system, with a DEC Microvax II as host machine. With this computer graphics system crystal structures of molecules may be displayed, and van der

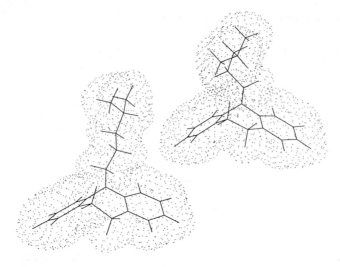

Fig. 1. Crystal structure of imipramine hydrochloride (Post et al. 1975). The two molecules in the asymmetric unit are shown after addition of hydrogen atoms and van der Waals surfaces. *Lines* connect the positions of the center of each atom; *dots* show the van der Waals surfaces

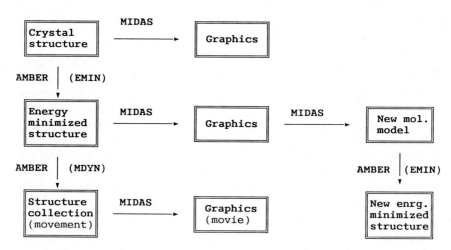

Fig. 2. Procedure for molecular modelling. The *MIDAS* (Molecular Interactive Display And Simulation) computer graphics programs were used to display three-dimensional molecular structures from X-ray crystallographic studies, energy minimizations and molecular dynamics simulations. New models may be built with the computer graphics system by rotation of bonds and substitution of atoms or groups. The *AMBER* (Assisted Model Building with Energy Refinement) programs were used for energy minimizations (*EMIN*) and molecular dynamics simulations (*MDYN*)

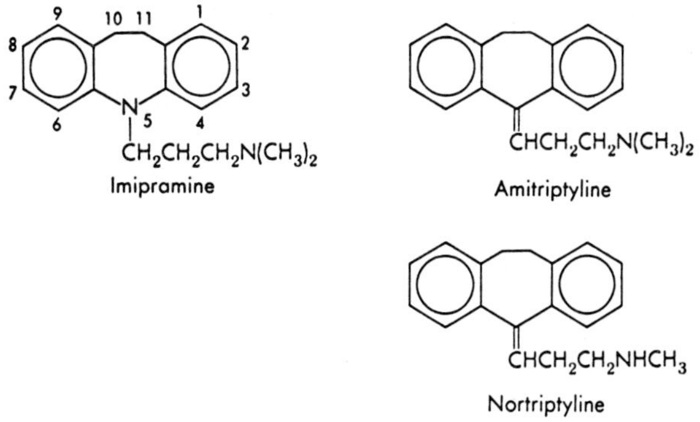

Fig. 3. Chemical formulas of imipramine, amitriptyline and nortriptyline

Waals or water accessible surfaces may easily be added, as shown in Fig. 1 for the crystal structure of imipramine hydrochloride (Post et al. 1975).

Molecular mechanics calculations of drug molecules are often based on their three-dimensional crystal structures, determined by X-ray diffraction techniques. However by combining molecular mechanics calculations and computer graphics, such calculations may be based on the crystal structure of a chemically related compound in cases where no crystal structure of the drug is available. A procedure for such calculations is outlined in Fig. 2.

This procedure was used to calculate three-dimensional molecular structures of amitriptyline, nortriptyline and 10-hydroxynortriptyline, compounds for which to our knowledge no crystal structures have been reported. The calculations started from the coordinates of one of the imipramine structures shown in Fig. 1. As a first step, the nitrogen atom of the central ring of the imipramine structure was replaced by carbon, and one hydrogen was removed from the adjacent CH_2 group of the side chain. The energy of this structure was minimized with suitable parameters for each atom type, for instance, corresponding to a double bond with high rotational barrier between the two carbons of the exocyclic bond. In this way a model of the structure of amitriptyline (Fig. 3) was produced. The amitriptyline structure was used for further calculations of a nortriptyline structure by replacement of one of the dimethylamino methyl groups by a hydrogen atom and subsequent energy minimization. Finally, each of the four hydrogens at the CH_2 groups of the central ring in nortriptyline was replaced by a hydroxyl group, and energy minimizations produced the four 10-hydroxynortriptyline structures shown in Fig. 4.

10-Hydroxynortriptyline has four enantiomers, $(+)$-E-10-OH-NT, $(-)$-E-10-OH-NT, $(+)$-Z-10-OH-NT and $(-)$-Z-10-OH-NT. As discussed by Bertilsson et al. (this volume), these compounds differ both in their pharmacokinetic and in their pharmacodynamic properties. The plasma concentrations of E-10-OH-NT in man are higher than those of Z-10-OH-NT after therapeutic doses of nortriptyline, and the plasma levels of $(-)$-E-10-

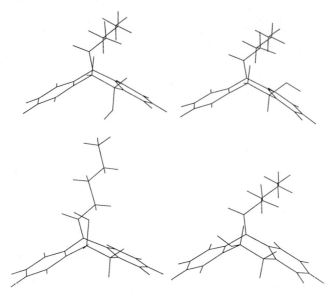

Fig. 4. Three-dimensional molecular structures of *R-Z-* (*upper left*), *S-Z-* (*upper right*), *R-E-* (*lower left*) and *S-E-*10-hydroxynortriptyline (*lower right*)

OH-NT are higher than the levels of (+)-*E*-10-OH-NT. Compared to nortriptyline, racemic *E*-10-OH-NT has about 50% of the potency in inhibiting noradrenaline uptake in brain slices, about 5% of the potency in muscarinic cholinergic receptor binding, and significantly fewer anticholinergic effects in man.

As shown in Fig. 4, the hydroxyl groups have different positions in the four enantiomers. The difference between the *E* and *Z* isomers lies in which of the two CH_2 groups, relative to the orientation of the side chain, is substituted with a hydroxyl group. The *R* and *S* forms, and (+) and (−) forms, correspond to substitutions of different hydrogen atoms at the same CH_2 group. The orientation of the hydrogen of each hydroxyl group shown in Fig. 4 is probably less significant, due to its rotational freedom. The absolute configurations of the four 10-hydroxynortriptyline enantiomers have not been determined, and it is not known therefore which of the two *E*-10-OH-NT enantiomers shown in Fig. 4 is identical to the (+) and which to the (−) enantiomer, and similar ambiguity exists for the two *Z* enantiomers. Although the exocyclic double bond effectively prevents rotation between *Z* and *E* isomers, the arrangement of the side chain and the tricyclic system is far from the planarity that formulas such as the ones shown in Fig. 3 might lead one to imagine. Electronic interactions and steric hindrance forces the side chain of each structure out of the plane of the ring system, and places it "above" the tricyclic system when viewed in the perspective shown in Fig. 4.

From atomic charges, calculated by quantum mechanics, the electrostatic potentials around each of the four 10-hydroxynortriptyline molecules was calculated. These potentials could be displayed together with the molecular structure on the screen of the graphics system, using different colouring of the molecular surfaces, as previously reported by Weiner et al. (1982) for other compounds. The electrostatic potential surfaces demonstrated that the electronic structure of the tricyclic region of the molecules differs according to the position of the hydroxyl groups. This might offer one explanation for the difference in pharmacological activity between the 10-hydroxynortriptyline enantiomers.

4 Molecular Dynamics of 10-Hydroxynortriptyline

The method of molecular dynamics treats each atom of a molecule as a particle which moves according to Newton's equations. Together with an energy function described by the terms of molecular mechanics, this method makes it possible to simulate the movements of molecular systems in a computer. Such movements occur in the femtosecond (10^{-15} s) time scale, and simulations are usually performed over a time span of 1–100 ps (10^{-12} s), which is often sufficiently long to observe collective movements in the molecule, i.e. between different conformations.

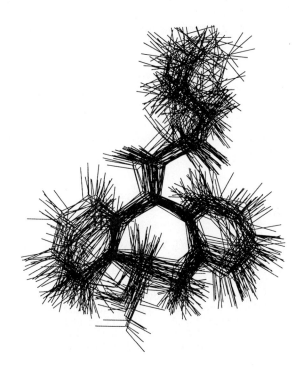

Fig. 5. Superposition of 50 different *S-E*-10-hydroxynortriptyline structures obtained during a 5 ps molecular dynamics simulation in vacuo

Molecular dynamics simulations have shown that unlike the static structures in a crystal, proteins in the biophase must be considered as flexible entities, which have freedom to move between different conformational states (Karplus and McCammon 1983). Similar flexibility of psychotropic drug molecules was observed by molecular dynamics simulations of phenothiazine drug molecules dissolved in water at physiological temperature (Dahl et al. 1987). This demonstrates the importance of the dynamic aspect for understanding the mechanisms of drug-receptor interactions at the molecular level.

Figure 5 shows the molecular dynamics of S-E-10-hydroxynortriptyline during a 5 ps molecular dynamics simulation in vacuo. The 50 superimposed structures were sampled at 0.1 ps intervals. Both the tricyclic ring system and the dimethylamino side chain moved considerably during the simulation, and the hydroxyl group rotated 360°. The ring system attained various degrees of folding along the central axis during the simulation, and the dimethylamino group at the side chain moved between different conformations.

5 Conclusions

Information about three-dimensional molecular structures from X-ray crystallographic studies alone can only partly explain the molecular mechanisms of drug interactions with receptors or enzymes. Molecular modelling based on quantum mechanical calculations of electrostatic potentials, energy minimizations by molecular mechanics methods, molecular dynamics simulations of the movements of molecules, combined with computer graphics, may increase our understanding of the mechanisms of such interactions. Molecular dynamics simulations of four hydroxymetabolites of nortriptyline and calculations of their electronic structures may explain the differences in their pharmacological activities. Both the position of the hydroxyl group and the contribution from the hydroxyl group to the electrostatic potential around the molecule may affect the pharmacological activity of each metabolite.

References

Bonner TI, Buckley NJ, Young AC, Brann MR (1987) Identification of a family of muscarinic acetylcholine receptor genes. Science 237:527–532
Dahl SG, Hals P-A, Johnsen H, Morel E, Lloyd KG (1983) Possible role of hydroxymetabolites in the action of neuroleptics. In: Gram LF, Usdin E, Dahl SG, Kragh-Sørensen P, Sjöqvist F, Morselli PL (eds) Clinical pharmacology in psychiatry. Bridging the experimental-therapeutic gap. Macmillan, London, pp 136–149
Dahl SG, Hough E, Hals P-A (1986) Phenothiazine drugs and metabolites: molecular conformation and dopaminergic, alpha adrenergic and muscarinic cholinergic receptor binding. Biochem Pharmacol 35:1263–1269

Dahl SG, Kollman PA, Rao SR, Singh UC (1987) Molecular graphics of neuroleptics: new perspectives in neuro-psychopharmacology and drug design. Nord Psykiatr Tidsskr 41:473–474

Eccles JR, Saldanha JW (1988) GENPRO: Automatic generation of PROLOG clause files for knowledge-based systems in molecular biology. Proceedings of the 7th annual conference of the Molecular Graphics Society, 10–12 Aug, San Francisco, pp 45–46 (Available from Molecular Graphics Society, c/o Thomas Ferrin, UCSF, CA 94143-0446)

Jarvis L, Huang C, Ferrin T, Langridge R (1986) UCSF MIDAS. Molecular interactive display and simulation. School of Pharmacy, University of California, San Francisco

Johnson CK (1971) ORTEP. Report ORNL-3794, revised. Oak Ridge National Laboratory, Tennessee

Karplus M, McCammon JA (1983) Dynamics of proteins: elements and function. Annu Rev Biochem 53:263–300

Kobilka BK, Dixon RAF, Frielle T, Dohlman HG, Bolanowski MA, Sigal IS, Yang-Feng TL, et al. (1987) cDNA for the human β_2-adrenergic receptor: a protein with multiple membrane-spanning domains and encoded by a gene whose chromosomal location is shared with that of the receptor for platelet-derived growth factor. Proc Natl Acad Sci USA 84:46–50

Langridge R (1988) Molecular graphics: reflections on the last thirty years and speculation on the next five. Proceedings of the 7th annual conference of the Molecular Graphics Society, 10–12 Aug, San Francisco, p 22 (Available from Molecular Graphics Society, c/o Thomas Ferrin, UCSF, CA 94143-0446)

Noda M, Furutani Y, Takahashi H, Toyosato M, Tanabe T, Shimizu H, Kikyotani S, et al. (1983) Cloning and sequence analysis of calf cDNA and human genomic DNA encoding alpha-subunit precursor of muscle acetylcholine receptor. Nature 305:818–823

Post ML, Kennard O, Horn AS (1975) The tricyclic antidepressants: imipramine hydrochloride. The crystal and molecular structure of 5-(3-dimethylaminopropyl)-10,11-dihydro-5H-dibenz[b,f]azepine hydrochloride. Acta Crystallogr B31:1008–1013

Shibahara S, Kubo T, Perski HJ, Takahashi H, Noda M, Numa S (1985) Cloning and sequence analysis of human genomic DNA encoding gamma subunit precursor of muscle acetylcholine receptor. Eur J Biochem 146:15–22

Stewart DE, Weiner PK, Wampler JE (1987) Prediction of the structure of proteins using related structures, energy minimization and computer graphics. J Mol Graphics 5:133–140

Weiner PK, Langridge RL, Blaney JM, Schaefer R, Kollman PA (1982) Electrostatic potential molecular surfaces. Proc Natl Acad Sci USA 79:3754–3758

Weiner SJ, Kollman PA, Case DA, Singh UC, Ghio C, Alagona G, Profeta S Jr, Weiner P (1984) A new force field for molecular mechanics simulation of nucleic acids and proteins. J Am Chem Soc 106:765–874

Weiner SJ, Kollman PA, Nguyen DT, Case DA (1986) An all atom force field for simulations of proteins and nucleic acids. J Comput Chem 7:230–252

Negative Symptoms in Schizophrenia: A Target for New Drug Development *

H. Y. Meltzer and J. Zureick [1]

1 Introduction

Delusions, hallucinations, and certain types of thought disorders, e.g., incoherence and illogicality, constitute the so-called positive symptoms in schizophrenia. It is unclear whether other kinds of thought disorder, e.g., looseness of associations, are also positive symptoms. The most important clinical effect of the current major classes of antipsychotic drugs, e.g., phenothiazines, butyrophenones, and thioxanthenes, is their ability to eliminate or significantly diminish positive symptoms in psychiatric patients, including those who meet narrow diagnostic criteria for schizophrenia. Positive symptoms are thought to be readily rated in most patients, at least in those who are not so guarded that they deny them or are mute and unable to confirm their presence or absence. The ability of antipsychotic drugs to diminish positive symptoms correlates highly with their ability to block dopamine D_2 receptors (Seeman and Lee 1975), a characteristic which is readily ascertainable preclinically through a variety of methods. Because of these three factors – effectiveness, ease of clinical evaluation and preclinical predictability – much of the search for novel drug treatments in schizophrenia has focused on the alleviation of positive symptoms by dopamine receptor blockers which have a favorable side effect profile, desirable pharmacokinetic features, or both. Putative antipsychotics are then tested in patients, with the major focus on the rapid alleviation of positive symptoms. The net result is that antipsychotic drugs have a similar efficacy profile, with little to choose between them except side effects (Rifkin and Siris 1987).

This emphasis on the alleviation of positive symptoms in the development of new drugs for the treatment of schizophrenia is fostered by the view, held by many, that the sort of features generally considered as constituting the negative symptoms of schizophrenia, e.g., flat affect, withdrawal, loss of motivation, and apathy, is less likely to respond to the existing classes of antipsychotic drugs, and, moreover, that their etiology may be not only qualitatively different from that of positive symptoms but, in fact, not

* Supported, in part, by USPHS MH 41594, MH 41684, and grants from the Cleveland and Sawyer Foundations. H. Y. M. is recipient of USPHS Research Career Scientist Award USPHS MH 47808
[1] Dept. of Psychiatry, Case Western Reserve University, School of Medicine, Cleveland, OH 44106, USA

Clinical Pharmacology in Psychiatry
Editors: S. G. Dahl and L. F. Gram
(Psychopharmacology Series 7)
© Springer-Verlag Berlin Heidelberg 1989

amenable to treatment of any kind because of their basis in structural brain damage (Crow 1980). Finally, there have been, until recently, no specific scales for rating negative symptoms, and there is still a lack of consensus as to what these are. For these and other reasons, there has been little focus on developing drugs for negative symptoms. Since negative symptoms are a major factor in the impairment of the quality of life of schizophrenics, since they augment the burden of those who care for or live with schizophrenics, over and above the impairments and burdens which result from positive symptoms, the alleviation of negative symptoms, if possible, must be a primary goal of any therapies which hope to be superior to the typical neuroleptics in more than side effects alone.

2 Identification of Negative Symptoms

The historical origins of the terms positive and negative symptoms have been reviewed by Berrios (1985) and Trimble (1986) and need not be further discussed here. Strauss et al. (1974) reawakened interest in negative symptoms such as withdrawal and apathy and included certain kinds of formal thought disorder, e.g., blocking, in their concept of negative symptoms. Wing (1978) grouped together "emotional apathy, slowness of thought and movement, underactivity, lack of drive, poverty of speech and social withdrawal" under the rubric of the clinical "poverty syndrome." As will be seen, our data suggest that some types of thought disorder such as poverty of thought content and looseness of associations cluster with the symptoms identified by Wing (1978) and can be separated from positive symptoms by cluster analysis (Meltzer et al., in preparation).

The concept of negative symptoms has been refined through factor analytic studies to better determine what they are, whether they are unitary in nature, and the relationship between negative and positive symptoms, i.e., whether they are independent (Lewine et al. 1983) or are part of a single dimension, as suggested by Andreasen (1982). Nearly all other factor-analytic studies of schizophrenic psychopathology (Spitzer et al. 1967; Fleiss et al. 1971; Everitt et al. 1971; Gibbons et al. 1985; Liddle 1987) have identified two or three dimensions of negative symptoms.

The lack of homogeneity of negative symptoms has potentially important clinical implications. Different types of negative symptoms may appear at different stages of schizophrenia or may respond differentially to pharmacological or psychosocial treatments. A cluster analysis of negative symptoms in 165 schizophrenic patients identified three clusters of negative symptoms:

- *Cognitive impairment/inappropriate affect:* incoherence, poverty of thought content, loosening of associations, inappropriate affect.
- *Anhedonia/anergia:* loss of interest, loss of sexual interest, depressed appearance, fatigue.
- *Retardation/flat affect:* slowed speech, slowed body movement, blunted affect.

These items were obtained from the Schedule for Affective Disorders in Schizophrenia-Change (SADS-C; Endicott and Spitzer 1978) or the Present State Examination (9th edition; Wing et al. 1974). None of the positive symptoms on the SADS-C clustered with these items. Thus, in addition to the symptoms identified by Strauss et al. (1974) and Wing (1978), our studies suggest that a broader range of affective and cognitive symptoms, e.g., inappropriate affect and loose associations, are independent of positive symptoms. It is unclear whether they should be considered negative symptoms or a third class of symptoms. I suggest the latter since they are independent of both positive and classical negative symptoms.

Carpenter et al. (1985) have proposed a distinction between primary and secondary negative symptoms. This distinction is based only on presumptive etiology, not on type of behavior. Secondary negative symptoms are proposed to be: (a) the direct result of the acute onset of or an increase in positive symptoms (e.g., withdrawal in response to a paranoid idea); (b) extrapyramidal side effects (e.g., motor retardation due to drug-induced akinesia); (c) apathy and flat affect due to a coexisting reactive depression or the so-called postpsychotic depression; or (d) as a response to an understimulating environment. Secondary, negative symptoms are expected to respond to appropriate treatments of the etiological factors.

Negative symptoms not due to clearly identified factors are considered by Carpenter et al. (1985) to be primary negative symptoms and constitute what they call the deficit state. They relate these symptoms to the type II schizophrenia of Crow (1980). They suggest that the treatment of primary and secondary negative symptoms may differ because of their differences in etiology.

3 Effect of Typical Neuroleptics on Negative Symptoms

Crow (1980) proposed that negative symptoms were largely unresponsive to neuroleptic treatment because they were manifestations of irreversible structural changes in the central nervous system. He subsequently suggested abnormalities in the temporal lobe to be the cause of negative symptoms based on neuropathological and neuropeptide abnormalities (Crow 1985). It is noteworthy that the cerebral atrophy and dilated ventricles which have been cited as evidence for the structural changes underlying negative symptoms have also been demonstrated in bipolar patients (Pearlson and Veroff 1981) and may also be found in schizophrenic patients who have few or no negative symptoms (see Meltzer 1987 for review). However, some authors believe that there is a correlation between negative symptoms and enlarged lateral ventricles (e.g., Williams et al. 1985).

There is considerable empirical evidence for the proposition that negative symptoms, while not as responsive to neuroleptic treatment as positive symptoms, do diminish during the course of treatment with neuroleptic drugs and may worsen in the absence of such treatment. The literature supporting this conclusion has been critically reviewed elsewhere (Meltzer et al. 1986; Meltzer 1986). A similar conclusion was also reached by Goldberg (1985). Preliminary results of a study in which we found that treatment with typical neuroleptics differentially affected positive and negative symptoms have been previously published (Meltzer 1985, 1986). We have now found that typical neuroleptics produce as much improvement in cognitive impairment/inappropriate affect as in positive symptoms. Significant improvement was also noted in anhedonia/anergia and retardation/flat affect but to a much lesser extent. No overall effect of paranoid as opposed to undifferentiated schizophrenia or of sex, age, or duration of illness was found. Improvement in negative symptoms was present even after controlling for improvement in positive symptoms (Meltzer et al., in preparation).

4 Clozapine and Negative Symptoms

Despite these results, clinical experience indicates that better treatments of negative symptoms are needed. There is now a strong body of evidence from controlled clinical trials which suggests that clozapine, an atypical neuroleptic (Meltzer 1988) may be superior to typical neuroleptics in treating negative symptoms as well as positive symptoms (Meltzer 1987, 1989; Kane et al. 1988). One early study indicated that clozapine was superior to chlorpromazine in treating negative symptoms (Fischer-Cornelssen and Ferner 1975), two showed a strong trend in that direction (Gerlach et al. 1974; Gelenberg and Doller 1979), and two others showed equal effectiveness for clozapine and CPZ (Niskanen et al. 1974; Guirgius et al. 1977).

Claghorn et al. (1987) compared chlorpromazine and clozapine in 151 schizophrenics (DSM-II criteria), none of whom had been hospitalized for more than 6 months. Negative symptoms were rated in terms of the anergia subscale of the Brief Psychiatric Rating Scale (BPRS; Overall and Gorham 1962), which includes the following mainly negative symptoms: emotional withdrawal, blunted affect, psychomotor retardation, and disorientation. Clozapine produced significantly greater improvement in this subscale compared to chlorpromazine at weeks 1, 2, 3, 5, 6, 8 as well as with an end-point analysis.

In a recently completed multicenter trial, we studied the effect of clozapine versus chlorpromazine in nearly 300 treatment-resistant chronic schizophrenics (Kane et al. 1989). Schizophrenic patients with a history of failure to respond to at least three neuroleptics of two different classes over a period of 5 years were included. These patients were then prospectively treated with haloperidol at doses up to 60 mg/day for 6 weeks. Those with no clinical improvement (99%) were then randomly assigned to a 6-week trial with chlorpromazine or clozapine. The mean peak dose of clozapine was 600 mg/day, and that of chlorpromazine was 1200 mg/day. Significant advantages of clozapine over chlorpromazine in decreasing total BPRS and BPRS anergia scores were noted from weeks 1 to 6. Of the clozapine-treated patients, 30% were considered responders ($\geq$ 20% decrease in BPRS plus other criteria based mainly on changes in positive symptoms) versus 4% of the chlorpromazine-treated patients. Nurses' ratings on the NOSIE scale (Honigfeld et al. 1966) indicated significant improvement in social competence, social interest, personal neatness, and retardation at weeks 2–6, with the social interest factor ratings showing the greatest improvement. There was no significant difference in EPS between the two groups because of the use of an anticholinergic with chlorpromazine. Side effects such as sedation or extrapyramidal side effects did not account for the difference.

We have administered clozapine on an open basis to 43 treatment-resistant chronic patients for periods of up to 27 months. A total of 17 (40%) patients were dropped because of side effects (including two cases of agranulocytosis), noncompliance, or failure to respond. Of the remaining 26 patients, 19 (13%) showed improvement in positive symptoms of at least 20% on the BPRS, as well as increased affective arousal and responsivity, increased intellectual content, spontaneous speech, social drive, interest in activities and independence. Improvement in some types of symptoms was dramatic in some cases. Thus, of the original 43 patients, 19 (44.2%) improved on clozapine. Improvement in negative symptoms was, if anything, more striking than improvement in positive symptoms. All three SADS-C negative symptoms factors – cognitive impairment/inappropriate affect, anhedonia/anergia, and retardation/flat affect – responded to clozapine treatment. We included only those subjects who initially had symptoms of a particular kind in our analysis. Some patients were too ill to be reliably rated. As indicated in Table 1, for 23 of the subjects for whom SADS-C data for at least 3 months of treatment was available at the time of this writing, neither the overall improvement in positive symptoms nor any of the negative symptom subscales was significantly different. When data from those subjects who improved by at least 20% in the total BPRS was examined separately, there again was no difference in the percentage of im-

Table 1. End-point analysis of effect of clozapine on positive, cognitive, and negative symptoms

Symptom cluster	Total subjects[a]		Subjects who improved	
	n	Mean $\pm$ SEM (%)	n (%)	Mean $\pm$ SEM (%)
Positive	20	19.9 $\pm$ 14.3	15(75)	48.4 $\pm$ 9.7
Cognitive impairment/ inappropriate affect	20	47.4 $\pm$ 13.8	16(80)	70.8 $\pm$ 10.1
Retardation/flat affect	22	24.9 $\pm$ 24.2	19(86)	63.1 $\pm$ 5.7
Anhedonia/anergia	23	33.3 $\pm$ 20.7	19(83)	72.1 $\pm$ 8.2

[a] Six subjects dropped out because of lack of effect or side effects.

provement in positive and negative symptoms. Nevertheless, there were trends for the percentage of improvement in negative symptoms to exceed that in positive symptoms. The proportion of patients with negative symptoms who improved ranged from 80% to 86% versus 75% for positive symptoms. Again, there was no significant difference. The proportion of patients with improvement in positive or negative symptoms of at least 20% over baseline also did not differ. Of interest is the fact that improvement in negative symptoms occurred in seven of eight patients with no improvement in positive symptoms. Since our treatment program included psychosocial treatments along with clozapine, and there was no drug comparison group, such improvement cannot definitely be attributed to clozapine.

Lindström (1988) recently reported that employment increased from 3% to 39% in patients who remained on clozapine for 2 years. We have noted a similar trend in our patients.

These studies make it clear that clozapine can produce significant improvement in negative symptoms and in social and work functioning. However, a number of questions remain with regard to clozapine and the treatment of negative symptoms. These questions would also be relevant for any drug treatment of negative symptoms. What is the relationship between improvement in positive symptoms and negative symptoms, especially the temporal relationship? Does improvement in negative symptoms depend upon improvement in positive symptoms? Can it occur in residual schizophrenics without prominent positive symptoms? Will it improve secondary negative symptoms due to other neuroleptics, affective disturbance, postpsychotic depression, or lack of stimulation in the environment, as well as primary negative symptoms which are part of the deficit state? How much can psychosocial interventions, e.g., family therapy, supportive psychotherapy, enhance the effect of clozapine on negative symptoms and social functioning? Finally, what is the biological basis for the ability of clozapine to produce a degree of improvement in negative symptoms not produced by typical neuroleptics? This will be considered subsequently.

5 Negative Symptoms – Target of Drug Therapy

As mentioned in the "Introduction," there is clearly a need for more effective treatments of negative symptoms. Affective blunting, lack of motivation, diminished ideation, marked dependency, and psychomotor retardation impair many schizophrenics who might have much better social functioning or quality of life were it not for their negative symptoms. Nonschizophrenic patients with delusional disorder or chronic auditory hallucinations do not usually have prominent negative symptoms. Their generally much better social functioning may be an indication of the deleterious effect that negative symptoms can have on overall social function. Negative symptoms rarely occur alone, except in the deficit state, which is characteristic of residual schizophrenics. The treatment of negative symptoms is generally necessary in patients who also have positive symptoms. Drugs such as clozapine which have an effect on both types of symptoms will have a broader application than drugs which act on negative symptoms alone, but there may be a place for the latter as well.

It is clear that negative symptoms in schizophrenics can respond to treatment with typical neuroleptics, but even more to clozapine, an atypical neuroleptic. The pessimistic view on the potential responsiveness of negative symptoms based on a relationship to structural abnormalities in the brain proposed by Crow (1980) is unsustainable, whatever the fate of the controversy as to whether there is an inverse relationship between response to neuroleptic drugs and computed tomography evidence of cerebral atrophy, as reported by some authors (Weinberger et al. 1980; Luchins et al. 1984; Andreasen et al. 1982) but not by others (Boronow et al. 1985; Williams et al. 1985; Smith et al. 1987). Negative symptoms can be ameliorated and are therefore a legitimate target of drug development.

To develop effective treatments of negative symptoms, at least five factors will have to be considered. It will have to be appreciated that there may more than be one type of negative symptoms, as found by us and others (Gibbons et al. 1985). Each of these may respond differently to drug treatment. A standard, reliable, sensitive rating scale of negative symptoms which has been psychometrically validated will be needed. Multivariate analyses which covary for course of illness, sex, age, changes in positive symptoms, effects of psychosocial interventions, and other factors may be necessary to identify the effect of treatments on negative symptoms. It would undoubtedly be helpful to have animal models of negative symptoms. These will be far more difficult to develop than those for positive symptoms, e.g., amphetamine-induced locomotor activity. They are not likely to be forthcoming until progress has been made on understanding the etiopathology of negative symptoms. Until it is known which biological phenomena are related to negative symptoms, e.g., decreased (or increased) dopaminergic activity, increased serotonergic activity, decreased cholecystokinin, and perhaps some change in the organization of neuronal activity (e.g., decreased frontal blood flow), progress will be slow in developing animal models of negative symptoms. Carnoy et al. (1986) have proposed that a deficient response to rewarding stimuli might be the rodent equivalent of negative symptoms and noted that low doses of apomorphine, which have been shown to decrease dopamine release, induced a reward deficit when rats were shifted from continuous reinforcement to a fixed ratio (FR4) schedule of food delivery. There are, however, many candidate atypical drugs, drugs with clozapine-like properties, e.g., melperone, amperozide, setoperone (Meltzer 1989). It is of great importance to learn whether these drugs share the ability of clozapine to diminish negative symptoms. It may then be possible to correlate specific biological characteristics of these drugs with the average clinical dose needed to treat negative symptoms. Once it is possible quantitatively to assess the ability of these and other drugs to treat both positive and negative symptoms, it will be possible to ascertain whether the biological basis for the two types of effects is shared or independent.

In conclusion, the treatment of negative symptoms most certainly is the legitimate target of the next generation of antipsychotic drugs.

Acknowledgement. The authors thank Mrs. Diane Mack for her secretarial assistance in preparing this manuscript.

References

Andreasen NC (1982) Negative symptoms in schizophrenia: definition and reliability. Arch Gen Psychiatry 39:784–788

Andreasen NC, Olsen S (1982) Negative vs positive schizophrenia: definition and validation. Arch Gen Psychiatry 39:789–794

Angrist B, Rotrosen J, Gershon S (1980) Differential effects of amphetamine and neuroleptics on negative vs positive symptoms in schizophrenia. Psychopharmacology (Berlin) 72:17–19

Bartko JJ, Carpenter WT (1976) On the methods and theory of reliability. J Nerv Ment Dis 163:307–312

Berrios GE (1985) Positive and negative symptoms and Jackson: a conceptual history. Arch Gen Psychiatry 42:95–97

Boronow J, Pickar D, Ninan PT, Roy A, Hommer D, Linnoila M, Paul SM (1985) Atrophy limited to IIIrd entricle only in chronic schizophrenic patients: report of a controlled series. Arch Gen Psychiatry 43:266–271

Carnoy P, Soubrie P, Puech AJ, Simon P (1986) Performance deficit induced by low doses of dopamine agonists in rats: toward a model for approaching the neurobiology of negative schizophrenic symptomatology? Biol Psychiatry 2:11–22

Carpenter WT, Heinrichs DW, Alphs LD (1985) Treatment of negative symptoms. Schizophr Bull 11:440–452

Claghorn J, Honigfeld G, Abuzzahab PS, Wang R, Steinbook R, Tuason V, Klerman G (1987) The risks and benefits of clozapine versus chlorpromazine. J Clin Psychopharmacol 7:377–384

Crow TU (1980) Molecular pathology of schizophrenia: more than one disease process? Br Med J 280:66–68

Crow TJ (1985) The two syndrome concept: origins and current status. Schizophr Bull 11:471–486

Endicott J, Spitzer RL (1978) A diagnostic interview: the schedule for affective disorders and schizophrenia. Arch Gen Psychiatry 35:837–844

Everitt BS, Gourlay A, Kendell R (1971) An attempt at validation of traditional psychiatric syndromes by cluster analysis. Br J Psychiatry 119:399–412

Fischer-Cornelssen KA, Ferner VJ (1976) An example of European multicenter trials: multispectral analysis of clozapine. Psychopharmacol Bull 12:34–39

Fleiss JL, Gurland BJ, Cooper JE (1971) Some contributions to the treatment of psychopathology. Br J Psychiatry 119:647–656

Gelenberg AJ, Doller JC (1979) Clozapine versus chlorpromazine for the treatment of schizophrenia: preliminary results from a double blind study. J Clin Psychiatry 40:238–240

Gerlach J, Koppelhus P, Helweg E, Mourad A (1974) Clozapine and haloperidol in a single-blind cross-over trial: therapeutic and biochemical aspects in the treatment of schizophrenia. Acta Psychiatr Scand 50:410–424

Gibbons RD, Lewine RJ, Davis JM, Schooler NR, Cole JO (1985) An empirical test of a Kraepelianan vs a bleulerian view of negative symptoms. Schizophr Bull 11:390–396

Goldberg SC (1985) Negative and deficit symptoms in schizophrenia do respond to neuroleptics. Schizophr Bull 11:453–456

Guirgius E, Voinesko G, Gray J, Schlieman E (1977) Clozapine (Leponex) vs Chlorpromazine (Largactil) in acute schizophrenia. (A double-blind controlled study). Curr Ther Res 21:707–719

Honigfeld G, Gillis R, Klett J (1966) A treatment-sensitive ward behavior scale. Psychol Rep 19:180–182

Jackman H, Luchins D, Meltzer HY (1983) Plasma serotonin levels in schizophrenia: relationship to race and psychopathology. Biol Psychiatry 18:887–902

Kane J, Honigfeld G, Singer J, Meltzer H (1988) Clozapine for the treatment-resistant schizophrenic: a double-blind comparison versus chlorpromazine/benztropine. Arch Gen Psychiatry 48:789–796

Lewine RJ, Fogg L, Meltzer HY (1983) Assessment of negative and positive symptoms in schizophrenia. Schizophr Bull 9:368–376

Liddle PF (1987) The symptoms of chronic schizophrenia: a reexamination of the positive-negative dichotomy. Br J Psychiatry 151:145–151

Lindstrom LH (1988) The effect of long-term treatment with clozapine in schizophrenia: a retrospective study in 96 patients treatment with clozapine for up to 13 patients. Acta Psychiatr Scand 17:524–529

Luchins DJ, Lewine RJ, Meltzer HY (1984) Lateral ventricular size, psychopathology, and medication response in the psychoses. Biol Psychiatry 19:29–44

Meltzer HY (1985) Dopamine and negative symptoms in schizophrenia: critique of the type I–type II hypothesis. In: Alpert M (ed) Controversies in schizophrenia: changes and constances. Guilford, New York, pp 110–136

Meltzer HY (1986) Effect of neuroleptics on the schizophrenia syndrome. In: Dahl SG, Gram LF; Paul SM, Potter WZ (eds) Clinical pharmacology in psychiatry. Selectivity in psychotropic drug action – promises or problems? Springer, Berlin Heidelberg New York, pp 255–265

Meltzer HY (1987) Biology of schizophrenia: an update. Schizophr Bull 13:77–111

Meltzer HY (1988) Clozapine: clinical advantages and biological mechanisms. In: Schulz C, Tamminga C (eds) Schizophrenia: a scientific focus. International Conference on Schizophrenia. University of Oxford Press, New York

Meltzer HY, Sommers AA, Luchins DJ (1986) The effect of neuroleptics and other psychotropic drugs on negative symptoms in schizophrenia. J Clin Psychopharmacol 6:329–338

Mita T, Hanada S, Nishino N, Kuno T, Nakai H, Yamadori T, Mizoi Y, Tanaka C (1986) Decreased serotonin S_2 and increased dopamine D_2 receptors in chronic schizophrenics. Biol Psychiatry 21:1407–1414

Niskanen P, Achte K, Jaskari M, Karesga M, Melsted B, Nilsson LB, Rontavaara M, et al. (1974) Results of a comparative double-blind study with clozapine and chlorpromazine in the treatment of schizophrenic patients. Psychiatr Fenn 307–313

Ota T, Maeshiro H, Ishido H, Shimizu Y, Uchida R, Toyoshima R, Ohshima H, et al. (1987) Treatment resistant chronic psychopathology and CT scans in schizophrenia. Acta Psychiatr Scand 75:415–427

Overall JE, Gorham D (1962) The Brief Psychiatric Rating Scale. Psychol Rep 10:799–812

Pearlson JD, Veroff AE (1981) Computerized tomographic scan changes in manic-depressive illness. Lancet 2:470

Prien RF, Cole JO (1968) High dose chlorpromazine therapy in chronic schizophrenia. Arch Gen Psychiatry 18:482–495

Rifkin A, Siris S (1987) Drug treatment of schizophrenia. In: Meltzer HY (ed) Psychopharmacology: the third generation of progress. Raven, New York, pp 1095–1101

Seeman P, Lee T (1975) Antipsychotic drugs: direct correlation between clinical potency and presynaptic action on dopamine neurons. Science 188:1217–1219

Smith RC, Baumgartner R, Ravichandran GK, Largen J, Calderon M, Burd A, Mauldin M (1987) Cortical atrophy and white matter density in the brains of schizophrenics and clinical response to neuroleptics. Acta Psychiatr Scand 75:11–19

Spitzer RL, Fleiss JL, Endicott J, Cohen J (1967) Mental Status Schedule: properties of factor analytically derived scales. Arch Gen Psychiatry 16:479–493

Strauss JS, Carpenter WT Jr, Bartko JJ (1974) The diagnosis and understanding of schizophrenia. III. Speculations on the processes that underlie schizophrenic symptoms and signs. Schizophr Bull 1:61–69

Trimble MR (1986) Positive and negative symptoms in schizophrenia. Br J Psychiatry 148:587–589

Weinberger DR, Bigelow LB, Kleinman JL, Klein ST, Rosenblatt JE, Wyatt RT (1980) Cerebral ventricular enlargement in chronic schizophrenia: an association with poor response to treatment. Arch Gen Psychiatry 37:11–13

Williams AO, Reveley MA, Kolakowska T, Andern M, Mandlebrote BM (1985) Schizophrenia with good and poor outcome. II. Cerebral ventricular size and its clinical significance. Br J Psychiatry 147:239–246

Wing JK (1978) Clinical concepts of schizophrenia. In: Schizophrenia: toward a new synthesis. Academic, London, pp 1–30

Wing JK, Cooper JE, Sartorius N (1974) Measurement and classification of psychiatric symptoms. An instructional manual for the PSE and Catego Program. Cambridge University Press, Cambridge

Clinical Significance of Receptor-Selective Drugs

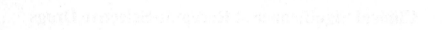

Clinical Effects of Selective Serotonin Reuptake Inhibitors

P. BECH [1]

1 Meta-Analytic Reviews and On-File Data Studies

Meta-analysis of controlled clinical trials has recently been established as a discipline that critically reviews and statistically combines the results of new treatment modalities. The objectives of a meta-analysis are to increase statistical power in detecting differences between treatments and to resolve uncertainties in the case of conflicting results. A meta-analytic literature review takes the trial itself as unit of analysis and consequently gives equal weight to each trial. A study of on-file data calculates the central tendency of the pooled data set, in which the individual patient in the trial is the unit for calculation of means, standard deviations, etc.

In a previous overview (Bech 1988a) of controlled clinical trials of serotonin reuptake inhibitors it was shown that there are many scientific problems in reviewing the research on clinical trials. Among the factors that were found to vary from trial to trial are outcome criteria, duration of treatment, dosage, and the setting (inpatient versus outpatients). The same review reported that most studies found no difference between tricyclic antidepressants and serotonin reuptake inhibitors in antidepressive effect. However, whereas tricyclic antidepressants in some trials were found superior to serotonin reuptake inhibitors, no trial found serotonin reuptake inhibitors superior to tricyclic antidepressants. Although such a literature review is not very powerful in a statistical sense, it was argued (Bech 1988a) that the results seemed powerful enough logically to classify serotonin reuptake inhibitors as weaker antidepressants than tricyclic antidepressants.

Statistically, 5% of trials should report significant superiority of serotonin reuptake inhibitors over tricyclic antidepressants due to change alone (using a 5% probability of type I error). In comparative trials on antidepressants versus placebo, placebo was found superior in only 4% (Smith et al. 1969) and 0% of patients (Morris and Beck 1974). On the other hand, no negative outcome trials of serotonin reuptake inhibitor effects compared to those with placebo has been published. In the present on-file data analysis of serotonin reuptake inhibitors, divergent trials will be compared to the meta-analytically determined central tendency of the pooled data.

---

[1] Department of Psychiatry, Frederiksborg General Hospital, 3400 Hillerød, Denmark

Clinical Pharmacology in Psychiatry
Editors: S. G. Dahl and L. F. Gram
(Psychopharmacology Series 7)
© Springer-Verlag Berlin Heidelberg 1989

So far, meta-analyses of serotonin reuptake inhibitors have concentrated on only short-term studies, i.e. studies of 4–6 weeks duration. However, a substance is generally accepted (e.g. EC 1987) as an antidepressant drug if it can be shown to be effective not only in short-term but also in medium-term studies, i.e. those of 2–6 months duration, corresponding to the total duration of a melancholic episode. Unfortunately, the number of medium-term studies with serotonin reuptake inhibitors is still too small for meta-analysis. This review is, therefore, an on-file data analysis of short-term studies of serotonin reuptake inhibitors, and a literature analysis of the few medium-term studies. Of the six serotonin reuptake inhibitors previously reviewed only citalopram, fluoxetine and fluvoxamine will be examined here.

2 Measures of Clinical Antidepressive Effect in Short-Term Studies

In this analysis of controlled trials it has not been possible systematically to control for diagnosis (no measure of endogenous depression), setting (many mixed cases), or dosage (no plasma measurements of drug concentration). The large number of patients included in the analysis may compensate for these shortcomings – in total, around 400 patients have been analysed for each drug. On the other hand, however, such a large number of cases may present statistical problems in that the null hypothesis might then be rejected facilely. To limit the statistical testing only few measures of outcome have been used, and only pretreatment and post-treatment (4–6 weeks) observations have been analysed. It should be emphasized that outcome evaluation is based only on patients who completed the planned short-term study (4–6 weeks of treatment). Fewer than 30% of patients in the various treatment groups, however, have been classified as non-completers.

2.1 The Hamilton Depression Scale

In combining individual trials on serotonin reuptake inhibitors for drawing overall conclusions as to antidepressive effect, the following aspects of the Hamilton Depression Scale (HDS; Hamilton 1967) have been found relevant (Bech 1988a): (a) the total 17-item HDS; (b) the 6-item melancholia subscale, including the most valied items for melancholic states (depressed mood, guilt, work and interests, retardation, psychic anxiety, and general somatic symptoms; Bech et al. 1975); and (c) the 3-item sleep subscale (Hamilton 1967). Statistically the HDS can be used to measure both improvement and recovery (Bech et al. 1984). In this analysis the weekly mean scores on the HDS measures have been used to indicate improvement over time. The reduction in final HDS score over pretreatment score has been used as a supplemental improvement measure. Recovery has been defined by use of the total HDS score after 4–6 weeks of treatment (≤ 7, complete recovery; 8–14, partial recovery; ≥ 15, non-recovery).

2.2 Global Improvement Scale

Previous meta-analytic studies on tricyclic antidepressants (e.g. Wechsler et al. 1965; Smith et al. 1969) have used only the Global Improvement Scale (GIS). To test the consistency of modern controlled tricyclic antidepressant studies the GIS has been considered as part of this meta-analysis.

3 On-File Data Analysis of Citalopram

The results shown in Table 1 are based on controlled clinical trials in which citalopram was compared to tricyclic antidepressants or placebo. In total, 422 patients have been evaluated, using amitriptyline (Shaw 1986), clomipramine (DUAG 1986), imipramine (Johnson, unpublished), and placebo (Fabre et al., unpublished; Herrington, unpublished). Among the trials comparing the effects of citalopram and tricyclic antidepressants, only that by DUAG found a

Table 1. On-file data analysis of total HDS

	Pre-treatment	Week 1	Week 2	Week 3	Week 4	Week 5	Week 6
Citalopram							
Subsample ($n=219$)							
Citalopram ($n=111$)	22.8	18.8	16.1	14.1	12.4		8.9
TCA ($n=108$)	22.8	17.6	13.6	11.6	9.7[a]		7.8
DUAG (1986) subsample ($n=102$)							
Citalopram ($n=50$)	22.5	18.9	16.5	14.9	13.2	12.1	
TCA ($n=52$)	22.1	18.1	13.4	10.8	9.2[a]	8.8[a]	
Non-DUAG subsample ($n=117$)							
Citalopram ($n=61$)	23.1	18.7	15.8	13.3	11.7		
TCA ($n=56$)	23.4	17.2	13.9	12.3	10.3		
Subsample ($n=203$)							
Citalopram ($n=96$)	24.1	19.8	16.7	14.8	12.6[a]		
Placebo ($n=107$)	23.7	20.4	19.3	16.3	15.5		
Total Sample ($n=422$)							
Fluvoxamine							
Amin et al. (1984)							
Fluvoxamine ($n=161$)	22.4	17.7	14.9	12.8	11.7[a]		
Imipramine ($n=152$)	22.6	18.0	15.1	12.7	12.3[a]		
Placebo ($n=148$)	22.7	18.1	16.3	15.9	15.4		
Itil et al. (1983) subsample ($n=53$)							
Fluvoxamine ($n=15$)	21.2				12.7		
Imipramine ($n=21$)	21.7				10.4[a]		
Placebo ($n=17$)	19.9				16.0		
Total Sample ($n=461$)							

TCA, Tricyclic antidepressant.
[a] $p \leq 0.05$.

Table 2. On-file data analysis of HDS melancholia subscale

	Pre-treatment	Week 1	Week 2	Week 3	Week 4	Week 5	Week 6
Citalopram							
Subsample ($n=219$)							
Citalopram ($n=111$)	11.8	9.9	8.7	7.5	6.9		4.6
TCA ($n=108$)	11.6	9.8	7.7	6.5	5.5[a]		4.1
DUAG (1986) subsample ($n=102$)							
Citalopram ($n=50$)	12.2	10.5	9.4	8.3	7.3	6.9	
TCA ($n=52$)	11.9	10.8	8.2	6.7	5.7[a]	5.4	
Non-DUAG subsample ($n=117$)							
Citalopram ($n=61$)	11.4	9.4	8.2	6.9	6.6		
TCA ($n=56$)	11.2	8.9	7.2	6.4	5.3		
Subsample ($n=203$)							
Citalopram ($n=96$)	11.8	9.7	8.4	7.4	6.3[a]		
Placebo ($n=107$)	11.8	10.2	9.7	8.0	7.5		
Total Sample ($n=422$)							
Fluvoxamine							
Fluvoxamine ($n=161$)	11.2	9.1	7.8	6.6	5.9[a]		
Imipramine ($n=152$)	11.3	9.1	8.1	6.6	6.2[a]		
Placebo ($n=148$)	11.4	9.4	8.3	8.3	7.9		
Norton et al. (1984) ($n=91$)							
Fluvoxamine ($n=35$)	9.5	7.9	6.6	6.6	5.5[a]		
Imipramine ($n=31$)	9.3	7.2	6.6	5.8	5.3[a]		
Placebo ($n=25$)	9.7	8.0	6.4	7.0	6.8		
Dominguez et al. (1985) ($n=94$)							
Fluvoxamine ($n=33$)	10.5	8.9	6.3	5.3	5.3[a]		
Imipramine ($n=30$)	11.5	9.5	8.3	5.8	5.5[a]		
Placebo ($n=31$)	11.1	8.6	7.8	8.1	7.0		
Lapierre et al. (1987) ($n=60$)							
Fluvoxamine ($n=21$)	13.0	9.0	7.1	5.4	4.7[a]		
Imipramine ($n=20$)	12.9	9.0	7.4	6.7	5.7[a]		
Placebo ($n=19$)	12.2	8.9	8.1	8.5	8.9		
Remaining sample ($n=215$)							
Fluvoxamine ($n=72$)	11.9	9.9	8.9	7.6	6.9[a]		
Imipramine ($n=71$)	11.6	9.8	8.9	7.1	6.9[a]		
Placebo ($n=73$)	11.9	10.5	9.3	8.9	8.4		
Total Sample ($n=461$)							

TCA, Tricyclic antidepressant.
[a] $p \leqq 0.05$.

difference. The DUAG study is shown separately in Table 1 because this is the divergent citalopram study. A previous review (Bech 1988 a) concluded that a 17-item HDS mean score of no higher than 10 should be obtained after 4–5 weeks of treatment with an antidepressant against a mean score of 15 for placebo. The citalopram results in Table 1 show that after 6 weeks of treatment both citalopram and tricyclic antidepressants have an acceptable effect. Whereas tricyclic antidepressants were superior to citalopram after 4 weeks of treatment in the total data set, when the DUAG results were excluded, no differences were obtained. In contrast to the other citalopram trials the DUAG study used a fixed dosage (40 mg citalopram versus 150 mg clomipramine), and treatment in this study lasted for only 5 weeks. Finally, citalopram was found superior to placebo.

Table 2 presents the results of citalopram trials using the HDS subscale on melancholic state. The difference between tricyclic antidepressants and citalopram in the DUAG study after 4 weeks of treatment seems due to a weak citalopram effect rather than a strong tricyclic antidepressant effect, indicating that a fixed dosage of citalopram of 40 mg daily is not recommendable. For the whole data set on citalopram versus tricyclic antidepressant the results in Table 2 on melancholic state are similar to those in Table 1 on the overall HDS scores. The most consistent difference between tricyclic antidepressants and citalopram was found in the sleep factor, the former showing a better effect than the latter (Table 3). However, compared to placebo the effect of citalopram on sleep was also statistically significant after 4 weeks of treatment.

Table 4 shows the improvement rates in short-term studies of tricyclic antidepressants and placebo compared to citalopram. The most important European study on tricyclic antidepressants (imipramine) versus placebo is the British multicentre study (Medical Research Council 1965). This study found a 72% improvement after 4 weeks of treatment with tricyclic antidepressants compared to a 45% improvement with placebo. This result is in harmony with the review study of Smith et al. (1969; see Table 4). The citalopram data using the GIS showed no difference between citalopram and tricyclic antidepressants after 4 weeks or after 6 weeks. Both drugs were superior to placebo. These results are consistent with the MRC study and the Smith et al. (1969) study. The low placebo response after 6 weeks (only 24 patients) is similar to the findings of Quitkin et al. (1984).

The measure of improvement on the HDS in Table 4 is a dichotomization on the basis of whether or not an improvement of 50% or more was observed in post-treatment rating scores compared to corresponding pretreatment scores. Because the HDS has not been used in all citalopram studies, the trials using another scale, the Montgomery-Åsberg Depression Rating Scale (MADRS; Montgomery and Åsberg 1979), have been included. In the study by Shaw (1986) both scales were included, and the HDS seemed here more sensitive than MADRS in measuring 50% improvement in citalopram-treated patients. The measure based on rating scale improvement of 50% or more gives a pattern similar to that using GIS scores, although it is a more conservative estimate.

Table 3. On-file data analysis of HDS sleep items

	Pre-treatment	Week 1	Week 2	Week 3	Week 4	Week 5	Week 6
Citalopram							
Subsample (n=219)							
Citalopram (n=111)	3.6	3.3	2.5	2.4	2.1		1.4
TCA (n=108)	3.7	1.9	1.4	1.2	1.1*		0.8*
DUAG (1986) subsample (n=102)							
Citalopram (n=50)	3.5	3.3	2.6	2.5	2.3	2.0	
TCA (n=52)	3.7	1.8	1.4	0.9	1.1*	1.2*	
Non-DUAG subsample (n=117)							
Citalopram (n=61)	3.7	3.3	2.4	2.3	1.8		
TCA (n=56)	3.8	2.0	1.5	1.4	1.1*		
Subsample (n=203)							
Citalopram (n=96)	3.9	3.1	2.3	1.9	1.5*		
Placebo (n=107)	4.0	3.4	3.2	2.6	2.5		
Total Sample (n=422)							
Fluvoxamine							
Fluvoxamine (n=161)	3.7	2.8	2.3	2.1	1.9*		
Imipramine (n=152)	3.7	2.8	2.1	1.9	1.9*		
Placebo (n=148)	3.8	2.9	2.8	2.5	2.4		
Norton et al. (1984) subsample (n=91)							
Fluvoxamine (n=35)				2.5	2.1*		
Imipramine (n=31)				1.7	1.7		
Placebo (n=25)				1.7	1.3		
Dominguez et al. (1985) subsample (n=94)							
Fluvoxamine (n=33)				1.4	1.2		
Imipramine (n=30)				1.6	1.8		
Placebo (n=31)				2.6	2.4*		
Lapierre et al. (1987) subsample (n=60)							
Fluvoxamine (n=21)				1.9	1.7		
Imipramine (n=20)				2.1	2.0		
Placebo (n=19)				2.7	3.1*		
Total sample (n=461)							

TCA, Tricyclic antidepressant.
* $p \leq 0.05$.

4 On-File Data Analysis of Fluvoxamine

The analysis of fluvoxamine, in contrast to that of citalopram, is not based on all controlled fluvoxamine trials as collected by Benfield and Ward (1986). The HDS data that have been analysed are from a large multicentre study involving eight centres in North America and the United Kingdom. A total of 461 patients with major depression were treated for 4 weeks with fluvoxamine, imipramine or placebo. These data have previously been described by Amin et

Table 4. Improvement on GIS (moderate to excellent) and HDS/MADRS ($\geq$50%): percentage of patients (and confidence limits)

Treatment	GIS				HDS/MADRS		
	Smith et al 1969	Medical research Council (1965)	Citalopram data on file (Feb. 1988)		DUAG (1986)	Citalopram on file (Feb. 1988)	
	Week 4	Week 4	Week 4	Week 6	Week 4	Week 4	Week 6
TCA	64 (62–66) $n=2548$	72 (59–83) $n=58$	76 (61–86) $n=49$	85 (72–93) $n=53$	73 (59–84) $n=52$	67 (52–80) $n=49$	73 (59–84) $n=52$
Citalopram			66 (60–72) $n=243$	72 (64–78) $n=155$	44 (30–59) $n=50$	59 (53–65) $n=269$	70 (62–77) $n=157$
Placebo	45 (41–49) $n=780$	45 (31–60) $n=51$	47 (36–59) $n=74$	29 (13–51) $n=24$		30 (20–42) $n=73$	24 (10–46) $n=25$

TCA, Tricyclic antidepressant.

al. (1984). Approximately one-third of subjects were treated as inpatients, the ratio of men to women was 1:3, and ages ranged from 19 to 70 years (mean, 42). The mean doses employed were 155 mg fluvoxamine and 156 mg imipramine (flexible dosage regime).

Among the controlled trials with fluvoxamine reviewed by Benfield and Ward (1986), that with divergent negative results was the trial conducted by Itel et al. (1983), which used a design similar to that with the pooled data of 461 patients analysed by Amin et al. (1984; see Table 1). This trial is also similar to that in using only the first 16 items of HDS, thereby excluding the item of weight loss, as recommended by Coppen et al. (1978). Whereas the imipramine effect after 4 weeks was of similar order in the pooled data and in the data of Itel et al. (1983), the effects of fluvoxamine and placebo were weaker in the latter trial than in the pooled sample. Compared to the citalopram results, the effects of fluvoxamine and of placebo were more pronounced after 4 weeks of treatment.

Table 2 presents results using the HDS subscale on melancholia – for the pooled sample and for the subsamples of Norton et al. (1984), Dominguez et al. (1985), and Lapierre et al. (1987). Whereas the outcome differences after 4 weeks treatment with fluvoxamine or imipramine is more pronounced in these three subsamples than in the pooled sample, the placebo effect in the trial by Lapierre et al. (1987) is weak. This trial, in contrast to those by Norton et al. (1984) and Dominguez et al. (1985), is on inpatients, and the mean daily dose of fluvoxamine (180 mg) and imipramine (173 mg) is significantly higher than that in the trial by Norton et al. (1984; 133 mg and 153 mg, respectively). In general, the placebo effect on the melancholia subscale is weaker than that on the 16-item HDS, and the placebo effect in the fluvoxamine sample is similar to that in the citalopram sample. The pretreatment severity of depression is highest in the inpatient study by Lapierre et al. (1987), but for the pooled fluvoxamine data the pretreatment means are comparable to those for the pooled citalopram data. On the other hand, the outcome with tricyclic antidepressants after 4 weeks is slightly better in the citalopram analysis, which includes amitriptyline and clomipramine.

The effect of fluvoxamine on the HDS factor of sleep (Table 3) demonstrates the divergence of the Norton et al. (1984) subsample, which found fluvoxamine weaker than placebo on sleep items than in trials by Dominguez et al. (1985) and Lapierre et al. (1987). In all three trials the imipramine effect was rather similar. Again, the tricyclic antidepressant effect on sleep in the citalopram trials is more pronounced than the imipramine effect obtained in the fluvoxamine trials, whereas the placebo effect is rather identical in the two serotonin reuptake inhibitor trials.

5 Recovery Rates with Serotonin Reuptake Inhibitors

For the treating doctor the rates of recovery are more meaningful than the rates of improvement. In Table 5 the findings of the meta-analysis of citalopram and fluvoxamine effects are compared to the effects of tricyclic antidepressant and placebo. There seems to be general agreement that tricyclic antidepressant after 4 weeks of treatment has a non-recovery rate of around

Table 5. Percentage recovery rates of HDS[a]

	Week 4			Week 5			Week 6		
	Complete	Partial	Non-recovery	Complete	Partial	Non-recovery	Complete	Partial	Non-recovery
Citalopram total sample ($n=422$)									
Citalopram ($n=207$)	24	40	36				47	20	32
TCA ($n=108$)	44	34	23				53	32	19
Placebo ($n=107$)	14	32	55				8	24	68
Citalopram Duag subsample ($n=102$)									
Citalopram ($n=50$)	20	40	40	28	42	30			
TCA ($n=52$)	46	38	15	61	16	24			
Fluvoxamine total sample ($n=461$)									
Fluvoxamine ($n=161$)	34	42	24						
Imipramine ($n=152$)	37	37	26						
Placebo ($n=148$)	29	32	39						

TCA, Tricyclic antidepressant.
[a] Complete recovery, ≤ 7; partial recovery, 8–14; non-recovery, ≥ 15.

25%. The fluvoxamine data also show a non-recovery rate of 25% after 4 weeks, whereas citalopram after 4 weeks has a non-recovery rate of 36% and after 6 weeks of around 30%. In contrast, placebo results are inconsistent. In the citalopram sample placebo has a non-recovery rate after 4 weeks of 55%, compared to that in the fluvoxamine sample of 39% for placebo. After 6 weeks the placebo rate has increased to 68%. The relatively good outcome with placebo in the fluvoxamine sample is also reflected in the high rate of complete recovery.

6 Discussion and Conclusions Regarding Clinical Effect of Serotonin Reuptake Inhibitors in Short-Term Studies

In a previous review (Bech 1988 a) it was concluded that the antidepressive effect of serotonin reuptake inhibitors was slightly less pronounced than that of tricyclic antidepressants, but significantly better than with placebo. This on-file data analysis has reconsidered the trials that diverged, showing a superiority of tricyclic antidepressants over serotonin reuptake inhibitors – DUAG (1986) concerning citalopram and Itel et al. (1983) and Norton et al. (1984) concerning fluvoxamine. The overall effect of citalopram, when evaluated with the most valid HDS subscale, showed that the DUAG trial identified a weak citalopram effect after 4 weeks rather than a strong tricyclic antidepressant effect. The other controlled tricyclic antidepressant studies in the citalopram sample showed no difference to the citalopram effect after 4 weeks. However, the pooled data set found citalopram inferior to tricyclic antidepresssants after 4 weeks, but not after 6 weeks of treatment. After 4 weeks citalopram was superior to placebo.

The overall effect of fluvoxamine measured on the HDS subscale of melancholic states showed that the trial by Norton et al. (1984) identified a strong placebo effect. In the pooled data set no difference was obtained between fluvoxamine and imipramine after 4 weeks of treatment.

On the HDS factor of sleep, citalopram was found to be consistently inferior to tricyclic antidepressant, but superior to placebo. The effect of fluvoxamine was similar to that of imipramine and superior to placebo in the pooled data, but also in this respect the Norton et al. (1984) trial was divergent. The difference between citalopram and fluvoxamine may be due to the fact that fluvoxamine trials have used imipramine as tricyclic antidepressant whereas citalopram trials have employed amitriptyline. Trials on fluoxetine have found amitriptyline superior on the HDS factor of sleep (e.g. Chouinard 1985).

The exclusion of patients in this on-file meta-analysis who failed to complete the planned short-term trial may have influenced the improvement rates with serotonin reuptake inhibitors compared to those with tricyclic antidepressants. The tolerance of serotonin reuptake inhibitors has varied from trial to trial; Lapierre et al. (1987), for example, found a rather high tolerance of fluvoxamine, but Itel et al. (1983) and Dominguez et al. (1985) found the reverse. In conclusion, the short-term trials of citalopram and fluvoxamine indicate that these drugs can be classified as non-sedating antidepressants, with no anticholinergic side effects but with an action that is not earlier in onset than that of tricyclic antidepressants, i.e. rather delayed.

7 Measures of Outcome in Medium-Term Studies

As discussed elsewhere (Bech 1988 b), the states of melancholia should be considered as a disability dimension relevant for short-term studies, whereas the dimensions of distress (the subjective acceptance of treatment with reference to side effects) and of discomfort (the subjective acceptance of illness with reference to demoralization) are relevant for medium-term studies. Self-rating scales should be considered for the measurement of distress and discomfort (Bech 1988 b). In this connection it is of interest that fluvoxamine was found inferior to imipramine on the Beck self-rating scale (Itel et al. 1983) and inferior to clomipramine (Dick and Ferrero 1983), whereas fluoxetine on the Zung self-rating scale was found inferior to amitriptyline (Chovinard 1985). So far these self-rating scales have not been used in citalopram trials.

7.1 Relapse Percentage with Serotonin Reuptake Inhibitors

The rate of relapse with electroconvulsive therapy and with amitriptyline in a medium-term (7-month) trial by Kay et al. (1970) was 47% and 24%, respectively. Other medium-term trials (6–8 months) on depressed patients who had initially recovered have confirmed an approximately 50% relapse with ECT and 20% with tricyclic antidepressants (amitriptyline or imipramine), as reviewed by Schou (1976). In an open but controlled study (Wernicke and Brenner 1986) it was found that fluoxetine had a relapse rate of 14% ($n = 112$) whereas imipramine ($n = 85$) had a relapse rate of 16%. In a controlled double-blind medium-term trial Guelfi et al. (1987) treated 15 patients on fluvoxamine and 21 patients on imipramine. The relapse rate in these patients was globally defined (J. Wakelin 1988, personal communication) and showed a 13% relapse with fluvoxamine and 19% with imipramine. Finally, in an open and non-controlled citalopram study (data on file, June 1988) a relapse rate of 6% in 93 patients was obtained.

7.2 Distressful Side Effects of Serotonin Reuptake Inhibitors

Distressful reactions of hypersensitivity as were found with the first serotonin reuptake inhibitor, zimeldine, have not been found for any of the serotonin reuptake inhibitors mentioned in this analysis. The most consistent subjective report of side effects with serotonin reuptake inhibitors has been nausea (Amin et al. 1984), which typically is an immediate side effect. As a tardive side effect nausea is rarely seen. It may well be that subclinical nausea is responsible for the absence of weight gain in medium-term trials with SRIs. Weight gain is one of the main reasons for non-acceptance of maintenance treatment with tricyclic antidepressants or lithium in manic-melancholic patients (Bech et al. 1976). Furthermore, dry mouth, sweating and other anti-cholinergic side effects of tricyclic antidepressants introduce a moderate distress in maintenance therapy with these drugs.

7.3 Discomfort of Serotonin Reuptake Inhibitors

It is undoubtful that patients who have received electroconvulsive therapy retrospectively consider their illness more negatively than do patients who have received only drugs. In general, patients with manic-melancholic disorder have a dissimulating attitude to their illness (Bech et al. 1980), but it is obvious that a specific drug, blocking only relevant dysfunctional impairment, psychologically should have a minimal influence on patients' acceptance of their illness.

8 Conclusion

This review of studies on citalopram and fluvoxamine has shown that these drugs can be classified as non-sedating antidepressants, as they have been found active both in short-term and in medium-term trials. Data from the short-term studies with divergent findings regarding citalopram and fluvoxamine have been pooled to permit a meta-analysis of the effects of drugs. Using the core symptoms in the HDS as outcome measurement, serotonin reuptake inhibitors were found to be superior to placebo and comparable to tricyclic antidepressants. However, the trials with divergent results and some trials using self-rating scales have found that serotonin reuptake inhibitors have a delayed action compared to tricyclic antidepressants. This feature is shared by the other serotonin reuptake inhibitors, fluoxetine.

The side effects of citalopram and fluvoxamine have been very restricted; only nausea at the beginning of treatment may be distressful. Also in this respect, fluoxetine resembles citalopram and fluvoxamine. This relative lack of side effects combined with the promising medium-term trials that have found a relapse rate in patients treated with serotonin reuptake inhibitors comparable to that in patients treated with tricyclic antidepressants, and thereby superior to electroconvulsive therapy, seems to indicate that SRIs may be useful in long-term relapse-preventive trials. However, more studies are needed to evaluate whether the basic action of serotonin reuptake inhibitors reestablishes the biological mechanisms that are necessary for developing a depressive state. Comparative short-term studies testing the onset of action with citalopram versus fluvoxamine are needed.

References

Amin MM, Ananth JV, Coleman BS, Darcourt G, Farkes T, Goldstein B, Lapierre YD, et al. (1984) Fluvoxamine: antidepressant effects confirmed in a placebo-controlled international study. Clin Neuropharmacol [Suppl 1] 7:580–581

Bech P (1988a) A review of the antidepressant properties of serotonin reuptake inhibitors. In: Gastpar M, Wakelin JS (eds) Selective 5-HT reuptake inhibitors: novel or commonplace agents? Karger, Basel, pp 58–69

Bech P (1988b) Rating scales for mood disorders: applicability, consistency and construct validity. Acta Psychiatr Scand [Suppl 345] 78:45–55

Bech P, Gram LF, Dein E, Jacobsen O, Vitger J, Bolwig TG (1975) Quantitative rating of depressive states. Acta Psychiatr Scand 51:161–170

Bech P, Vendsborg PB, Rafaelsen OJ (1976) Lithium maintenance treatment of manic-melancholic patients: its role in the daily routine. Acta Psychiatr Scand 53:70–81

Bech P, Shapiro RW, Sihm F, Nielsen BM, Sørensen B, Rafaelsen OJ (1980) Personality in unipolar and bipolar manic-melancholic patients. Acta Psychiatr Scand 62:245–257

Bech P, Allerup P, Reisby N, Gram LF (1984) Assessment of symptom change from improvement curves on the Hamilton Depression Scale in trials with antidepressants. Psychopharmacology (Berlin) 84:276–281

Benfield P, Ward A (1986) Fluvoxamine: a review of its pharmacodynamic and pharmacokinetic properties and therapeutic efficacy in depressive illness. Drugs 32:313–334

Chovinard G (1985) A double-blind controlled clinical trial of fluoxetine and amitriptyline in the treatment of outpatients with major depressive disorder. J Clin Psychiatry 46:32–37

Coppen A, Ghose K, Baily J, Christensen J, Mikkelsen PL, van Praag HM, van de Poel F et al. (1978) Amitriptyline plasma-concentration and clinical effect. Lancet 1:63–66

Dick P, Ferrero E (1983) A double-blind comparative study of the clinical efficacy of fluvoxamine and clomipramine. Br J Clin Pharmacol 15:419–425

Dominguez RA, Goldstein BJ, Jacobson AF, Steinbook RM (1985) A double-blind placebo-controlled study of fluvoxamine and imipramine in depression. J Clin Psychiatry 46:84–87

DUAG, Danish University Antidepressant Group (1986) Citalopram: clinical effect profile in comparison with clomipramine. A controlled multicenter study. Psychopharmacology (Berlin) 90:131–138

EC, European Community (1987) Clinical investigation of antidepressant drugs. EC Brussels No 111/476/87

Guelfi JD, Dreyfus JF, Pichot P, GEPECEP (1987) Fluvoxamine and imipramine: results of a long-term controlled trial. Int Clin Psychopharmacol 2:103–109

Hamilton M (1967) Development of a rating scale for primary depressive illness. Br J Soc Clin Psychol 6:278–296

Itil TM, Shrivastava RK, Mukherjee S, Coleman BS, Michael ST (1983) A double-blind placebo-controlled study of fluvoxamine and imipramine in out-patients with primary depression. Br J Clin Pharmacol 15:433–438

Kay DWK, Fahy T, Garside RF (1970) A seven-month double-blind trial of amitriptyline and diazepam in ECT-treated depressed patients. Br J Psychiatry 117:667–671

Klok CJ, Brouwer GJ, van Praag HM, Doogan D (1981) Fluvoxamine and clomipramine in depressed patients. Acta Psychiatr Scand 65:1–11

Lapierre YD, Browne M, Horn E, Oyewumi LK, Sarantidis D, Roberts N, Badoe K, Tessier P (1987) Treatment of major affective disorder with fluvoxamine. J Clin Psychiatry 48:65–68

Medical Research Council (1965) Clinical trial of the treatment of depressive illness. Br Med J 1:881–886

Montgomery SA, Åsberg M (1979) A new depression scale designed to be sensitive to change. Br J Psychiatry 134:382–389

Morris JB, Beck AT (1974) The efficacy of antidepressant drugs. Arch Gen Psychiatry 30:667–674

Norton KRW, Sireling LI, Bhat AV, Rao B, Paykel ES (1984) A double-blind comparison of fluvoxamine, imipramine and placebo in depressed patients. J Affect Dis 7:297–308

Quitkin FM, Rabkin JG, Ross D, McGrath PJ (1984) Duration of antidepressant drug treatment. Arch Gen Psychiatry 41:238–245

Schou M (1976) Prophylactic and maintenance therapy in recurrent affective disorders. In: Gallant DM, Simpson GM (eds) Depression: behavioral biochemical, diagnostic and treatment concept. Spectrum, New York, pp 309–326

Shaw DM (1986) A comparison of the antidepressant action of citalopram and amitriptylin. Br J Psychiatry 149:515–517

Smith A, Traganza E, Harrison G (1969) Studies of the effectiveness of antidepressant drugs. Psychopharmacol Bull [Special issue]:1–21

Stark P, Hardison DC (1985) A review of multicenter controlled studies of fluoxetine vs imipramine and placebo in outpatients with major depressive disorder. J Clin Psychiatry 46:53–58

Wechsler H, Grosser GH, Greenblatt M (1965) Research evaluating antidepressant medications on hospitalized mental patients: a survey of published reports during a five-year period. J Nerv Ment Dis 141:231–239

Wernicke JF, Brenner JD (1986) Fluoxetine effective in the long term treatment of depression. Br J Clin Pract [Suppl 46] 40:17–23

Effects of Serotonergic Agonists on Neuroendocrine Responses of Rhesus Monkeys and Patients with Depression and Anxiety Disorders

G. R. Heninger, D. S. Charney, L. H. Price, P. Delgado,
S. Woods, and W. Goodman [1]

1 Introduction

The role of the serotonergic (5-HT) system in the etiology and treatment of neuropsychiatric disorders has been a focus of considerable research for many years. Recent progress in biochemical neuropharmacology has resulted in the delineation of a variety of serotonin receptor subtypes. More specific agonists and antagonists for the serotonin receptor subtypes are available, and a few are available for clinical use. One research strategy has been to administer "challenge" doses of a serotonin receptor agonist to patients and compare the behavioral and neuroendocrine response to that of healthy controls. At times it has been possible to utilize this strategy both before and after pharmacologic treatment in order to allow an evaluation of the treatment on the sensitivity of the receptor system.

There is considerable data indicating that serotonin is stimulatory to prolactin release. However, the nature of the serotonin receptor subtypes involved in this response is not fully understood, particularly in primates (Van de Kar et al. 1985). In order to delinate more clearly the type of serotonin receptor subtype that might be involved in stimulating prolactin, cortisol, and growth hormone release, studies were conducted in rhesus monkeys.

2 Serotonin Agonists in Rhesus Monkeys

Four to eight adult male rhesus monkeys were chaired daily and had intravenous catheters placed in a lower leg vein once weekly. This allowed for the infusion of a serotonin agonist and antagonist as well as the withdrawal of blood for hormone assays. In order more fully to understand the relative potency of the serotonin agonists, two dopamine receptor antagonists (SCH 23390 for D_1 and haloperidol for D_2) were also studied. Monkeys received from three to eight different doses of each compound spaced at least 1 week apart. The specific serotonin S_2 antagonist ritanserin and the non-

[1] Abraham Ribicoff Research Facilities, Department of Psychiatry, Yale University School of Medicine, and the Connecticut Mental Health Center, DMH, 34 Park St., New Haven, CT 06508, USA

Table 1. Effects of dopamine D_1 and H_2 receptor antagonists and 5-HT receptor agonists and antagonists on prolactin release in rhesus monkeys

	Halo-periodol	Bus-pirone	SCH 23390	8-OHDPAT	Ge-prione	Ipsa-pirone	MCPP	Mes-ca-line	Tryp-tophan
Relative[a] potency	0.02	0.2	0.5	1	1	2	4	13	1000
Antagonism (%)									
Ritanserin	0	0	–	0	0	–	50	90	18
Metergoline	72	95	–	96	90	–	100	100	97

[a] In µmol/kg to produce a peak prolactin response of 20 ng/ml over baseline.

specific serotonin antagonist metergoline were used to block the response (Heninger et al. 1987, 1988).

For all of the drugs studied prolactin gave a consistent dose response curve, but growth hormone and cortisol changes were much more variable. In terms of prolactin release, in Table 1, the dopamine D_2 receptor antagonist haloperidol is over 50 times more potent than the specific serotonin S_{1A} agonist 8-OHDPAT. The dopamine D_1 receptor antagonist SCH 23390 was only twice as potent. Haloperidol, buspirone, and SCH 23390 all produced catatonia at the higher doses. *m*-Chlorophenylpiperazine (MCPP) is four times less potent than 8-OHDPAT while the serotonin S_2 agonist mescaline is 13 times less potent. Obviously tryptophan is many orders of magnitude less potent. Metergoline antagonized all the serotonin agonists studied, as well as producing some antagonism of the effects of haloperidol. Ritanserin did not block the effects of haloperidol, buspirone, 8-OHDPAT, or gepirone, but it produced an almost complete antagonism of mescaline and a 50% block of MCPP. A partial (18%) antagonism of tryptophan was also observed. The data suggest that, in terms of the regulation of prolactin release, the serotonin S_{1A} receptors are much more relevant than the serotonin S_{1B} or the S_2 receptor systems. The high potency of haloperiodol and buspirone suggests that the dopaminergic inhibition is relatively more important than the stimulatory effects of serotonin on prolactin. Since buspirone and gepirone differ very little in chemical structure, it is of considerable interest that there is this strong evidence of dopamine D_2 receptor antagonism with buspirone.

3 Neuroendocrine Response to Intravenous Tryptophan in Depressed Patients: Effects of Treatment

Substantial data from animal studies suggest that one of the major mechanisms of antidepressant treatment is the facilitation of serotonergic function (Blier et al. 1987). The data support the hypothesis that long-term but not short-term treatment with serotonin uptake inhibitors and monoamino oxidase (MAO) inhibitors reduces the sensitivity of serotonin S_{1A} presynaptic receptors located on cell bodies and/or dendrites and possibly some nerve terminals. A slow desensitization of these receptors results in an increase in the firing rate of serotonin neurons and an overall increased efficacy of serotonin release. Tricyclic antidepressants such as desipramine produce a postsynaptic increased sensitivity at some serotonin receptors. Thus, even though serotonin uptake inhibitors, MAO inhibitors, and tricyclic antidepressants may differ in their mechanisms, they all appear to increase serotonergic function.

In order to obtain clinical data revelant to this hypothesis, the prolactin response to infused tryptophan was studied in a large number of depressed patients, before and during active treatment with various antidepressant drugs (Price et al. 1985, 1988, 1989a, b). In Table 2 the results are summarized. It can be seen that both short-term and long-term fluvoxamine treatment produces a very robust increase in the prolactin response to the infused tryptophan. With desipramine the percentage change is much less and is statistically significant only following long-term treatment. With tranylcypromine the prolactin response was increased approximately equally following short-term and long-term treatment. Trazodone was not studied in the short term, but in the long term there was no change from pretreatment levels. Of considerable interest is the fact that lithium produced a much more reliable increase in prolactin response when patients were treated for less than 10 days than when they were treated over 3–4 weeks.

Taken together, the data for fluvoxamine and desipramine suggest that overall serotonergic function is increased more during longer term treatment, and it is not as effectively increased when treatment is less than 10–14 days. This provides some support to the findings in laboratory rats of the relatively slow desensitization of the serotonin 5_{1A} receptors and the similarly slow in-

Table 2. Effects of short- and long-term antidepressant treatment on the prolactin response to intravenous tryptophan

Treatment	Short-term treatment				Long-term treatment			
	n	Dose (mg/day)	Treatment duration (days $\pm$ SD)	Percent of baseline[a]	n	Dose (mg/day)	Treatment duration (days $\pm$ SD)	Percent of baseline[a]
Fluvoxamine	16	203	7.9 ± 2.8	250[c]	22	264	33 ± 8	344[c]
Desipramine	13	188	6.8 ± 2	150	16	197	28 ± 4	184[c]
Tranylcypromine[b]	5	25	9 ± 2	135	4	30	24 ± 2	157
Trazodone[b]	–	–	–	–	9	311	33 ± 10	96
Lithium	13	1015	5.6 ± 1.5	150[c]	13	1200	31 ± 10	110

[a] Peak response minus baseline after treatment divided by peak minus baseline before treatment.

[b] Area under the curve instead of peak response minus baseline.

[c] $p < 0.05$, paired t test.

crease in postsynaptic sensitization following the standard tricyclic drugs such as desipramine. It is of interest that trazodone, which has been reported to be an effective antidepressant, does not produce changes in serotonergic function even following long-term treatment. Lithium has offered a less effective acute antidepressant treatment, but it has been found to be efficacious in about 70% of refractory patients when added to ongoing treatment with other drugs (Heninger et al. 1983). The early augmentation of serotonergic function with lithium and the adaptation of this back toward baseline levels does not directly correlate with clinical observations since relapse of depression during lithium treatment is not common, indeed lithium has been used as an effective long-term prophylactic treatment of unipolar depression.

4 The Effect of Serotonin Agonists on Fear/Anxiety Behavior in Laboratory Animals

A review of the multitude of behavioral effects of serotonin agonists is beyond the scope of this brief report, but the heterogeneity of the effects is of some interest, especially as it applies to neuropsychiatric syndromes. In Table 3 the

Table 3. Effects of drugs that modify 5-HT function on laboratory animal behaviors that are thought to model fear/anxiety

Class of drug	Efficacy and consistency in reducing fear/anxiety behaviors
5-HT neurotoxins	+ + + +
5-HT synthesis inhibitors	+ + + +
5-HT receptor antagonists	
Nonselective	+ +
Selective	
5-HTS$_1$	0
5-HTS$_2$	+ + + +
5-HTS$_3$	+ + +
5-HTS$_{1A}$ receptor agonists/antagonists	
Buspirone	+ +
Gepirone	+ +
Isapirone	+ + +
5-HTS$_{1A}$ receptor agonists	+ +
5-HTS$_{1B}$ receptor agonists	0
5-HT uptake inhibitors	0
MAO-A and MAO-B inhibitors	0

+ + + +, Very reliable effect; + + +, moderate reliable effect; + +, mild reliable effect; +, slight or questionably reliable effect; 0, no effect.

variety of drugs that alter serotonergic function are listed relative to their effects on fear/anxiety behavior in animals (Chopin and Briley 1987; Traber and Glaser 1987). The increased efficacy of serotonin neurotoxins and synthesis inhibitors has been thought to represent the disinhibition of punished behavior and therefore may not be as relevant to clinical anxiety situations as some of the other drugs, such as the selective serotonin S_2 antagonists, the serotonin S_3 antagonists, or the mixed agonist-antagonists for the serotonin S_{1A} receptors. It is of some interest that the serotonin uptake inhibitors and the MAO-A and MAO-B inhibitors are without effect in these animal models. It has been well known that MAO inhibitors and, more recently, the selective serotonin uptake inhibitors (Evans et al. 1986; Kahn et al. 1988) may be useful in the treatment of panic disorder. Patients with obsessive-compulsive disorder have been found to respond to both of these classes of drugs, particularly the specific serotonin uptake inhibitors. Thus, the differential sensitivity of animal behavior to the various drugs listed in Table 3 illustrates the specificity of the serotonin receptor subtype systems on behavioral effects. However, this does not have a direct one-to-one correlation to the use of these compounds in the treatment of anxiety disorders.

5 Studies of the Serotonergic Agonist MCPP in Patients with Major Depression and Anxiety Disorders

There has been considerable progress in understanding the role of the various serotonin receptor subtypes in regulating autonomic function and behavior in laboratory animals. It would be extremely useful to be able to apply drugs with specific effects on serotonergic function in a clinical situation to investigate the possible abnormalities in serotonergic function in patients as well as to assess the effects of treatments. There is a great limitation, however, due to the lack of clinically available specific compounds for this purpose, and most clinical investigators have been restricted to one or two available drugs. One drug which has been studied for a number of years has been tryptophan, administered intravenously at a dose of approximaltey 100 mg/kg, which stimulates prolactin and growth hormone release. There is no stimulation of cortisol release with this method. 5 Hydroxytryptophan stimulates cortisol but not prolactin; space limitations, however, do not allow a full discussion of this problem here. Another available compound has been MCPP. Since MCPP is a metabolite of the widely used antidepressant trazodone (Caccia et al. 1981), it is felt by these authors to be safe for administration to human subjects. Several studies have been conducted investigating MCPP in healthy subjects, where it has been found to produce some increases in anxiety, nervousness, and somatic symptoms, as well as the stimulation of prolactin, cortisol, and growth hormone release (Mueller et al. 1986). In Table 4, the neuroendocrine effects of intravenous tryptophan, intravenous MCPP, and

Table 4. Neuroendocrine response to tryptophan and MCPP in psychiatric patients

	Intravenous Tryptophan[a]		Intravenous MCPP[a]			Oral MCPP[a]		
	Pro-lactin	Growth Hormone	Pro-lactin	Growth Hormone	Cor-tisol	Pro-lactin	Growth Hormone	Cor-tisol
Major depression	↓	↓	N	↓	N	–	–	–
Panic disorder	N	N	N	N	N	–	–	–
Obsessive-compulsive disorder	N	N	↓[b]	N	N	N	–	↓

N, Not statistically different than healthy controls; ↓, statistically significant ($p < 0.05$) decreased response compared to healthy controls.
[a] Increase in hormone concentration following tryptophan intravenously at 100 mg/kg or MCPP 0.1 mg/kg intravenously or 0.5 mg/kg oral.
[b] Only in women.

oral MCPP have been listed for the studies of patients with major depression, panic disorder, and obsessive-compulsive disorder (Charney and Heninger 1986; Charney et al. 1987, 1988; Heninger et al. 1984; Zohar et al. 1987). It can be seen that there is a blunting of the prolactin and growth hormone release to intravenous tryptophan in depressed patients which has not been seen in patients with panic disorder or obsessive-compulsive disorder. With intravenous MCPP (infused over 20 min) there is a rapid increase in anxiety symptoms, and this is accompanied by a clear-cut increase in prolactin, cortisol, and growth hormone. However, in patients with panic disorder the neuroendocrine response to MCPP is not statistically different to that in healthy controls. In patients with obsessive-compulsive disorder the prolactin response in female patients following intravenous MCPP was blunted. This contrasts with an essentially normal prolactin response to oral MCPP in patients with obsessive-compulsive disorder, who in this study also had a blunting to the cortisol response, which was normal following intravenous MCPP. These data clearly indicate some difference in patients' responses to the intravenous versus the oral forms of MCPP, since, in addition, the patients with obsessive-compulsive disorder had an increase in obsessive-compulsive symptoms following oral MCPP but not following intravenous MCPP. It is of interest that with intravenous administration of MCPP the maximal effects occur at the end of the infusion, i.e., after 20 min, peak somewhere between 20 and 30 min, and then rapidly dissipate. The symptomatic and neuroendocrine effects following oral administration of MCPP slowly increased to a peak response at about 3 h. Thus, marked differences in the rate of systemic availability of the compound could account for some of the differences in these results. The data do indicate, however, that abnormalities in the neuroendocrine response of patients to stimulation of the serotonergic system do exist, and that there are differences between diagnostic groups. It would be very important to be able to utilize more specific and pure agonists, since MCPP has been reported to have high affinity for a number of other receptor systems (Hamik and Peroutka 1987), and serotonin S_{1B} receptors are reported to be nonexistent or at very low numbers in human brain. Thus, the pharmacologic specificity of both tryptophan and MCPP infusion could be questioned, and it would be much more useful to utilize more specific compounds.

6 Recent Studies on the Effects of Tryptophan Depletion on the Symptoms of Depressed Patients

There are considerable data indicating that brain serotonin levels are, to some degree, dependent on plasma tryptophan concentrations. Thus, there are a number of studies which have shown that there are mild to moderate correlations between lowered plasma tryptophan levels and dysphoric moods. There has been some problem, however, in the robustness of this relationship and in demonstrating the physiologic and behavioral relevance of the changes in plasma tryptophan levels relative to changes in mood and behavior of patients. Recent studies have shown that there is a statistically significant greater prolactin release following intravenous tryptophan in healthy subjects receiving a diet of 200 mg tryptophan each day than in those on a regular diet. This difference was not seen when a diet of 700 mg/day was given (Delgado et al. 1987).

    More recently, Delgado et al. (1988) have presented evidence that a severe depletion of plasma tryptophan markedly alters the mood and behavior of previously depressed patients who have recently responded to antidepressant treatment. In this procedure patients ingest a diet low in tryptophan (160 mg) for 24 h and then ingest a tryptophan-free 16 amino acid drink, which produces a 90% reduction in plasma tryptophan levels. In the initial report 12 patients on a variety of antidepressant treatments were studied. Within 24 h of this severe depletion of plasma tryptophan, 8 of the 12 patients had an increase of 10 or more points on the Hamilton Depression Scale before gradually returning to predrink status. Four of the patients did not have marked changes in scale ratings. These data are listed in Table 5. Also in Table 5 it can be seen that there is a tendency for those patients who are on lithium plus fluvoxamine or desipramine to be somewhat more resistant to the increase in depressive symptoms following the amino acid drink. A larger number of subjects will need to be studied to assess more fully whether lithium could protect against this effect. This would be of considerable interest since a number of lines of evidence indicate that lithium augments serotonergic function, much of this being related to presynaptic effects, including increased uptake of tryptophan. Also in Table 5 it can be seen that when the same subjects are given a control diet and drink which includes the same diet and a low-tryptophan

Table 5. Effects of a 24 h low-tryptophan diet and a tryptophan-deficient amino acid drink on depressive symptoms of patients who recently responded to antidepressant treatment

	Relapse[a]	No relapse
Antidepressant treatment		
Fluvoxamine	3	1
Tranylcypromine	3	0
Desipramine	1	1
Lithium plus fluvoxamine or desipramine	1	2
Control diet and drink	0	8

[a] A greater than 10-point increase in Hamilton Depression Scale ratings within 24 h following the drink.

amino acid drink, but with 1500 mg oral tryptophan added to the diet and 2.3 g of L-tryptophan added to the drink, there is no change in any of the eight patients in whom this procedure was studied.

These data provide evidence in support of earlier studies in which the condition of depressed patients became worse following the serotonin synthesis inhibitor parachlorophenylalanine (Shopsin et al. 1976). Taken together, the results of the parachlorophenylalanine study and of this plasma tryptophan depletion study suggest that adequate function of the serotonergic system is necessary (but possibly not sufficient) for effective antidepressant treatment.

7 Discussion

Major advances in the understanding of the multiple receptor subtypes of the serotonergic system have led to the use of a number of new compounds for the treatment of neuropsychiatric disorders. Thus, a recent report on induction of migraine-like headaches by MCPP (Brewerton et al. 1988) can be evaluated in the context of the very recent report on improvement in migraine following the novel serotonin S_1-like receptor agonist, GR 431175 (Doenicke et al. 1988). This compound was quite effective in the acute treatment of severe migraine. Whether the exacerbation of headache by MCPP involves its agonist or antagonist actions on different serotonin receptors remains to be demonstrated. Hopefully the improved specificity of available compounds for clinical use will permit these effects increasingly to be sorted out.

The most consistent and simple unified hypothesis of antidepressant drug action involves the multiple mechanisms of augmenting the overall serotonergic function. This hypothesis remains to be fully tested clinically. However, the data in Table 2 provide some support for this idea, since it was the longer term treatment with fluvoxamine and desipramine that produced the greatest augmentation of prolactin response to infused tryptophan. The more rapid action of lithium in augmenting this type of serotonergic function could possibly relate to the very rapid improvement in mood seen when lithium is added to the ongoing treatment of nonresponding patients (Heninger et al. 1983). Thus, the data in Table 2 provide some clinical support for the serotonin augmentation hypothesis of antidepressant drug action.

Results regarding neuroendocrine response following MCPP are somewhat conflicting, depending on the route of MCPP administration. The pharmacokinetic effects could be a large determinant of this. In addition, MCPP has been reported to have a number of other effects besides its stimulation of serotonin S_1 receptors (which may not exist in human brain). Thus, it is not clear which receptor subtypes are being stimulated by MCPP. It would be important to replicate the studies reported in Table 4, using a more specific serotonin S_{1A} receptor agonist such as 8-OHDPAT or possibly gepirone (Harto et al. 1988) or ipsapirone.

The tryptophan depletion studies provide very interesting and provocative data relative to the role of serotonergic function in the maintenance of antidepressant drug effects. Thus, the original studies with parachlorophenylalanine (Shopsin et al. 1976) were never extended with published reports. The rapid and large increase in depressive symptoms following the tryptophan-deficient amino acid drink suggest very strongly that intact serotonergic function is an essential ingredient in the antidepressant response. This, too, would be in support of the augmented serotonergic function hypothesis of antidepressant treatment.

There is a great deal of current and very active research directed at the neuropharmacology of serotonin receptor systems. A whole additional dimension not currently discussed is the receptor-effector coupling and the postsynaptic effects of the variety of serotonin receptor subtypes. It has been postulated that lithium may act through some of these mechanisms, including actions on the cyclic AMP and the phosphotidylinositol cycles (Worley et al. 1988). We should be optimistic that through continued research in this area much more progress can be made regarding the role of the serotonergic system in the mediation of psychotropic drug response and possible abnormalities in patients with neuropsychiatric disorders.

References

Blier P, deMontigny C, Chaput Y (1987) Modifications of the serotonin system by antidepressant treatments: implications for the therapeutic response in major depression. J Clin Psychopharmacol 7(6):24–35

Brewerton TD, Murphy DL, Mueller EA, Jimerson DC (1988) Induction of migraine-like headaches by the serotonin agonist m-chlorophenylpiperazine. Clin Pharmacol Ther (in press)

Caccia S, Ballabio M, Samanin R, Zanini MG, Garattini S (1981) (−) M-chlorophenylpiperazine, a central 5-hydroxytryptamine agonist, is a metabolite of trazodone. J Pharmacol 33:477–478

Charney DS, Heninger GR (1986) Serotonin function in panic disorders: the effect of intravenous tryptophan in healthy subjects and panic disorder patients before and during alprazolam treatment. Arch Gen Psychiatry 43:1059–1065

Charney DS, Woods SW, Goodman WK, Heninger GR (1987) Serotonin function in anxiety. II. Effects of the serotonin agonist, MCPP, in panic disorder patients and healthy subjects. Psychopharmacology (Berlin) 92:14–24

Charney DS, Goodman WK, Price LH, Rasmussen SA, Heninger GR (1988) Serotonin function in obsessive compulsive disorder: a comparison of the effects of tryptophan and MCPP in patients and healthy subjects. Arch Gen Psychiatry 45:177–185

Chopin P, Briley M (1987) Animal models of anxiety: the effect of compounds that modify 5-HT neurotransmission. Trends Pharmacol Sci 8:383–388

Delgado PL, Charney DS, Price LH, Anderson G, Landis H, Heninger CR (1987) Dietary tryptophan restriction produces an upregulation of the neuroscience response to infused tryptophan in healthy human subjects. Soc Neurosci Abstr 1:227

Delgado PL, Price L, Charney DS, Aghajanian GK, Landis H, Heninger GR (1988) Tryptophan depletion alters mood in depression. Annu Meet Am Psychiatr Assoc 141:189

Doenicke A, Brand J, Perrin VL (1988) Possible benefit of GR43175, A novel 5-HT1-like receptor agonist, for the acute treatment of severe migraine. Lancet II:1309–1311

Evans L, Kenardy J, Schneider P, Hoey H (1986) Effect of a selective serotonin uptake inhibitor in agoraphobia with panic attacks. Acta Psychiatr Scand 73:49

Hamik A, Peroutka SJ (1987) 1-(m-Chlorophenyl) piperazine (mCPP) interactions with neurotransmitter receptors in human brain. Soc Neurosci Abstr 13:1237

Harto NE, Branconnier RJ, Spera KF, Dessain EC (1988) Clinical profile of gepirone, a nonbenzodiazepine anxiolytic. Psychopharmacol Bull 24(1):154–160

Heninger GR, Charney DS, Sternberg DE (1983) Lithium carbonate augmentation of antidepressant treatment: an effective prescription for treatment-refractory depression. Arch Gen Psychiatry 40:1335–1342

Heninger GR, Charney DS, Sternberg DE (1984) Serotonergic function in depression: prolactin response to intravenous tryptophan in depressed patients and healthy subjects. Arch Gen Psychiatry 41:398–402

Heninger GR, Charney DS, Smith A (1987) Effects of serotonin receptor agonists and antagonists on neuroendocrine function in Rhesus monkeys. Soc Neurosci Abstr 1:801

Heninger G, Charney D, Price L, Woods S, Goodman W (1988) Neuroendocrine and behavioral effects of 5HT agonists in rhesus monkeys, and patients with major depression or anxiety disorders. Can Coll Neuropsychopharmacol Abstr 1:28

Kahn RS, van Praag HM, Wetzler S, Asnis GM, Barr G (1988) Serotonin and anxiety revisited. Biol Psychiatry 23:189

Mueller EA, Murphy DL, Sunderland T (1986) Further studies of the putative serotonin agonist, m-chlorophenylpiperazine: evidence for a serotonin receptor mediated mechanism of action in humans. Psychopharmacology (Berlin) 89:388–391

Price LH, Charney DS, Heninger GR (1985) Effects of tranylcypromine treatment on neuroendocrine, behavioral and autonomic responses to tryptophan in depressed patients. Life Sci 37:809–818

Price LH, Charney DS, Delgado PL, Anderson GM, Heninger GR (1988) Effects of desipramine and fluvoxamine treatment on the prolactin response to L-tryptophan: a test of the serotonergic function enhancement hypothesis of antidepressant action. Arch Gen Psychiatry

Price LH, Charney DS, Heninger GR (1989a) Effects of trazodone treatment on serotonergic function in depressed patients. Psychiatry Res (in press)

Price LH, Charney DS, Delgado PL, Heninger GR (1989b) Lithium treatment and serotonergic function: neuroendocrine behavioral and physiologic responses to intravenous L-tryptophan in affective disorder patients. Arch Gen Psychiatry (in press)

Shopsin B, Friedman E, Gershon S (1976) Parachlorophenylalanine reversal of tranylcypromine effects in depressed patients. Arch Gen Psychiatry 33:811–819

Traber J, Glaser T (1987) 5-H-1A receptor-related anxiolytics. Trends Pharmacol Sci 8:432

Van de Kar LD, Karteszi M, Bethea CL, Ganong WF (1985) Serotonergic stimulation of prolactin and corticosterone secretion is mediated by different pathways from the mediobasal hypothalamus. Neuroendocrinology 41:380–384

Worley PF, Heller WA, Snyder SH, Baraban JM (1988) Lithium blocks a phosphoinositide-mediated cholinergic response in hippocampal slices. Science 239:1428–1429

Zohar J, Mueller EA, Insel TR, Zohar-Kadouch RC, Murphy DL (1987) Serotonergic responsivity in obsessive-compulsive disorder: comparison of patients and health controls. Arch Gen Psychiatry 44:946–951

Zohar J, Insel TR, Zohar-Kadouch RC, Hill JL, Murphy DL (1988) Serotonergic responsivity in obsessive-compulsive disorder: effects of chronic clomipramine treatment. Arch Gen Psychiatry 45:167–172

Theoretical and Practical Implications of a Controlled Trial of an α_2-Adrenoceptor Antagonist in the Treatment of Depression

S. A. MONTGOMERY [1]

1 Mechanisms of Antidepressant Action

The simple monoamine deficit hypothesis of depressive illness proposed that a disturbance in the serotonin or the noradrenaline neurotransmitter system is an important factor in the pathogenesis of depression. It was presumed that the activity of tricyclic antidepressants in inhibiting the reuptake of monoamines and a consequent increase in monoamines in the synaptic cleft would facilitate neurotransmission, and that this was the mechanism mediating their antidepressant effect. The theory has been of great value in stimulating research and for more than 20 years has formed the basis for investigations into the aetiology of depression and into the development of possible antidepressants. While there is agreement that the catecholamines and/or the indoleamines are likely to play an important part in the mechanisms underlying depressive illness, there are a number of challenges to the theory and inconsistencies in the studies (Montgomery et al. 1987).

The original hypothesis postulated a deficiency in monoamines associated with depression (Schildkraut 1965; Bunney and Davis 1965), and research was directed towards establishing deficits in depressed patients compared with controls. The results from these studies have not led to a consistent pattern of deficiency in depressed patients, and both hyperactivity and hypoactivity of neurotransmitter systems have been postulated in the aetiology of depression. More recent attention has focussed on functional abnormalities in the regulatory activity of neurotransmitter systems, and one model (Siever and Davis 1985) proposes dysregulation of noradrenaline release as the defect associated with depression.

It is possible that in depression there is enhanced presynaptic α_2-adrenergic receptor activity with decreased noradrenaline release. It has been shown in a number of animal studies that chronic administration of tricyclic antidepressant drugs produces a reduction in the number of α_2-adrenoceptors in the brain. Similar effects have been observed peripherally in depressed patients, and these changes have been related by some investigators to response to antidepressants (Garcia-Sevilla 1981). It is well established that presynaptic α_2-adrenoceptors have an important role in the feedback regulatory system of noradrenaline release, and manipulation of these receptors seems a possible area for the search for antidepressant intervention.

[1] St. Mary's Hospital Medical School, Academic Department of Psychiatry, Praed Street, London W2 1NY, England

Clinical Pharmacology in Psychiatry
Editors: S. G. Dahl and L. F. Gram
(Psychopharmacology Series 7)
© Springer-Verlag Berlin Heidelberg 1989

The most direct challenge to the simple view of amine reuptake blockade as the mechanism of antidepressant effect was the development of new atypical antidepressants which are without clear monoamine uptake inhibiting properties. Similarly, not all antidepressants have the same effect on α_2-adrenoceptors, and a simple explanation of antidepressant effect is unlikely. It is accepted that several interacting neurotransmitter systems are likely to be involved in the pathophysiology of depression. It is nevertheless useful to investigate the effects of changes in particular systems in order to estimate their role in depressive illness.

2 Specific α_2-Adrenoceptor Antagonists

The earlier atypical antidepressants such as mianserin did not provide useful pharmacological tools as they were "impure compounds". With mianserin, for example, it has not been possible to determine which of its pharmacological actions contribute most to the antidepressant effect. One of its actions of interest, however, is that it acts as an α_2-adrenoceptor antagonist. It is possible that its antidepressant effect is mediated by this inhibitory activity on the feedback mechanism, which would increase the release of noradrenaline.

The test of the relevance of the theory had to wait for the appearance of compounds with selective effects in antagonising α_2-adrenoceptors, several of which are now in development. It these compounds are shown to have antidepressant effect, it will be of considerable theoretical interest.

The first of this series of compounds in development to be tested for antidepressant efficacy in the clinic is idazoxan, which has been shown to be a potent and selective antagonist for α_2-adrenoceptors in vitro and in vivo, although its selectivity in relation to α_2-adrenoceptors is not as clear-cut as with later compounds. Radiological binding studies have confirmed the high affinity of the drug for α_2-adrenoceptors in the brain.

The initial test of this compound was to establish whether it had antidepressant efficacy. The appropriate test of this is to compare it with reference antidepressants and to reject the compound if there is significantly less antidepressant efficacy in a carefully conducted trial. Idazoxan was therefore compared in a double-blind trial with amitriptyline in a large group-comparison multicentre study. This study was not designed to fully assess the antidepressant efficacy of the new compound but to answer the question of whether it was significantly worse than amitriptyline. If this were the case, it would cast doubt on the role of α_2-adrenoceptors in depression.

The study was conducted in two parts, using the same protocol, and including patients suffering from major depression satisfying the research diagnostic criteria of Spitzer et al. (1975) and who remained moderately or severely depressed following a placebo washout period. The dose of idazoxan was 20 mg three times per day in the first study and 40 mg three times per day in the second study; the effects were compared to those with 50 mg amitriptyline three times per day. In the first study, in 97 patients completing 3 weeks treatment and 88 completing 4 weeks treatment, response to idazoxan was significantly worse than that to amitriptyline. This advantage for amitriptyline was more apparent in the more severely depressed patients. In the second, higher dose study in 65 patients there was no difference in apparent efficacy between amitriptyline and idazoxan. A transient advantage for idazoxan in the moderately depressed patients seen early in treatment is intriguing in view of the theoretical predictions of early onset of action with α_2-antagonists, although the numbers in this substratification are too small to be sure of the effect.

3 Conclusion

The results from this study are of great theoretical interest. The lack of efficacy of the lower doses and the probable efficacy of the higher dose suggest a dose-response relationship with α_2-antagonists in the treatment of depression. Clearly the numbers in this study are too small to give more than an indication of the efficacy of idazoxan, but they are sufficient to pursue this concept further.

The most intriguing feature of this study is the apparent lack of efficacy in the group suffering from severe depression, which is evident in both studies. This is the first study to reveal a differential response between those with moderate and those with severe depression, and this might, if replicated, indicate a separate pathogenesis of severe and moderate depression. The differential response is normally seen between mild depression, which has not been shown reliably to respond to antidepressant treatment (Montgomery 1987), and moderate and severe depression, where antidepressant response is generally seen to be equal.

Further full testing of the antidepressant properties of idazoxan is needed. These preliminary results should now be tested in a large multicentre placebo-controlled study.

References

Bunney WE, Davis JM (1965) Norepinephrine in depressive reactions: a review. Arch Gen Psychiatry 13:483–494

Garcia-Sevilla JA, Zis AP, Zelnik TC, Smith CB (1981) Tricyclic antidepressant drug treatment decreases alpha$_2$ adrenoceptors on human platelet membranes. Eur J Pharmacol 69:121–123

Montgomery SA (1987) Common errors in clinical trials. In: Biziere K, Garattini S, Simon P (eds) Diagnosis and treatment of depression: quo vadis? Sanofi, Montpellier

Montgomery SA, James D, Montgomery DB (1987) Pharmacological specificity is not the same as clinical selectivity. In: Dahl SG, Gram LF, Paul SM, Potter WZ (eds) Clinical pharmacology in psychiatry. Springer, Berlin Heidelberg New York

Schildkraut JJ (1965) The catecholamine hypothesis of affective disorders: a review of supporting evidence. Am J Psychiatry 122:509–522

Siever LJ, Davis KL (1985) Overview: toward a dysregulation hypothesis of depression. Am J Psychiatry 142:1017–1031

Spitzer R, Endicott J, Robins E (1975) Research diagnostic criteria. NY State Psychiatric Institute, New York

Selective Dopamine D_1 and D_2 Receptor Antagonists

J. Hyttel [1], J. Arnt [1], and M. van den Berghe [2]

1 Introduction

The concept of selective dopamine D_1 and D_2 receptor antagonists is rather new. Previously, dopamine receptor antagonism was evaluated simply as the ability to inhibit dopamine- or dopamine agonist-mediated behaviour or biochemical responses. In 1979 Kebabian and Calne introduced the dopamine D_1 and D_2 receptor concept based on differential linkage to adenylate cyclase. At that time receptor binding techniques had already been introduced, and more or less selective ligands were available (Iversen 1978). Today, very selective ligands are used to differentiate the two dopamine receptor populations.

The selective D_1 antagonist SCH 23390 (Hyttel 1983) has been labelled with tritium and has replaced [³H]cis-(Z)-flupentixol and [³H]piflutixol (Hyttel 1978, 1981, 1982) as the ligand of choice (Billard et al. 1984; Andersen et al. 1985; Hyttel and Arnt 1987). [³H]Spiperone has replaced [³H]haloperidol as the ligand of choice for D_2 receptor binding studies, although [³H]raclopride may be considered a better choice, since the inclusion of a serotonin S_2 receptor antagonist in the assay – mandatory for the [³H]spiperone assay – is unnecessary with [³H]raclopride.

2 Selectivity of Dopamine Antagonists In Vitro

The receptor binding affinities of a series of dopamine antagonists listed in Table 1 have been obtained in our laboratories using [³H]SCH 23390 and [³H]spiperone (plus mianserin) as ligands for dopamine D_1 and D_2 receptors, respectively. For a smaller number of compounds, the profiles of dopamine receptor antagonism in vitro and in vivo are shown as pie charts in Fig. 1.

In fact, only a few selective dopamine D_1 receptor antagonists have been found, e.g. SCH 23390 and the bromine analog SK&F 83566 C, which have selectivity ratios ($K_i D_2/K_i D_1$) of 3100 and 580, respectively. Many neuroleptics – including the thioxanthenes (i.e. zuclopenthixol, cis-(Z)-flupentixol, cis-

[1] Department of Pharmacology, H. Lundbeck A/S, Ottiliavej 7-9, 2500 Copenhagen, Denmark
[2] Lundbeck NV, Luchthavenlaan 20, 1800 Vilvoorde, Belgium

Clinical Pharmacology in Psychiatry
Editors: S. G. Dahl and L. F. Gram
(Psychopharmacology Series 7)
© Springer-Verlag Berlin Heidelberg 1989

Table 1. Effect of Dopamine antagonists on dopamine D_1, D_2 and 5-HT$_2$ Receptors

Drug	K_i(nM) – in vitro receptor binding studies			ED$_{50}$ (µmol/kg) – in vivo behavioural studies		
	D_1	D_2	5-HT$_2$	D_1	D_2	5-HT$_2$
Thioxanthenes						
cis(Z)-chlorprothixene	1.5	1.2	0.63	1.8	0.63	0.092
cis(Z)-flupentixol	0.91	0.36	4.2	0.15	0.032	0.037
cis(Z)-piflutixol	0.16	0.26	0.63	0.051	0.0062	0.014
cis(Z)-thiothixene	4.9	0.63	51	> 5.6	0.080	1.0
Zuclopenthixol	0.45	0.65	1.8	1.3	0.050	0.30
Phenothiazines						
Chlorpromazine	11	2.6	3.0	8.4	0.97	0.37
Perphenazine	9.1	1.0	5.0	1.1	0.018	0.32
Thioridazine	3.4	5.5	8.4	> 49	4.8	6.7
Trifluoroperazine	3.2	0.57	8.4	> 10	0.040	0.29
Fluphenazine	0.70	0.49	5.8	2.0	0.010	0.088
Butyrophenones						
Haloperidol	15	0.84	29	7.0	0.036	0.99
Spiperone	86	0.067	0.49	> 13	0.039	0.12
Diphenylbutylpiperidines						
Penfluridol	12	0.60	99	—	> 2.4	> 4.8
Pimozide	220	0.11	5.2	> 11	0.27	1.1
Benzamides						
Clebopride	6200	1.8	150	> 41	0.029	3.9
Metoclopramide	11000	82	2800	>230	7.8	36
Raclopride	30000	17	7300	> 20	0.17	7.0
Remoxipride	>41000	1300	14000	> 94	0.56	28
Sulpiride	17000	92	37000	>230	11	>230
YM 08050	4900	0.66	99	> 11	0.019	0.55
YM 09151-2	1200	0.054	26	> 13	0.0041	0.32
Piperazino-6-7-6-tricyclics						
Clothiapine	6.2	2.2	2.3	5.6	0.48	0.26
Clozapine	53	46	4.1	8.0	3.7	1.1
Fluperlapine	91	150	6.8	22	5.5	2.4
Loxapine	13	4.6	2.0	3.9	0.16	0.072
Methiothepin	2.4	0.29	0.36	0.31	0.053	0.024
Octoclothepin	0.91	0.27	0.30	0.25	0.033	0.016
Perlapine	120	260	13	> 34	11	7.7
Zotepine	2.2	1.0	0.58	2.8	0.55	0.14
Miscellaneous						
(+) Butaclamol	1.6	1.1	2.4	1.3	0.052	0.46
Pirenperone	190	9.3	0.32	36	0.40	0.051
Ritanserin	82	1.3	0.21	> 21	>21	0.078
Setoperone	230	5.9	0.58	20	0.20	0.090
SCH 23390	0.12	360	7.3	0.0092	>14	1.8
SK&F 83566C	0.37	210	13	0.013	> 3.0	0.81
Tefludazine	9.5	1.8	1.6	2.2	0.018	0.029

[^{3}H]-SCH 23390, [^{3}H]-spiperone and [^{3}H]-ketanserine were used as ligands for D_1, D_2 and 5-HT$_2$ receptor binding in vitro, respectively. For the in vivo data unilaterally 6-OH-dopamine-lesioned rat model was used for dopamine D_1 and D_2 receptors. Rotation was induced by SK&F 38393 or pergolide, respectively. Inhibition of quipazine-induced head twitches was used for 5-HT$_2$ receptors. Drugs were tested after subcutaneous administration.

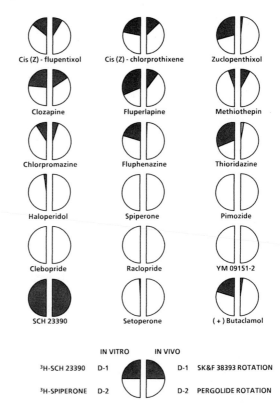

Fig. 1. Dopamine D_1 and D_2 profile of neuroleptics in vitro (*left*) and in vivo (*right*). The affinities for D_1 and D_2 receptors – for in vitro and in vivo results, respectively – are shown as percentages of the total calculated from: $(1/K_i D_1) + (1/K_i D_2)$ $= 100\%$; and $(1/ED_{50} D_1)$ $+ (1/ED_{50} D_2) = 100\%$. K_i and ED_{50} values from Table 1

(Z)-chlorprothixene and teflutixol), some phenothiazines (e.g. fluphenazine) and some piperazino-6-7-6-tricyclics (i.e. perlapine, fluperlapine, clozapine, clothiapine and octoclothepin) – have similar affinities for dopamine D_1 and D_2 receptors.

The benzamides, diphenylbutylpiperidines, butyrophenones and some phenothiazines have selective affinity for dopamine D_2 receptors. The most selective are the benzamides, with YM 09151-2 as the most extreme (ratio K_i $D_1/K_i D_2 = 21\,000$). The phenothiazines have ratios from 1.4 to 20, the butyrophenones from 14 to 1300, the diphenylbutylpiperidines from 20 to 2000, and the benzamides from > 30 to 21 000.

The affinities for dopamine D_1 receptors, using [³H]SCH 23390 as a ligand, correlate closely to those obtained using [³H]piflutixol and cis-(Z)-flupentixol and to data for the inhibition of dopamine-stimulated adenylate cyclase. Likewise, the [³H]spiperone binding data closely correlate to those obtained using [³H]haloperidol (Andersen et al. 1985; Hyttel and Arnt 1987; Leysen et al. 1978).

3 Behavioural Effects in Animals

Antipsychotic and behavioural potencies of neuroleptics, including the antistereotypic, cataleptogenic and avoidance-inhibitory effects, have been known for several years to correlate closely with binding affinities for dopamine D_2 receptors (Creese et al. 1976; Niemegeers and Janssen 1979; Peroutka and Snyder 1980; Seeman 1980; Arnt 1982, 1983; Hayashi and Tadokoro 1984). Some of the test models are summarized in Table 2, with approximate potencies shown for a selective dopamine D_1 (SCH 23390) and D_2 receptor antagonist (spiperone) and for a mixed D_1/D_2 antagonist (cis-(Z)-flupentixol or clozapine). The correlation between dopamine D_2 receptor affinity and behavioural potency, together with the lack of behavioural effects of the D_1 agonist SK&F 38393, initially led to doubt about the functional significance of dopamine D_1 receptors. Surprisingly, SCH 23390 had behavioural effects almost similar to those of dopamine D_2 and D_1/D_2 receptor antagonists, as shown in the upper part of Table 2. Of particular interest was that SCH 23390 and spiperone equally well blocked the effects of D_2 agonists (pergolide, quinpirole, RU 24213), regardless of whether stereotypy or circling was the behavioural response (O'Boyle et al. 1984; Arnt 1985). A similar profile has been observed with another selective dopamine D_1 receptor

Table 2. Effect of dopamine receptor antagonists (D_1 selective, D_2 selective and mixed D_1/D_2) in various in vivo models of neuroleptic activity

Model	D_1	D_2	D_1/D_2
Normosensitive dopamine receptors			
Inhibition conditioned avoidance, rats	S	S	S
Catalepsy, rats	S	S	S
Antistereotypic effects, pergolide (D_2), rats	S	S	S
Antistereotypic effects, apomorphine (D_1/D_2), rats	S	S	S
Circling (6-OH-dopamine) amphetamine, rats	S	S	S
Circling (hemitransection), apormorphine, rats	S	S	S
Inhibition of cue, amphetamine (D_1/D_2), rats	S	S	S
Inhibition of cue, SK&F 38393 (D_1), rats	S	N	W
Inhibition of cue, (−)-NPA (D_2), rats	N	S	S
Supersensitive dopamine receptors			
Circling (6-OH-dopamine) SK&F 38393 (D_1), rats	S	N	S
Circling (6-OH-dopamine) pergolide (D_2), rats	N	S	S
Circling (6-OH-dopamine) apomorphine (D_1/D_2), rats	W	W	S
Hyperactivity, chronic reserpine, SK&F 38393 (D_1), rats	S	W	S
Hyperactivity, chronic reserpine, pergolide (D_2), rats	N	S	S

Comparison is made between the dopamine D_1 receptor antagonist SCH 23390, a dopamine D_2 receptor antagonist, either spiperone or YM 09151-2, and a D_1/D_2 antagonist, either *cis* (Z)-flupentixol or clozapine. The effect is graduated as strong (S), weak (W) or as no effect (N).

antagonist, SK&F 83566 C (O'Boyle and Waddington 1984; Molloy and Waddington 1985 b; Arnt 1985; for review see Clark and White 1987).

The precise neuronal localization of dopamine D_1 and D_2 receptor is unknown, but it must be assumed that they are present at the same or closely connected output systems. This does not exclude the presence of separate efferent systems for specific dopamine D_1 or D_2 receptor-mediated behaviour, e.g. the sniffing and grooming responses induced by SK&F 38393, which were blocked by SCH 23390 but not affected by metoclopramide (Molloy and Waddington 1984 a). Indeed, studies with intracerebral injections of SK&F 38393, SCH 23390, and ($-$)-sulpiride have indicated a similar functional effect of dopamine D_1 and D_2 receptor manipulation within the same site (for review see Clark and White 1987).

Water-deprived rats can be trained to discriminate between a dopamine D_1 agonist (SK&F 38393) and saline or a dopamine D_2 agonist ($-$)-N-propylnorapomorphine, or ($-$)-NPA, and saline in a two-lever operant chamber (Arnt and Hyttel 1988). Dopamine D_1 agonists readily induced the SK&F 38393-like stimulus whereas D_2 agonists did not. The SK&F 38393 stimulus was antagonized by SCH 23390, but not by YM 09151-2. Conversely, dopamine D_2 agonists induced the ($-$)-NPA-like stimulus, which was readily antagonized by YM 09151-2, while SCH 23390 had no inhibitory effect.

In spite of the similar antistereotypic and cataleptogenic activities of SCH 23390 and dopamine D_2 antagonists, it has been possible to differentiate between these compounds in interaction studies with the antimuscarinic compound scopolamine and with diazepam. In mice it was found that the inhibitory potencies of dopamine D_2 antagonists against methylphenidate-induced gnawing were markedly reduced by either substance, while the effects of mixed dopamine D_1/D_2 antagonists or SCH 23390 were almost unchanged (Christensen et al. 1984 a). Similar differentiation was obtained in rats by investigating anti-amphetamine and cataleptogenic activities with or without co-administration of scopolamine. The antistereotypic activity was unaltered for compounds with high dopamine D_1 receptor affinities, and cataleptogenic potencies were only moderately reduced. Greater shifts in ED_{50} values were obtained with selective dopamine D_2 receptor antagonists (Arnt and Christensen 1981; Christensen et al. 1984 a). Obviously, caution is needed in the interpretation of such studies, in particular because of the additional neuropharmacological properties of dopamine antagonists (Peroutka and Snyder 1980; Hyttel 1983). Still, these results suggest that dopamine D_1 receptor blockade makes the behavioural effects of neuroleptics less sensitive to interaction from other neurotransmitter systems.

The original article on SK&F 38393 (Setler et al. 1978 a) reported that a contralateral circling behaviour, with efficacy similar to that of apomorphine, was induced by SK&F 38393 in rats with unilateral 6-OH-dopamine lesions. The same authors also showed high efficacy of SK&F 38393 after intrastriatal injection (Setler et al. 1978 b; see also Gower and Marriott 1982). The latter authors noted that dopamine antagonists inhibited SK&F 38393-induced circling with a rank order of potencies which was significantly different from the rank order obtained by use of either apomorphine or dipropyl-5,6-ADTN as the agonist for circling behaviour. Haloperidol and pimozide were ineffective only against SK&F 38393-inducing circling. With the recent availability of a selective dopamine D_1 receptor antagonist (SCH 23390) and also of selective dopamine D_2 receptor agonists, it has been possible to characterize further the structure-activity relations of antagonistic effects at denervated dopamine receptors. Using the circling behaviour induced by SK&F 38393, pergolide, quinpirole, and apomorphine as test models, a range of antagonists have been studied, as shown in Table 1 against the behavioural effects of SK&F 38393 and pergolide. SCH 23390 was a very potent antagonist of SK&F 38393-induced circling whereas it was ineffective as an inhibitor of pergolide- or quinpirole-induced circling (Arnt and Hyttel 1984, 1985, 1986).

In contrast, selective dopamine D_2 receptor antagonists were potent inhibitors of pergolide- or quinpirole-induced circling but were at least 500-fold weaker in inhibiting SK&F 38393-induced circling (Arnt and Hyttel 1984, 1985, 1986). The apomorphine-induced rotations were partially antagonized by dopamine D_1 and D_2 antagonists (Coward 1983; Herrera-Marschitz and Ungerstedt 1984; Arnt and Hyttel 1985). Thioxanthenes having mixed dopamine D_1/D_2 receptor blocking activity, or a combination of SCH 23390 with clebopride or spiperone, showed dose-dependent blockade against all the above-mentioned agonists (Table 2; Arnt and Hyttel 1984, 1985; Herrera-Marschitz and Ungerstedt 1984). These results indicate that circling behaviour can be induced at separate D_1 and D_2 receptor sites.

As shown in Fig. 2 the in vivo data obtained using the 6-OH-dopamine lesioned rat model, where the rotation is mediated either via D_1 receptors (with SK&F 38393) or via D_2 receptors (with pergolide), in many respects resemble the in vitro data (Table 1, Fig. 1). SCH 23390 and SK&F 83566 C are selective antagonists at dopamine D_1 receptors. At the other extreme of the spectrum, YM 09151-2 is found to be a selective antagonist at dopamine D_2 receptors.

One interesting example of divergence is fluphenazine, which is a highly selective antagonist of dopamine D_2 receptors in vivo but much less so in vitro. Using receptor binding techniques ($[^3H]$SCH 23390 and $[^3H]$raclopride) in vivo and in vitro, Andersen (1988) found that compounds exhibiting dopamine D_1/D_2 receptor selectivity in vitro retain this selectivity in vivo. In other words, the in vitro and in vivo data for both $[^3H]$SCH 23390 and $[^3H]$raclopride correlate closely. Interestingly, Andersen (1988) found that fluperlapine and fluphenazine were nonselective in vitro but were D_1 and D_2 selective, respectively, in vivo. However, the difference was not as great as reported here for fluphenazine. Furthermore, rats were used for in vitro and mice for in vivo experiments.

The general impression from Fig. 1 is that the selectivity ratio obtained in vitro is retained or changed in favour of D_2 selectivity when tested in vivo. The most outstanding examples are fluphenazine, thioridazine, zuclopenthixol and (+)-butaclamol. The apparent D_2 selectivity in vivo of, for example,

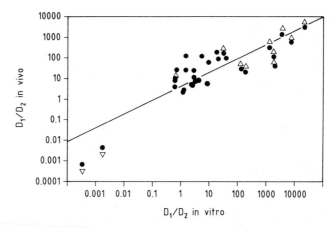

Fig. 2. Relationship of in vitro and in vivo data on the selectivity of antagonists to dopamine D$_1$ and D$_2$ receptors. Values from Table 1 are shown. *Abscissa*, ratio of K_i-values; *ordinate*, ratio of ED$_{50}$ values. *Symbols with arrowhead*, values for which one of the ED$_{50}$ values was not attained, i.e. ED$_{50}$ values smaller or greater than the values given in Table 1. Pearson's product-moment correlation coefficient is 0.865; omitting values with arrowhead the correlation coefficient in 0.587, whereas the coefficient for the arrowhead values is 0.953

zuclopenthixol should be born in mind if this compound is used (in animal experiments or in the clinic) to reveal the influence of dopamine D$_1$ and D$_2$ receptors in different aspects of behaviour, biochemistry, etc.

The importance of relative dopamine D$_1$ and D$_2$ receptor affinities for the development of tolerance to methylphenidate-inhibitory effects of dopamine antagonists, has been studied in mice after daily administration of the same dopamine antagonist (homologous tolerance) or another one (cross-tolerance). In this species, tolerance phenomena are readily observed (Christensen and Møller Nielsen 1980; Christensen et al. 1984b, c). Administration of selective dopamine D$_2$ receptor antagonists for 12 days led to marked homologous tolerance in the withdrawal phase, i.e. increase of ED$_{50}$ values on the order of 25–50 times. Mixed dopamine D$_1$/D$_2$ receptor antagonists induced less homologous tolerance and also less cross-tolerance to 12 days of treatment with dopamine D$_2$ receptor antagonists. SCH 23390, administered twice daily, did not induce such tolerance (Christensen et al. 1984b, c). Furthermore, concomitant treatment with SCH 23390 and haloperidol for 12 days prevented the marked tolerance development observed with haloperidol alone (Christensen et al. 1985). Zuclopenthixol also had the ability to prevent haloperidol-induced tolerance during 12 days of combined treatment. These results indicate an effect of dopamine D$_1$ receptor antagonism against tolerance development at dopamine D$_2$ receptors.

However, it should be noted that a similarly clear differentiation between the long-term effects of mixed dopamine D$_1$/D$_2$ and selective dopamine D$_2$ receptor antagonists in rats has not been shown so far (Waddington and Gamble 1980; Waddington et al. 1981; Fleminger et al. 1983).

Studies by Rosengarten et al. (1983, 1986) indicate that SK&F 38393 induces a characteristic pattern of repetitious opening and closing of the mouth and clonic jaw movements. This effect is also seen after blockade of D_2 receptors (e.g. with sulpiride, spiperone), whereas blockade of dopamine D_1 receptors by SCH 23390 antagonizes the perioral movements. The likelihood that dopamine D_1 receptors are involved in this phenomenon is strengthened by studies in which selective loss of either dopamine D_1 or D_2 receptors is induced by N-ethoxycarbonyl-2-ethoxy-1,2-dihydroquinoline (EEDQ) (Arnt et al. 1988 a). When the density of D_2 receptors is lowered to 25%, an increased frequency of perioral movements is seen. This effect is further increased by treatment with the dopamine D_1 receptor agonist SK&F 38393. Should these perioral movements in any way be related to tardive dyskinesia, one might expect neuroleptics with potent dopamine D_1 receptor-blocking properties to have a better chance of alleviating these symptoms than neuroleptics inhibiting solely dopamine D_2 receptors.

It has been suggested that inhibition of the spontaneous activity of the dopamine neurons in substantia nigra observed after chronic tretment with neuroleptics should account for the development of extrapyramidal side effects, while inhibition of the activity in the ventral tegmental area should indicate the antipsychotic potential of a compound (Bunney 1984). After treatment for 21 days with SCH 23390, the number of spontaneously active neurons in substantia nigra and the ventral tegmental area decreased to the same level. A similar result was seen after treatment with haloperidol for the same period of time (Skarsfeldt 1988). Apparently, the differentiation of antipsychotic effect and side effect potential is coupled neither to dopamine D_1 nor to dopamine D_2 receptor blockade.

4 Effects of Dopamine Antagonists on Other Receptors

Selectivity of neuroleptics is usually referred to as the dopamine D_1/D_2 receptor selectivity, as described above. However, the drugs can be regarded as selective only when other effects are negligible as compared to their dopamine D_1 or D_2 receptor effect. In this respect only a few neuroleptics can be regarded as selective (Hyttel et al. 1985). Focus has mostly been on serotonin S_2 receptors, α_1-adrenoceptors, muscarinic acetylcholine receptors and histamine H_1 receptors.

Of special interest is the effect on serotonin S_2 receptors, since the recent development of neuroleptics has led to compounds with high affinity for these receptors, e.g. ritanserin, setoperone and tefludazine (Svendsen et al. 1986; Leysen et al. 1987). The affinity of neuroleptics for serotonin S_2 receptors, as measured in vitro with [^{3}H]ketanserin as a ligand, is shown in Table 1 and as pie charts in Fig. 3.

Induction of head twitches is a characteristic behavioural response to serotonin S_2 receptor stimulation in rats and can be induced by, for example,

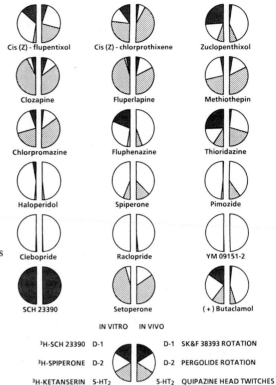

Fig. 3. Receptor profile of neuroleptics in vitro (*left*) and in vivo (*right*). The affinities for dopamine D$_1$, D$_2$ and 5-HT$_2$ receptors – for in vitro and in vivo results, respectively – are shown as percentages of the total calculated from: $(1/K_i D_1) + (1/K_i D_2) + (1/K_i 5\text{-HT}_2) = 100\%$; and $(1/ED_{50} D_1) + (1/ED_{50} D_2) + (1/ED_{50} 5\text{-HT}_2) = 100\%$. K_i and ED$_{50}$ values are taken from Table 1

1-5-hydrotryptophan, mescaline or quipazine (Niemegeers et al. 1983; Arnt et al. 1984, 1989). Antagonist studies indicate that serotonin S$_2$ receptor antagonists inhibit head twitches with high potencies, although α_1-adrenoceptor inhibition may also contribute to this inhibition, whereas dopamine antagonism is of less importance (Niemegeers et al. 1983; Arnt et al. 1984, 1989).

The effect of neuroleptics on quipazine-induced head twitches is shown in Table 1 and in pie charts in Fig. 3. For butyrophenones, benzamides and SCH 23390 the serotonin S$_2$ component is of minor importance (Fig. 3). For other compounds the serotonin S$_2$ component is most important. Setoperone is an example of this. For clozapine, fluperlapine, methiothepin, *cis-(Z)*-chlorprothixene and chlorpromazine the serotonin S$_2$ receptor blockade dominates.

With these receptor profiles in mind the number of selective dopamine D$_1$ and D$_2$ receptor antagonists is dramatically decreased. As judged from Fig. 3, only haloperidol and the benzamides can be regarded as dopamine D$_2$ receptor selective both in vitro and in vivo, whereas only SCH 23390 (and from Table 1 also SK&F 83566C) can be regarded as dopamine D$_1$ receptor selective compounds.

5 Clinical Significance of Selectivity

The pharmacological tolerance of a neuroleptic can be assessed either as an increase in the daily dose necessary for maintaining the clinical efficacy or as a decrease in the therapeutic effect using a repeated fixed dose.

In order to assess the clinical relevance of the pharmacological characteristics specific for thioxanthene neuroleptics (mixed dopamine D_1/D_2 receptor antagonists; lack of tolerance development), data from double-blind clinical trials in which thioxanthenes were compared with butyrophenones and phenothiazines have been analysed.

In a double-blind study by Kuny and Woggon (1984), zuclopenthixol was compared to haloperidol in patients with acute symptoms of schizophrenia, treated for 20 days. In this study, the dose increase at day 20 compared to the starting dose at day 1 was 100% for haloperidol and 60% for zuclopenthixol. The antipsychotic effect, measured at different occasions during the trial period with the AMP rating scale system, was similar for both neuroleptics. A similar difference in dose increase was observed in a double-blind trial by Heikkila et al. (1981) comparing zuclopenthixol with haloperidol in the treatment of chronic schizophrenic patients. At the end of the 12-week treatment period, the Brief Psychiatric Rating Scale (BPRS) total score showed an almost equal therapeutic effect for both drugs. However, the relative increase in mean daily dose was 42% of the starting dose for haloperidol and 11% for zuclopenthixol. In these two double-blind studies it was demonstrated that in order to achieve a similar therapeutic effect, the relative dose increase needed was significantly higher for haloperidol than for zuclopenthixol. This could be related to the above mentioned selectivity of zuclopenthixol and haloperidol for dopamine D_1 and D_2 receptors.

In another double-blind controlled study by Wistedt et al. (1984), flupentixol decanoate was compared with fluphenazine decanoate during 2 years of treatment in schizophrenic patients. It was shown that during the first 48 weeks of treatment, similar and stable therapeutic results were obtained with both depot medications. In the following period of 52 weeks patients were kept on a fixed effective dose. At the end of this period, the groups were significantly different, with flupentixol decanoate showing the greatest decrease in Comprehensive Psychopathological Rating Scale (CPRS) scores. This trial also demonstrated that at a fixed maintenance dose the therapeutic effect of flupentixol decanoate is stable while the efficacy of fluphenazine decanoate decreased with time and showed a pharmacological tolerance phenomenon.

6 Tardive Dyskinesia

The clinical pharmacology of tardive dyskinesia indicates that postsynaptic dopamine receptor supersensitivity, induced by long-term neuroleptic treatment, is one of the mechanisms involved in this serious extrapyramidal movement disorder. A large amount of evidence supports this concept. In agreement with this it was shown that the greater the dopamine receptor blockade, the greater is the dopamine receptor supersensitivity (Christensen et al. 1976). It has been shown that increasing the dose of the offending neuroleptic or administrating a more powerful neuroleptic temporarily suppresses tardive dyskinesia (Jenner and Marsden 1987).

In most studies, neuroleptics induce parkinsonism together with suppression of the tardive dyskinesia (Claveria et al. 1975; Gerlach and Simmelsgaard 1978; Pollak et al. 1985). The potential of neuroleptic drugs to induce tardive dyskinesia may be measured as the relative tardive dyskinesia aggravation seen after withdrawal of the neuroleptic drug (Gerlach and Simmelsgaard 1978).

This model for rebound-aggravation of tardive dyskinesia has recently been tested in patients with diagnosed tardive dyskinesia. During a double-blind cross-over study, patients received treatment with chlorprothixene, haloperidol or perphenazine (Nordic Dyskinesia Study Group 1986). The analysis of the overall results, expressed as a percentage of the number of aggravations, no change or improvements during the withdrawal periods after chlorprothixene, haloperidol and perphenazine treatments, showed a tendency ($p < 0.1$) in favour of chlorprothixene, implying the lowest risk of eliciting tardive dyskinesia in the long run.

Studies of positron emission tomography scans (Farde 1987) indicate that the occupancy of dopamine D$_1$ receptors is considerably lower than the D$_2$ receptor occupancy in patients treated with thioxanthenes. This is in full accordance with the in vivo receptor binding profile of these drugs. Thus a sufficiently high blockade of dopamine D$_1$ receptors may not have been achieved under clinical conditions. It may very well turn out that a higher proportion of dopamine D$_1$ receptor blockade may be more advantageous than that obtained with the thioxanthene neuroleptics. Hopefully such drugs may be developed and tested clinically.

References

Andersen PH, Gronvald C (1986) Specific binding of ^{3}H-SCH 23390 to dopamine D1 receptors in vivo. Life Sci 38:1507–1515

Andersen PH, Grønvald FC, Aas Jansen J (1985) A comparison between dopamine-stimulated adenylate cyclase and ^{3}H-SCH 23390 binding in rat striatum. Life Sci 37:1971–1983

Arnt J (1982) Pharmacological specificity of conditioned avoidance response inhibition in rats. Inhibition by neuroleptics and correlation to dopamine receptor blockade. Acta Pharmacol Toxicol (Copenh) 51:321–329

Arnt J (1983) Neuroleptic inhibition of 6,7-ADTN-induced hyperactivity after injection into the nucleus accumbens. Specificity and comparison with other models. Eur J Pharmacol 90:47–55

Arnt J (1985) Behavioral stimulation is induced by separate D-1 and D-2 receptor sites in reserpine-pretreated but not in normal rats. Eur J Pharmacol 113:79–88

Arnt J, Christensen AV (1981) Differential reversal by scopolamine and THIP of the antistereotypic and cataleptic effects of neuroleptics. Eur J Pharmacol 69:107–111

Arnt J, Hyttel J (1984) Differential inhibition by dopamine D-1 and D-2 antagonists of circling behaviour induced by dopamine agonists in rats with unilateral 6-hydroxydopamine lesions. Eur J Pharmacol 102:349–354

Arnt J, Hyttel J (1985) Differential involvement of dopamine D-1 and D-2 receptors in the circling behaviour induced by apomorphine, SK&F 38393, pergolide and LY 171555 in 6-hydroxydopamine-lesioned rats. Psychopharmacology (Berlin) 85:346–352

Arnt J, Hyttel J (1986) Inhibition of SKF 38393- and pergolide-induced circling in rats with unilateral 6-OHDA lesion is correlated to dopamine D-1 and D-2 receptor affinities in vitro. J Neural Transm 67:225–240

Arnt J, Hyttel J (1988) Behavioral differentiation between effects elicited at dopamine D-1 and D-2 receptors in rats with normosensitive DA receptors. Pharmacopsychiatry 21:24–27

Arnt J, Hyttel J, Larsen J-J (1984) The citalopram/5-HTP-induced head shake syndrome is correlated to 5-HT$_2$ receptor affinity and also influenced by other transmitters. Acta Pharmacol Toxicol (Copenh) 55:363–372

Arnt J, Bøgesø KP, Hyttel J (1988a) Dopamine D-1 and D-2 receptor differentiation revealed by behavioural studies in rats. In: Beart P, Jackson D, Woodruff GN (eds) Pharmacology and functional regulation of dopaminergic neurons. Macmillan, London, p 110–116

Arnt J, Bøgesø KP, Boeck V, Christensen AV, Dragsted N, Hyttel J, Skarsfeldt T (1989) In vivo pharmacology of irindalone, a 5-HT$_2$ receptor antagonist with predominant peripheral effects. Drug Dev Res 16:59–70

Billard W, Ruperto V, Crosby G, Iorio LC, Barnett A (1984) Characterization of the binding of ^{3}H-SCH 23390, a selective D-1-receptor antagonist ligand, in rat striatum. Life Sci 35:1885–1893

Bunney BS (1984) Antipsychotic drug effects on the electrical activity of dopaminergic neurons. Trends Neurosci 7:212–215

Christensen AV, Møller Nielsen I (1980) On the supersensitivity of DA receptors after single and repeated administration of neuroleptics. In: Smith RC (ed) Tardive dyskinesia, research and treatment. Spectrum, New York, pp 35–50

Christensen AV, Fjalland B, Møller Nielsen I (1976) On the supersensitivity of dopamine receptors, induced by neuroleptics. Psychopharmacology (Berlin) 48:1–6

Christensen AV, Arnt J, Hyttel J, Larsen J-J, Svendsen O (1984a) Pharmacological effects of a specific dopamine D-1 antagonist SCH 23390 in comparison with neuroleptics. Life Sci 34:1529–1540

Christensen AV, Arnt J, Svendsen O (1984b) Animal models for neuroleptic-induced neurological dysfunction. In: Usdin E, Carlsson A, Dahlström A, Engel J (eds) Catecholamines: neuropharmacology and central nervous system – therapeutic aspects. Liss, New York, pp 99–109

Christensen AV, Arnt J, Hyttel J, Svendsen O (1984c) Behavioural correlates to the dopamine D-1 and D-2 antagonists. Pol J Pharmacol Pharm 36:249–264

Christensen AV, Arnt J, Svendsen O (1985) Pharmacological differentiation of dopamine D-1 and D-2 antagonists after single and repeated administration. Psychopharmacology (Berlin) [Suppl] 2:182–190

Clark D, White FJ (1987) Review: D1 dopamine receptor – the search for a function: a critical evaluation of the D1/D2 dopamine receptor classification and its functional implications. Synapse 1:347–388

Claveria LE, Teychenne PF, Calne DB, Haskayne L, Petrie A, Pallis CA, Lodge-Patch IC (1975) Tardive dyskinesia treated with pimozide. J Neurol Sci 24:393–404

Coward DM (1983) Apomorphine-induced biphasic–circling behaviour in 6-hydroxy-dopamine-lesioned rats. Naunyn Schmiedebergs Arch Pharmacol 323:49–53

Creese I, Burt DR, Snyder SH (1976) Dopamine receptor binding predicts clinical and pharmacological potencies of antischizophrenic drugs. Science 192:481–483

Farde L (1987) Dopamine receptor characteristics in the living human brain. Thesis, University of Stockholm

Fleminger S, Rupniak NMJ, Hall MD, Jenner P, Marsden CD (1983) Changes in apomorphine-induced stereotypy as a result of subacute neuroleptic treatment correlates with increased D-2 receptors, but not with increases in D-1 receptors. Biochem Pharmacol 32:2921–2927

Gerlach J, Simmelsgaard H (1978) Tardive dyskinesia during and following treatment with haloperidol, haloperidol + biperiden, thioridazine and clozapine. Psychopharmacology (Berlin) 59:105–112

Gower AJ, Marriott AS (1982) Pharmacological evidence for the subclassification of central dopamine receptors in the rat. Br J Pharmacol 77:185–194

Hayashi T, Tadokoro S (1984) Parallelism between avoidance-suppressing and prolactin-increasing effects of antipsychotic drugs in rats. Jpn J Pharmacol 35:451–456

Heikkila L, Laitinen J, Vartiainen H (1981) Cis(Z)-clopenthixol and haloperidol in chronic schizophrenic patients – a double-blind clinical multicentre investigation. Acta Psychiatr Scand [Suppl 294] 64:30–38

Herrera-Marschitz M, Ungerstedt U (1984) Evidence that apomorphine and pergolide induce rotation in rats by different actions on D1 and D2 receptor sites. Eur J Pharmacol 98:165–176

Hyttel J (1978) Effects of neuroleptics on ^{3}H-haloperidol and ^{3}H-cis(Z)-flupenthixol binding and on adenylate cyclase activity in vitro. Life Sci 23:551–556

Hyttel J (1981) Similarities between the binding of ^{3}H-piflutixol and ^{3}H-flupenthixol to rat striatal dopamine receptors in vitro. Life Sci 28:563–569

Hyttel J (1982) Preferential labelling of adenylate cyclase coupled dopamine receptors with thioxanthene neuroleptics. In: Kohsaka M, Shohmori T, Tsukada Y, Woodruff GN (eds) Advances in dopamine research. Pergamon, Oxford, pp 147–152 (Advances in the biosciences, vol 37)

Hyttel J (1983) SCH 23390 – the first selective dopamine D-1 antagonist. Eur J Pharmacol 91:153–154

Hyttel J, Arnt J (1987) Characterization of binding of ^{3}H-SCH 23390 to dopamine D-1 receptors. Correlation to other D-1 and D-2 measures and effect of selective lesions. J Neural Transm 68:171–189

Hyttel J, Larsen J-J, Christensen AV, Arnt J (1985) Receptor-binding profiles of neuroleptics. Psychopharmacology (Berlin) [Suppl] 2:9–18

Iversen LL (1978) More than one type of dopamine receptor in brain? Trends Neurosci 1:V–VI

Jenner P, Marsden D (1987) Neuroleptic-induced tardive dyskinesia. Acta Psychiatr Belg 87:566–598

Kebabian JW, Calne DB (1979) Multiple receptors for dopamine. Nature 277:93–96

Kuny S, Woggon B (1984) Cis(Z)-clopenthixol in the treatment of acute schizophrenia. In: Hall P (ed) Proceedings of the symposium "Modern trends in the chemotherapy of schizophrenia". VII World Congress of Psychiatry, Vienna. H. Lundbeck A/S, Copenhagen, pp 13–24

Leysen JE, Gommeren W, Laduron PM (1978) Spiperone: a ligand of choice for neuroleptic receptors. I. Kinetics and characteristics of in vitro binding. Biochem Pharmacol 27:307–316

Leysen JE, van Gompel P, Gommeren W, Laduron PM (1987) Differential regulation of dopamine-D$_2$ and serotonin-S$_2$ receptors by chronic treatment with the serotonin-S$_2$ antagonists, ritanserin, and setoperone. In: Dahl S, Gram L, Paul S, Potter W (eds) Clinical pharmacology in psychiatry. Springer, Berlin Heidelberg New York, pp 214–224 (Psychopharmacology series, vol 3)

Molloy AG, Waddington JL (1985a) Sniffing, rearing and locomotor responses to the D-1 dopamine agonist R-SK&F 38393 and to apomorphine: differential interactions with the selective D-1 and D-2 antagonists SCH 23390 and metoclopramide. Eur J Pharmacol 108:305–308

Molloy AG, Waddington JL (1985b) The enantiomer of SK&F 83566, a new selective D-1 dopamine antagonist, stereospecifically blocks stereotyped behaviour induced by apomorphine and by the selective D-2 agonist RU 24213. Eur J Pharmacol 116:183–186

Niemegeers CJE, Janssen PAJ (1979) A systematic study of the pharmacological activities of dopamine antagonists. Life Sci 24:2201–2216

Niemegeers CJE, Colpaert FC, Leysen JE, Awouters F, Janssen PAJ (1983) Mescaline-induced head-twitches in the rat: an in vivo method to evaluate serotonin S_2 antagonists. Drug Dev Res 3:123–135

Nordic Dyskinesia Study Group (1986) Effect of different neuroleptics in tardive dyskinesia and parkinsonism. A video-controlled multicenter study with chlorprothixene, perphenazine, haloperidol and haloperidol + biperiden. Psychopharmacology (Berlin) 90:423–429

O'Boyle K, Waddington JL (1984) Identification of the enantiomers of SK&F 83566 as specific and stereoselective antagonists at the striatal D-1 dopamine receptor: comparisons with the D-2 enantioselectivity of Ro 22-1319. Eur J Pharmacol 106:219–220

O'Boyle KM, Pugh M, Waddington JL (1984) Stereotypy induced by the D-2 agonist RU 24213 is blocked by the D-2 antagonist Ro 22-2586 and the D-1 antagonist SCH 23390. Br J Pharmacol 82:242 P

Peroutka SJ, Snyder SH (1980) Relationship of neuroleptic drug effects at brain dopamine, serotonin, α-adrenergic, and histamine receptors to clinical potency. Am J Psychiatry 137:1518–1522

Pollak P, Gaio J-M, Hommel M, Pellat J, Perret J (1985) Effect of tiapride in tardive dyskinesia. Psychopharmacology (Berlin) 85:236–239

Rosengarten H, Schweitzer JW, Friedhoff AJ (1983) Induction of oral dyskinesias in naive rats by D_1 stimulation. Life Sci 33:2479–2482

Rosengarten H, Schweitzer JW, Friedhoff AJ (1986) Selective dopamine D2 receptor reduction enhances a D1 mediated oral dyskinesia in rats. Life Sci 39:29–35

Seeman P (1980) Brain dopamine receptors. Pharmacol Rev 32:229–313

Setler PE, Sarau HM, Zirkle CL, Saunders HL (1978a) The central effects of a novel dopamine agonist. Eur J Pharmacol 50:419–430

Setler PE, Malesky M, McDevitt J, Turner K (1978b) Rotation produced by administration of dopamine and related substances directly into the supersentive caudate nucleus. Life Sci 1:1277–1284

Skarsfeldt T (1988) Effect of chronic treatment with SCH 23390 and haloperidol on spontaneous activity of dopamine neurones in SNC and VTA in rats. Eur J Pharmacol 145:239–243

Svendsen O, Arnt J, Boeck V, Bøgesø KP, Christensen AV, Hyttel J, Larsen J-J (1986) The neuropharmacological profile of tefludazine, a potential antipsychotic drug with dopamine and serotonin receptor antagonistic effects. Drug Dev Res 6:35–47

Waddington JL, Gamble SJ (1980) Neuroleptic treatment for a substantial proportion of adult life: behavioural sequelae of 9 months haloperidol administration. Eur J Pharmacol 67:363–369

Waddington JL, Gamble SJ, Bourne RC (1981) Sequelae of 6 months continuous administration of cis(Z)-and trans(E)-flupenthixol in the rat. Eur J Pharmacol 69:511–513

Wistedt B (1984) Effect of neuroleptic withdrawal during the maintenance treatment of chronic schizophrenics. In: Hall P (ed) Proceedings of the Symposium "Modern trends in chemotherapy of schizophrenia". VII World Congress of Psychiatry, Vienna. H. Lundbeck A/S, Copenhagen, pp 44–59

Animal Pharmacology of Raclopride, a Selective Dopamine D_2 Antagonist

H. HALL, S. O. ÖGREN, C. KÖHLER, and O. MAGNUSSON [1]

1 Introduction

The substituted benzamides constitute a group of substances which have been shown to be selective dopamine D_2 antagonists (Jenner and Marsden 1981), a property suggested to be associated with antipsychotic effects (Seeman 1980). Sulpiride and remoxipride are two typical compounds belonging to this group. In the present paper we present some pharmacological properties of raclopride (Fig. 1), a substituted benzamide structurally related to remoxipride, but with higher potency than that of sulpiride or remoxipride.

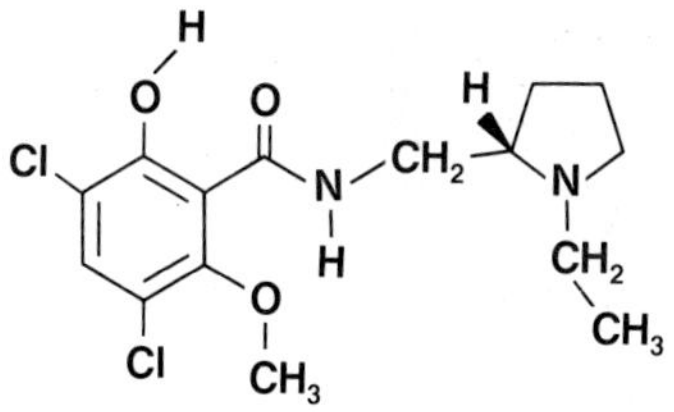

Fig. 1. Structural formula of raclopride, S-($-$)-3,5-dichloro-N-(1-ethyl-2-pyrrolidinyl)methyl-6-methoxy-salicylamide. The chemistry of raclopride is described by de Paulis et al. (1986)

2 Receptor Studies

Raclopride inhibits in vitro [^{3}H]spiperone binding to rat striatum with an IC_{50} value of 32 nM (Hall et al. 1986; $K_i = 7.5$ nM, Hall and Wedel 1986), while it is practically devoid of affinity for other receptors studied, including the dopamine D_1 receptor (Hall et al. 1986; Fig. 2). Using ^{3}H raclopride or ^{3}H sulpiride as radioligands, the affinity of raclopride is markedly higher than that seen with [^{3}H]spiperone ($K_i = 1$–2 nM, Hall and Wedel 1986). Raclopride has also been shown to bind to the dopamine D_2 receptors of human basal ganglia with a K_i value of approximately 1 nM (Hall et al. 1988; Table 1). Of the two isomeric forms, only the S-($-$)-enantiomer (i.e. raclopride) is an active dopamine antagonist, while the R-($+$)-enantiomer (FLB 472) is virtually inactive (Farde et al. 1988).

[1] Astra Research Centre AB, CNS 2 Research and Development, Neuropharmacology, 15185 Södertälje, Sweden

Clinical Pharmacology in Psychiatry
Editors: S. G. Dahl and L. F. Gram
(Psychopharmacology Series 7)
© Springer-Verlag Berlin Heidelberg 1989

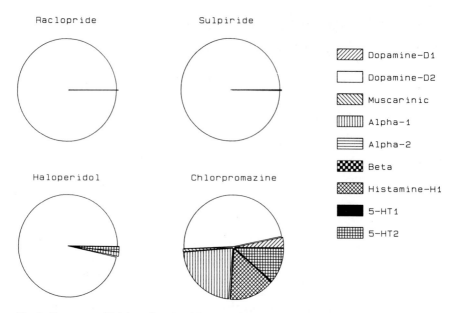

Fig. 2. Receptor affinities of raclopride, sulpiride, haloperidol and chlorpromazine for a number of rat brain receptors as determined with in vitro receptorbinding techniques. The proportion of the total affinity (expressed in $1/K_i$) for each receptortype is indicated. Data are obtained from Hall et al. (1986; K_i values recalculated from the IC_{50} values) and unpublished results. The following radioligands were used: dopamine D_1, [³H]flupenthixol; dopamine D_2, [³H]raclopride; muscarinic cholinergic, [³H]QNB; α_1-adrenergic, [³H]WB4101; α_2-adrenergic, [³H]p-aminoclonidine; β-adrenergic, [³H]dihydroalprenolol; histamine H_1, [³H]pyrilamine; 5-HT$_1$, [³H]5-HT; 5-HT$_2$, [³H]spiperone

Table 1. Effects of raclopride on dopamine receptors in the brain as studied with in vitro receptor-binding assays and on dopamine-stimulated adenylate cyclase

Receptor radioligand Compound	Human dopamine D_1 [³H]SCH 23390 K_i (nM)		Human dopamine D_2 [³H]raclopride K_i (nM)		Rat adenylate cyclase IC_{50} (nM)
Thioridazine	98.9	(79.9–130)	8.39	(6.90–10.7)	260
Chlorpromazine	158	(144–175)	4.04	(3.46–4.86)	390
Haloperidol	128	(103–168)	0.74	(0.60–0.98)	340
d-Sulpiride	47 300	(40 200–57 500)	253	(205–330)	
l-Sulpiride	> 50 000		9.44	(8.53–10.6)	> 100 000 [a]
Raclopride	> 50 000		0.99	(0.83–1.23)	> 100 000

Two or more binding experiments were performed with each compound, and the data were pooled and analysed together. Mean ± standard error range of the estimates (in parenthesis) as determined using the nonlinear iterative program Ligand (Munson and Rodbard 1980) are presented. The amount of cyclic AMP formed after 5 min incubation with ATP (2.5 μM) and dopamine (10 μM) in the presence of various concentrations of the compounds was used as a measure of activity of dopamine stimulated adenylate cyclase.
[a] Racemic form of sulpiride used in the assay of adenylate cyclase.

The marked selectivity of raclopride for the dopamine D_2 receptor has led to the use of [³H]raclopride in receptor binding assays in vitro (Köhler et al. 1985; Hall et al. 1986). Raclopride enters the brain rapidly, in contrast to, for example, sulpiride, and radiolabelled raclopride has thus also been shown to be suitable for receptor binding studies in vivo (Köhler et al. 1985; Köhler and Radesäter 1986), for autoradiography (Köhler and Radesäter 1986) and for positron-emission tomography (PET) studies (Farde et al. 1985, 1986). These studies show a distinct localization of raclopride in the basal ganglia, with very little accumulation in extrastriatal brain areas.

3 Studies on Monoamines and Monoamine Metabolites

Acute oral treatment of rats with raclopride produces large dose-dependent increases in the turnover of dopamine in the striatum and limbic system, as

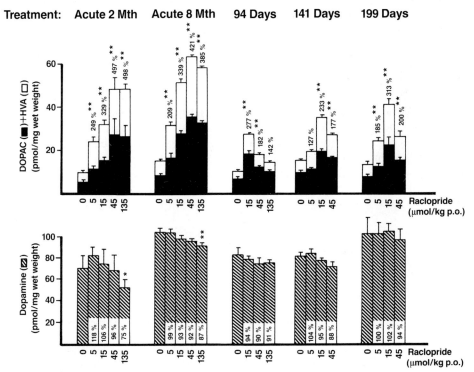

Fig. 3. Effects of acute and chronic treatment with raclopride on the concentrations of dopamine, DOPAC and HVA in rat striatum. The rats were sacrificed 2 h after intraperitoneal administration. *Acute 2 mth, acute 8 mth,* acute treatment in 2-month-old and 8-month-old rats. Values are given as means ±SEM of the concentrations for six to ten animals in each treatment group, expressed as picomoles per milligram wet weight. Mean values for the treatment groups are also expressed as percentage of the respective mean control values. Significance was calculated in terms of the Student-Newman-Keul multiple range test; *, $p < 0.05$; **, $p < 0.01$. (From Fowler et al. 1987)

seen by increases in the concentrations of dihydroxyphenyl acetic acid (DOPAC) and homovanillic acid (HVA; effects in striatal tissue shown in Fig. 3; Ögren et al. 1986; Fowler et al. 1987). Increased turnover of dopamine in the striatum and limbic system, measured 2 h after the final administration, has also been found after repeated oral treatment with raclopride (Fowler et al. 1987). However, after treatment for 3 months or longer, tolerance to the effects on the turnover of dopamine in the striatum and limbic system was obtained after large (45 and 135 µmol/kg) doses of raclopride. Repeated administration of the lower doses (5 and 15 µmol/kg) of raclopride resulted in relatively little tolerance for the turnover of dopamine.

The effect of raclopride on dopamine autoreceptors in striatal and limbic regions have been studied by use of the γ-butyrolactone model of Walters and Roth (1976). The results suggest that raclopride is able to act as an antagonist of dopaminergic autoreceptors coupled to dopamine synthesis (Magnusson et al. 1988).

Raclopride appears to produce only minor, if any, changes in the levels of noradrenaline, 5-hydroxytryptamine (5-HT) and the 5-HT metabolite 5-hydroxyindole acetic acid (5-HIAA) (Ögren et al. 1986; Fowler et al. 1987).

4 Behavioural Studies

In behavioural studies in the rat, raclopride discriminates between the motor behaviours induced by the dopamine agonist apomorphine (Ögren et al. 1986; Table 2, Fig. 4). Thus, unlike haloperidol, raclopride blocked the apomorphine-induced hyperactivity at considerably lower doses (ED_{50} = 0.13 µmol/kg i.p.) than those inhibiting oral stereotypics (ED_{50} = 1.70 µmol/kg i.p.). Moreover, raclopride induces catalepsy only at very high doses (ED_{50} = 27 µmol/kg i.p.; Table 2, Fig. 4). Since it has been suggested

Table 2. Potencies of raclopride, haloperidol and sulpiride in antagonizing apomorphine-induced hyperactivity and stereotypies and in inducing cataleptic behaviour in the male rat (ED_{50}, µmol/kg i.p.)

	Blockade of apomorphine induced		Induction of catalepsy	
	Stereotypies	Hyperactivity	Bar test	Vertical grid
Raclopride	1.70 (1.58–1.91)	0.13 (0.13–0.14)	27 (20–47)	28 (17–950)
Haloperidol	0.27 (0.26–0.29)	0.29 (0.27–0.35)	1.60 (1.13–2.32)	0.89 (0.70–1.25)
Sulpiride	212 (198–238)	65.6 (62.6–68.5)	>590	385 (280–1520)

The ED_{50} values (90% confidence limits in parentheses) refer to the calculated dose, which reduces the intensity of stereotypies by 50% over the observation period of 60 min compared to apomorphine controls, and which reduces the number of animals displaying hyperacitivity by 50%. In both models, catalepsy was defined as an inability of the rat to remove itself from the awkward position within 60 s. ED_{50} refers to the dose at which 50% of the rats displayed catalepsy. The ED_{50} values were calculated by probit analysis.

that apomorphine-induced stimulation of hyperactivity and stereotypies are due to stimulation of dopamine receptors in limbic and striatal systems, respectively (Costall et al. 1977), this may reflect a different functional effect on different systems in the brain. Moreover, there is a separation between apomorphine-induced stereotypies and induction of catalepsy, both suggested to be mediated through striatal dopaminergic systems. The reason for this separation, as well as its relevance for the clinical effects, remains to be elucidated. However, the separation between the doses mediating these behavioural parameters is hypothesized to indicate a separation between doses exerting antipsychotic effects and doses inducing extrapyramidal symptoms.

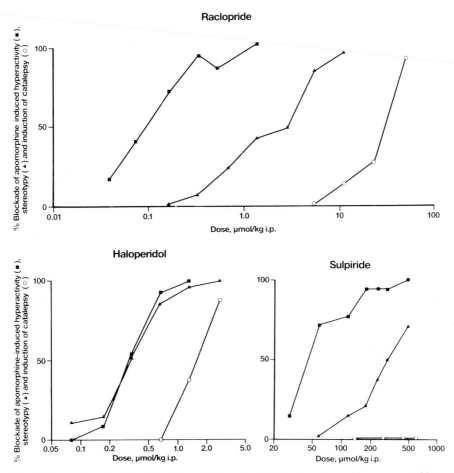

Fig. 4. Potencies of raclopride, haloperidol and sulpiride in antagonizing apomorphine-induced hyperactivity and stereotypies and in inducing cataleptic behaviour in the male rat. The compounds were injected intraperitoneally 60 min prior to apomorphine injection (1 mg/kg subcutaneously). The results on catalepsy are based on the peak-time effect of each compound in the bar test. Results are the means from eight rats in each group, in percentage of controls. (From Ögren et al. 1986).

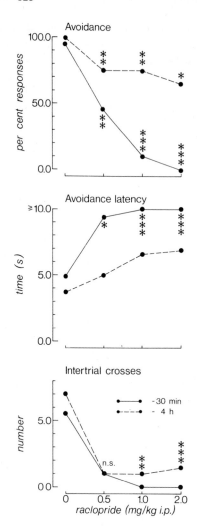

Fig. 5. Effects of raclopride on avoidance behaviour, avoidance latency and intertrial crosses. The results are based on eight animals per dose, and the animals were tested 10 min before and 30 min and 4 h after drug administration. Results are presented as medians, and the statistical analyses were performed by means of Friedman's two-way ANOVA, followed by Wilcoxon matched-pairs summed-ranks test for individual comparisons with saline-treated controls; *n.s.*, $p > 0.05$; ★, $p < 0.05$; ★★, $p < 0.02$; ★★★, $p < 0.001$. (From Hillegaart and Ahlenius 1987)

The effects of raclopride on the conditioned avoidance response have also been studied (Hillegaart and Ahlenius 1987). Raclopride showed a dose-dependent suppression of the avoidance responses with a significant effect at 0.5–2.0 mg/kg intraperitoneally (approximately 2–8 µmol/kg; Fig. 5). The avoidance latency was also increased, and the intertrial crosses were decreased. The interpretation of these effects on conditioned avoidance responses is unclear. Although this model has been regarded as predictive of antipsychotic efficacy, it may also reflect the propensity of the compound to induce side effects.

5 Conclusions

The results obtained with raclopride in animal pharmacodynamic studies show that this compound is a potent and selective antagonist of dopamine D_2 receptors in vitro as well as in vivo. The separation between different functional effects seen in the behavioural studies indicate that the compound may have an advantageous clinical profile.

References

Costall B, Naylor RJ, Cannon JG, Lee T (1977) Differentiation of the dopamine mechanisms mediating stereotyped behaviour and hyperactivity in the nucleus accumbens and caudate-putamen. J Pharm Pharmacol 29:337–342

de Paulis T, Kumar Y, Johansson L, Rämsby S, Hall H, Sällemark M, Ängeby-Möller K, Ögren SO (1986) Potential neuroleptic agents. 4. Chemistry, behavioural pharmacology, and inhibition of [^{3}H]spiperone binding of 3,5-disubstituted (N-[(1-ethyl-2-pyrrolidinyl)methyl]-6-methoxysalicylamides. J Med Chem 29:61–69

Farde L, Ehrin E, Eriksson L, Greitz T, Hall H, Hedström CG, Litton JE, Sedvall G (1985) Substituted benzamides as ligands for visualization of dopamine receptor binding in the human brain by positron emission tomography. Proc Natl Acad Sci USA 82:3863–3867

Farde L, Hall H, Ehrin E, Sedvall G (1986) Quantitative analysis of D2 dopamine receptor binding in the living human brain by PET. Science 231:258–261

Farde L, Pauli S, Hall H, Stone-Elander S, Eriksson L, Halldin C, Högberg T et al. (1988) Stereoselectivity of ^{11}C-raclopride binding – a search for extrastriatal D_2-dopamine receptors in man by PET. Psychopharmacology (Berlin) 94:471–478

Fowler CJ, Magnusson O, Thorell G, Mohringe B, Huang R-B (1987) Dopamine turnover and glutamate decarboxylase activity in the rat brain after acute and chronic treatment with raclopride, a dopamine D_2-selective antagonist. Neuropharmacology 26:339–345

Hall H, Wedel I (1986) Comparisons between the in vitro binding of two substituted benzamides and two butyrophenones to dopamine-D_2 receptors in the rat striatum. Acta Pharmacol Toxicol (Copenh) 58:368–373

Hall H, Sällemark M, Jerning E (1986) Effects of remoxipride and some related new substituted salicylamides on rat brain receptors. Acta Pharmacol Toxicol (Copenh) 58:61–70

Hall H, Farde L, Sedvall G (1988) Human dopamine receptor subtypes – in vitro binding analysis using ^{3}H-SCH 23390 and ^{3}H-raclopride. J Neural Transm 73:7–21

Hillegaart V, Ahlenius S (1987) Effects of raclopride on exploratory locomotor activity, treadmill locomotion, conditioned avoidance behaviour and catalepsy in rats: behavioural profile comparisons between raclopride, haloperidol and preclamol. Pharmacol Toxicol 60:350–354

Jenner P, Marsden CD (1981) Substituted benzamide drugs as selective neuroleptic agents. Neuropharmacology 20:1285–1293

Köhler C, Radesäter A-C (1986) Autoradiographic visualization of dopamine D-2 receptors in the monkey brain using the selective benzamide drug [^{3}H]raclopride. Neurosci Lett 66:85–90

Köhler C, Hall H, Ögren SO, Gawell L (1985) Specific in vitro and in vivo binding of ^{3}H-raclopride, a potent substituted drug with high affinity for dopamine D-2 receptors in the rat brain. Biochem Pharmacol 34:2251–2259

Magnusson O, Fowler CJ, Mohringe B, Wijkström A, Ögren S-O (1988) Comparison of the effects of haloperidol, remoxipride and raclopride on "pre"- and postsynaptic dopamine receptors in the rat brain. Naunyn Schmiedebergs Arch Pharmacol 337:379–384

Munson PJ, Rodbard D (1980) Ligand: a versatile computerized approach for characterization of ligand-binding systems. Anal Biochem 107:220–239

Ögren SO, Hall H, Köhler C, Magnusson O, Sjöstrand S-E (1986) The selective dopamine D_2 antagonist raclopride discriminates between dopamine-mediated motor functions. Psychopharmacology (Berlin) 90:287–294

Seeman P (1980) Brain dopamine receptors. Pharmacol Rev 32:229–313

Walters JH, Roth RH (1976) Dopaminergic neurons: in an vivo system for measuring drug interactions with presynaptic receptors. Naunyn Schmiedebergs Arch Pharmacol 296:5–14

Benzodiazepine Receptor Subtypes and Their Possible Clinical Significance

W. Sieghart[1]

1 Properties of the GABA-Benzodiazepine Receptors

Benzodiazepines such as diazepam, flunitrazepam or bromazepam belong to the most widely prescribed drugs in current therapeutic use because of their anxiolytic, anticonvulsant, muscle-relaxant and hypnotic effects. A large number of electrophysiological investigations indicate that benzodiazepines enhance the actions of γ-aminobutyric acid (GABA) on its receptor (Haefely et al. 1981). GABA is the quantitatively most important inhibitory neurotransmitter in the mammalian CNS. Approximately 30% of all synapses in the brain are estimated to be GABAergic. Since this GABA-enhancing effect was found in many different physiological systems, it is now generally assumed that benzodiazepines produce most of their actions by modulating the GABAergic system (Tallman et al. 1980).

Biochemical investigations have indicated that there are high-affinity binding sites for benzodiazepines in brain membranes (Braestrup and Squires 1977; Möhler and Okada 1977). These binding sites exhibit many properties that one would expect from a pharmacological receptor for these compounds. Thus, binding of radiolabelled benzodiazepines to brain membranes occurred rapidly at nanomolar concentrations, was reversible, stereospecific and saturable, and there was an excellent correlation between the clinical potency of a series of benzodiazepines and their ability to displace [^{3}H]diazepam or [^{3}H]flunitrazepam from their high-affinity binding sites. In addition, a close association of these binding sites with the GABA$_A$ receptor, a chloride ion channel and several different drug binding sites has been demonstrated (Olsen 1982). Since these benzodiazepine binding sites have been found in the central nervous system of all vertebrates investigated (Braestrup and Nielsen 1983), and since most actions of the classical benzodiazepines seem to be centrally mediated (Haefely et al. 1981), it is now generally assumed that these specific high-affinity binding sites for [^{3}H]flunitrazepam are the physiological receptors by which benzodiazepines exert their pharmacologically and clinically relevant actions.

Thus, combining electrophysiological and biochemical evidence, benzodiazepine receptors are allosteric modulatory sites on the GABA$_A$ receptor

[1] Department of Biochemical Psychiatry, Psychiatrische Universitätsklinik, Währinger Gürtel 18–20, 1090 Wien, Austria

Clinical Pharmacology in Psychiatry
Editors: S. G. Dahl and L. F. Gram
(Psychopharmacology Series 7)
© Springer-Verlag Berlin Heidelberg 1989

gated chloride ion channel. In recent years it has been demonstrated that, surprisingly, two exactly opposite effects could be mediated by these benzodiazepine receptors. Certain ligands for these receptors, the classical benzodiazepines and some newer non-benzodiazepine compounds (benzodiazepine receptor agonists) enhance GABA-induced chloride ion flux
across cell membranes and exhibit anticonvulsant, anxiolytic, muscle-relaxant
and sedative properties (Haefely and Polc 1986). However, other ligands of
the benzodiazepine receptors (inverse benzodiazepine receptor agonists) were
found which reduce GABA-induced chloride ion flux across cell membranes
and exhibit proconvulsant or convulsant, anxiogenic, vigilance and muscle
tone increasing effects. The first compounds discovered which act in this way
were esters of β-carboline-3-carboxylic acid, but similar properties were subsequently found in other classes of chemicals, including benzodiazepines
(Haefely et al. 1985). Finally, a third group of compounds was identified
which bound with high affinity to benzodiazepine receptors without producing relevant pharmacological effects by themselves. However, these compounds highly specifically blocked the effects of benzodiazepine receptor
agonists and of inverse benzodiazepine receptor agonists (Haefely et al. 1985).
These benzodiazepine receptor antagonists exhibited no or only minimal
modulatory effect on the GABA-induced chloride ion flux. Benzodiazepine
receptor antagonists, again, occur in several chemical classes, e.g. β-
carbolines, pyrazolopyridazines and imidazobenzodiazepines.

2 Other Benzodiazepine Binding Sites
and Their Possible Clinical Significance

In addition to these "central" benzodiazepine receptors, two other types of
benzodiazepine binding sites have been identified. The "peripheral" benzodiazepine binding sites exhibit a high affinity for some benzodiazepines and
are present in liver, kidney and other peripheral tissues (Braestrup and Squires
1977) as well as in brain (Schoemaker et al. 1981). The "micromolar" benzodiazepine binding sites so far have been found in brain tissue only and exhibit a rather low affinity for benzodiazepines (Bowling and de Lorenzo
1982). These two types of binding sites are not associated with GABA receptors and differ from central benzodiazepine receptors in their binding
properties, kinetics and pharmacological characteristics. Since there is no significant correlation between the clinical potency of benzodiazepines and their
affinity for the peripheral or micromolar benzodiazepine binding sites, the
physiological significance of these sites is presently not known. However, micromolar (Johansen et al. 1985) as well as peripheral benzodiazepine binding
sites (Mestre et al. 1986) seem to interact with voltage-sensitive Ca^{2+} channels. In addition, peripheral binding sites have been implicated in mediating
the direct neuromuscular effects of benzodiazepines (Wilkinson et al. 1982)
which are clinically used in anaesthesia, in modulating the proliferation or dif-

ferentiation of various cells (Morgan et al. 1985) and in modulating the humoral immune response (Zavala et al. 1984). Further investigation of these various actions could possibly lead to an application of peripheral benzodiazepine receptor ligands or drugs derived from them in the treatment of cardiovascular diseases, immune diseases and tumours. The use of peripheral benzodiazepine receptor ligands labelled with positron- or γ-emitting isotopes for imaging of human primary central nervous system tumours was recently suggested due to the presence of high concentrations of peripheral receptors on these tumours (Starosta-Rubinstein et al. 1987).

3 Subtypes of GABA-Benzodiazepine Receptors and Their Possible Clinical Significance

3.1 Evidence for Heterogeneity of GABA-Benzodiazepine Receptors from Reversible Binding Studies

Originally, it was assumed that there is only one type of the central high-affinity benzodiazepine receptor in the brain. Recently, however, several compounds with distinct chemical structures have been identified which seem differentially to interact with benzodiazepine receptors in various brain regions. Thus, the triazolopyridazine Cl 218872 (Klepner et al. 1979), some esters of β-carboline-3-carboxylate (Braestrup and Nielsen 1983), and some new benzodiazepines such as quazepam, SCH 15725 and cinolazepam (Iorió et al. 1984; Sieghart and Schuster 1984) have been shown to have affinity that is several times higher for benzodiazepine receptors in cerebellum than for those in hippocampus and other brain regions. Results from studies on the displacement of [^{3}H]flunitrazepam binding by these compounds indicated homogeneity and heterogeneity of benzodiazepine binding sites in cerebellum and hippocampus, respectively. Furthermore, these compounds not only in vitro at 0 °C or 37 °C (Gee and Yamamura 1982; Eichinger and Sieghart 1984) but also in vivo had a different affinity for benzodiazepine receptors in cerebellum and hippocampus (Lippa et al. 1982; Mazière et al. 1985). These results led to the hypothesis that in cerebellum a benzodiazepine receptor subtype (type I receptor, BZ_1 receptor) is enriched which exhibits a high affinity for Cl 218872 or the various selective benzodiazepines. In addition, it was concluded that at least one other benzodiazepine receptor subtype, a type II receptor (BZ_2 receptor) must exist which exhibits a low affinity for the above-mentioned compounds and is enriched in hippocampal membranes (Klepner et al. 1979). Other experiments suggested that both the BZ_1 and BZ_2 receptors are coupled to GABA and anion recognition sites (Stapleton et al. 1982).

3.2 Molecular Heterogeneity of GABA-Benzodiazepine Receptors

These data from reversible binding experiments are supported and supplemented by results from irreversible binding studies. [^{3}H]Flunitrazepam on irradiation with ultraviolet light has been shown irreversibly to bind to a membrane protein with an apparent molecular weight of 51 000 (P_{51}) in all brain regions investigated (Sieghart and Karobath 1980). Whereas in cerebellum only P_{51} was significantly labelled, in hippocampus and several other brain regions this compound irreversibly bound to several other proteins with apparent molecular weights of 51 000 (P_{51}), 53 000 (P_{53}), 55 000 (P_{55}) and 59 000 (P_{59}) (Sieghart and Karobath 1980; Lippa et al. 1982). All these proteins, specifically and irreversibly labelled by [^{3}H]flunitrazepam, seem to be associated with the central GABA receptor associated type of benzodiazepine receptors, since irreversible binding to these proteins was abolished by diazepam, was stimulated by GABA and was unaffected by the peripheral benzodiazepine receptor ligand Ro 5-4864 (Sieghart and Karobath 1980). Since in cerebellum BZ_1 receptors were most highly enriched, and only one protein (P_{51}) was significantly labelled by [^{3}H]flunitrazepam, and since labelling of P_{51} by [^{3}H]flunitrazepam was inhibited with higher potency by the BZ_1-selective ligands Cl 218872 or SCH 15725 than that of the other photolabelled proteins, P_{51} seems to be associated with BZ_1 receptors (Sieghart et al. 1983). The different and distinct regional distribution of the other photolabelled proteins and the differential interaction of the BZ_1 receptor selective compounds with [^{3}H]flunitrazepam binding to the individual proteins (Sieghart et al. 1983) seem to indicate that proteins P_{53}, P_{55} and P_{59} are associated with separate and different benzodiazepine receptor subtypes.

This conclusion was supported by several experiments indicating a difference in the molecular structure of benzodiazepine receptors associated with proteins P_{51} or P_{55} (Sieghart et al. 1987; Sieghart 1988).

3.3 Heterogeneity of the α and β Subunits of the GABA-Benzodiazepine Receptor Complex

Recently, the $GABA_A$-benzodiazepine receptor complex has been completely purified by affinity chromatography (Sigel et al. 1983). The purified receptor preparation seemed to contain only two major protein bands with apparent molecular weights of 53 000 (α subunit) and 57 000 (β subunit), as revealed by SDS polyacrylamide gel electrophoresis. Molecular mass determination suggested the complex to be a heterotetramer with an $\alpha_2\beta_2$ stoichiometry (Barnard et al. 1984). SDS polyacrylamide gels with higher resolution, however, revealed that the α and β subunits each consist of several different proteins with quite similar molecular weight (Fuchs and Sieghart 1989). Using monoclonal antibodies specific for α or β subunits, it was possible to demonstrate that all the various proteins irreversibly labelled by [^{3}H]flunitrazepam are different α subunits of the GABA-benzodiazepine receptor complex (Fuchs et al. 1988). In addition, the existence of several different β subunits was demonstrated. These subunits are specifically and irreversibly labelled by the GABA agonist [^{3}H]muscimol and are recognized by a β subunit selective antibody (Fuchs and Sieghart 1989). Assuming a molecular structure of $\alpha_2\beta_2$ for the $GABA_A$-benzodiazepine receptor complex, a large variety of structurally different GABA-benzodiazepine receptor subtypes could possibly arise by a combination of various α and β subunits. Thus, there could be receptors containing identical or different α or β subunits. Alternatively, there could be receptors containing different α but identical β subunits or identical α but different β subunits.

3.4 Possible Clinical Significance of Benzodiazepine Receptor Subtypes

Since the α subunits seem to contain the benzodiazepine binding site, whereas the β subunits seem to contain the GABA/muscimol binding sites, different combinations of α and β subunits could possibly lead to a different manner of interactions of benzodiazepines with various GABA$_A$-benzodiazepine receptors. Thus, it is quite possible that a compound acting as a benzodiazepine agonist on one receptor subtype could act as a partial agonist on another subtype. This of course could be one explanation for the differential spectrum of actions of different clinically used benzodiazepines.

The regional distribution of the various α subunits is different, as revealed by the regional distribution of the various proteins photolabelled by [^{3}H]flunitrazepam (Sieghart and Karobath 1980). So far no data are available on a possible difference in the regional distribution of β subunits. In any case, there are receptor subtypes which are differentially distributed in various brain regions, and there are compounds available which have some selectivity for one of these subtypes. Their selectivity, however, is rather weak and cannot be used for the investigation of functions of these specific receptors. If it were possible to develop highly selective ligands for these various receptors, one would certainly be able selectively to influence the function of different neuronal GABA systems. For instance, GABA neurons by influencing certain serotonin neurons in the raphe nuclei or norepinephrine neurons in locus coeruleus could produce anxiolytic actions. Other GABA systems, by influencing neurons in the midbrain reticular formation, could cause sedative-hypnotic effects, and could cause muscle-relaxant effects by influencing neurons in the spinal cord and cerebellum. Finally, GABA neurons in the cerebral cortex and limbic system could dampen increased excitability of neurons and thus produce an anticonvulsive action.

Selective benzodiazepine receptor ligands thus could lead to more selective anxiolytic, sedative, muscle-relaxant or anticonvulsant drugs with low toxicity and could also offer the possibility of pharmacologically influencing many different other neuronal systems via the GABA-benzodiazepine receptor complex. One of these systems, which could possibly be manipulated by way of benzodiazepine receptors, is the cholinergic system, which might be responsible for the memory deficits in the course of senile dementia. Recent evidence seems to indicate that partial inverse benzodiazepine receptor agonists, by disinhibiting remaining cholinergic neurons of the basal forebrain, might exert memory enhancing and general nootropic effects (Sarter et al. 1988). Non-selective partial inverse agonists obviously could exhibit serious side effects because of their proconvulsive, convulsive or anxiogenic actions. Therefore, the development of partial inverse benzodiazepine agonists, with highly selective actions on receptors modulating only certain and relevant cholinergic neurons could significantly enhance the value of such drugs in the treatment of senile dementia.

Because of the widespread distribution of the GABAergic system in the brain it is highly probable that still other applications for GABAergic drugs will arise as soon as more selective drugs are developed. It is quite reasonable to assume that many other actions of GABAergic drugs are covered and superimposed by the predominant sedative action of these compounds. Thus, it can be anticipated that the investigation of the structure and function of the various benzodiazepine receptor subtypes and the development of highly selective ligands for these receptors will have a broad clinical application in the future.

References

Barnard EA, Stephenson FA, Sigel E, Mamalaki C, Bilbe G, Constanti A, Smart TE, Brown DA (1984) Structure and properties of the brain GABA/benzodiazepine receptor complex. In: Kito S, Segawa T, Kuriyama K, Yamamura HI, Olsen RW (eds) Neurotransmitter receptors: mechanisms of action and regulation. Plenum, New York, pp 235–254

Bowling AC, de Lorenzo RJ (1982) Micromolar affinity benzodiazepine receptors identification and characterization in central nervous system. Science 216:1247–1250

Braestrup C, Nielsen MJ (1983) Benzodiazepine receptors. In: Iversen L, Iversen SD, Snyder SH (eds) Handbook of psychopharmacology, vol 17. Plenum, New York, pp 285–384

Braestrup C, Squires R (1977) Specific benzodiazepine receptors in rat brain characterized by high affinity [^{3}H]-diazepam binding. Proc Natl Acad Sci USA 74:3804–3809

Eichinger A, Sieghart W (1984) Photoaffinity labeling of different benzodiazepine receptors at physiological temperature. J Neurochem 43:1745–1748

Fuchs K, Möhler H, Sieghart W (1988) Various proteins from rat brain, specifically and irreversibly labeled by [^{3}H]-flunitrazepam are distinct α-subunits of the GABA-benzodiazepine receptor complex. Neurosci Lett 90:314–319

Fuchs K, Sieghart W (1989) Evidence for the existence of several different α- and β-subunits of the GABA/benzodiazepine receptor complex from rat brain. Neurosci Lett 97:329–333

Gee KW, Yamamura HI (1982) Regional heterogeneity of benzodiazepine receptors at 37 °C: an in vitro study in various regions of the rat brain. Life Sci 31:1939–1945

Haefely W, Polc P (1986) Physiology of GABA enhancement by benzodiazepines and barbiturates. In: Olsen RW, Venter JC (eds) Benzodiazepine-GABA receptors and chloride channels; structure and functional properties. Liss, New York, pp 97–133

Haefely W, Pieri L, Polc P, Schaffner R (1981) General pharmacology and neuropharmacology of benzodiazepine derivatives. In: Hoffmeister E, Stille G (eds) Handbook of experimental pharmacology, vol 55/II. Springer, Berlin Heidelberg New York, p 134

Haefely W, Kyburz E, Gerecke M, Möhler H (1985) Recent advances in the molecular pharmacology of benzodiazepine receptors and in the structure-activity relationships of their agonists and antagonists. Adv Drug Res 14:167–322

Iorió LC, Barnett A, Billard W (1984) Selective affinity of 1-N-trifluoroethyl benzodiazepines for cerebellar type I receptor sites. Life Sci 35:105–114

Johansen J, Taft WC, Yang J, Kleinhaus AL, de Lorenzo RJ (1985) Inhibition of Ca^{++} conductance in identified leech neurons by benzodiazepines. Proc Natl Acad Sci USA 82:3935–3939

Klepner CA, Lippa AS, Benson DI, Sano MC, Beer B (1979) Resolution of two biochemically and pharmacologically distinct benzodiazepine receptors. Pharmacol Biochem Behav 11:457–462

Lippa AS, Jackson D, Wennogle LP, Beer B, Meyerson LR (1982) Non-benzodiazepine agonists for benzodiazepine receptors. In: Usdin E, Skolnick P, Tallman JF, Greenblatt D, Paul SM (eds) Pharmacology of benzodiazepines. Macmillan, London, pp 431–440

Mazière M, Hantraye P, Kaijima M, Dodd R, Guibert B, Prenant C, Sastre J, et al. (1985) Visualization by positron emission tomography of the apparent regional heterogeneity of central type benzodiazepine receptors in the brain of living baboons. Life Sci 36:1609–1616

Mestre M, Belin C, Uzan A, Renault C, Dubroeucq MC, Gueremy C, Le Fur G (1986) Modulation of voltage operated, but not receptor operated, calcium channels in the rabbit aorta by PK 111 95, an antagonist of peripheral-type benzodiazepine receptors. J Cardiovasc Pharmacol 8:729–734

Möhler H, Okada T (1977) Benzodiazepine receptors – demonstration in the central nervous system. Science 198:849–851

Morgan JI, Johnson MD, Wang JKT, Sonnenfeld KH, Spector S (1985) Peripheral type benzodiazepines influence ornithinedecarboxylase levels and neurite outgrowth in PC12 cells. Proc Natl Acad Sci USA 82:5223–5226

Olsen RW (1982) Drug interactions at the GABA receptor ionophore complex. Annu Rev Pharmacol Toxicol 22:245–277

Sarter M, Schneider HH, Stephens DN (1988) Treatment strategies for senile dementia: antagonist β-carbolines. Trends Neurosci 11:13–16

Schoemaker H, Bliss M, Yamamura HI (1981) Specific high affinity binding of [^{3}H]-Ro 5-4864 to benzodiazepine binding sites in rat cerebral cortex. Eur J Pharmacol 71:173–175

Sieghart W (1988) Comparison of two different benzodiazepine binding proteins by peptide mapping after limited proteolysis. Brain Res 450:387–391

Sieghart W, Karobath M (1980) Molecular heterogeneity of benzodiazepine receptors. Nature 286:285–287

Sieghart W, Schuster A (1984) Affinity of various ligands for benzodiazepine receptors in rat cerebellum and hippocampus. Biochem Pharmacol 33:4033–4038

Sieghart W, Mayer A, Drexler G (1983) Properties of [^{3}H]-flunitrazepam binding to different benzodiazepine binding proteins. Eur J Pharmacol 88:291–299

Sieghart W, Eichinger A, Zezula J (1987) Comparison of tryptic peptides of benzodiazepine binding proteins photolabeled with [^{3}H]-flunitrazepam or [^{3}H]-Ro 15-4513. J Neurochem 48:1109–1114

Sigel E, Stephenson FA, Mamalaki C, Barnard E (1983) A γ-aminobutyric acid/benzodiazepine receptor complex of bovine cerebral cortex. Purification and partial characterization. J Biol Chem 258:6965–6971

Stapleton SR, Prestwich SA, Horton RW (1982) Regional heterogeneity of benzodiazepine binding sites in rat brain. Eur J Pharmacol 84:221

Starosta-Rubinstein S, Ciliax BJ, Penney JB, McKeever P, Young AB (1987) Imaging of a glioma using peripheral benzodiazepine receptor ligands. Proc Natl Acad Sci USA 84:891–895

Tallman JF, Paul SM, Skolnick P, Gallager DW (1980) Receptors for the age of anxiety: pharmacology of the benzodiazepines. Science 207:274–281

Wilkinson M, Grovestine D, Hamilton JT (1982) Flunitrazepam binding sites in rat diaphragm. Receptors for direct neuromuscular effects of benzodiazepines? Can J Physiol Pharmacol 60:1003–1005

Zavala F, Haumont J, Lenfant M (1984) Interaction of benzodiazepines with mouse macrophages. Eur J Pharmacol 106:561–566

Pharmacogenetics in Psychopharmacology

Genetic Polymorphisms of Drug-Metabolizing Enzymes: Molecular Mechanisms *

U. A. Meyer, U. Zanger, R. Skoda, and D. M. Grant [1]

1 Introduction

Genetic polymorphisms of drug-metabolizing enzymes give rise to distinct subgroups in the population which differ in their ability to perform a certain drug biotransformation reaction. Genetic polymorphisms thus contribute considerably to interindividual variation in drug response. Individuals with genetically impaired metabolism are usually designated as poor metabolizers, as compared to normal or extensive metabolizers.

The objective of the research of our laboratory is the elucidation of the molecular mechanisms at the protein and DNA level of common genetic polymorphisms of drug metabolism, namely: (a) the debrisoquine/sparteine-type polymorphism of drug oxidation, (b) the mephenytoin-type polymorphism, and (c) the polymorphism of arylamine N-acetyltransferase. These types of polymorphism have been extensively reviewed, e.g. by Küpfer and Preisig (1983), Eichelbaum (1984) and Meyer et al. (1986).

The debrisoquine/sparteine-type polymorphism occurs in 5%–10% of individuals in Caucasian populations and affects the metabolism of over 20 drugs, including antiarrhythmic agents, β-adrenoreceptor blocking drugs, antidepressants, dextromethorphan, codeine and many other clinically used agents. Recent studies have also indicated that a link may exist between this polymorphism and some forms of cancer or with early-onset Parkinson's disease, presumably related to environmental chemicals (for original references see Gonzalez et al. 1988).

A genetic polymorphism of deficient metabolism of the anticonvulsant mephenytoin is observed in 2%–8% of Caucasian and in over 20% of Japanese subjects (for review, see Küpfer and Preisig 1983). The deficiency is inherited as an autosomal recessive trait and is distinct from the debrisoquine polymorphism.

Marked variation in the disposition of a large number of primary arylamine and hydrazine drugs and chemicals such as isoniazid, clonazepam, phenelzine and sulfamethazine, has been linked to a genetic polymorphism in the activity of the cytosolic liver enzyme N-acetyltransferase. This defect,

* This research was supported by Swiss National Science Foundation grant 3.817.87 and by an MRC Canada fellowship to D. M. G.
[1] Department of Pharmacology, Biocentre of the University of Basel, 4056 Basel, Switzerland

Table 1. Possible mechanisms responsible for a deficiency of drug-metabolizing enzymes

---

Abnormal function of enzyme
   Decreased affinity for substrates (K_m)
   Decreased maximal velocity (V_{max})
   Combination of the two above
   Change in the stereoselectivity of the reaction

Decreased intracellular concentration or absence of enzyme protein
   Diminished rate of synthesis
   Accelerated degradation of labile enzyme variant

At DNA/RNA level
   Deletion, insertion or rearrangement of gene
   Defect in transcription, RNA processing or RNA stability

---

which displays an approximately 50% prevalence of the poor metabolizer (or acetylator) phenotype in Caucasian populations has been the subject of extensive investigations at the clinical level (for review, see Weber and Hein 1985). However, as yet our understanding of the underlying mechanism of the acetylation polymorphism is based almost entirely upon extrapolations from results obtained in animal model systems.

The present paper summarizes recent studies in our laboratory designed to elucidate the molecular mechanisms of these three polymorphisms at the microsomal, purified protein and RNA/DNA levels and provides initial insights into these mechanisms.

2 General Considerations in Regard to Molecular Mechanisms Causing Polymorphisms of Drug Metabolism

The principal mechanisms causing quantitative or functional deficiencies of drug-metabolizing enzymes in human liver are summarized in Table 1. It is evident from these considerations that elucidation of the molecular basis of these polymorphisms requires access to large quantities of human liver tissue for isolation and purification of proteins and RNA, but also access to tissue (liver, leucocytes) from subjects of families phenotyped in vivo in order to establish the causal relationship between in vitro and in vivo findings. Moreover, sensitive assays for the involved metabolic reactions are necessary to monitor the purification of enzymes with affinity for the substrates in question.

3 Methodological Aspects

In order to investigate these polymorphisms we have established a bank of human liver tissue. This bank presently contains 35 human livers collected immediately after circulatory arrest from kidney transplant donors. In addition, wedge biopsies of 0.5–2 g wet weight were obtained from the livers of patients during either diagnostic or therapeutic laparotomy. These patients were phenotyped during their hospital stay by means of the urinary metabolic ratio of debrisoquine, sparteine or dextromethorphan for the debrisoquine polymorphism, with mephenytoin for the mephenytoin polymorphism, and with caffeine for the N-acetyltransferase polymorphism (for references, see Meyer 1987; Grant et al. 1984). Sensitive assays for debrisoquine-4-hydroxylase, bufuralol-1'-hydroxylase and dextromethorphan-O-demethylase (Kronbach et al. 1987), for mephenytoin hydroxylation and demethylation (Meier et al. 1985), and for N-acetyltransferase activity (Grant and Meyer, submitted for publication) were developed.

4 Results and Discussion

4.1 Debrisoquine Polymorphism

Studies at the Microsomal Level. We first observed that more than one P450 isozyme may catalyse the microsomal metabolism of bufuralol, debrisoquine and the other substrates involved in this polymorphism. Thus, purification from human liver with activity monitoring resulted in two functionally different cytochrome P450 isozymes, both able to catalyse bufuralol-1'-hydroxylation (Gut et al. 1986a). Indirect studies indicated that only one of these isozymes, P450bufI, is affected by the debrisoquine polymorphism (Dayer et al. 1987). We have since discovered that P450bufI (now called P450db1 or P450II D1) and the corresponding microsomal activity can be uniquely assessed using the peroxygenase function of this isozyme in a cumene hydroperoxide (CuOOH) supported reaction, whereas at least two isozymes are active in the classical mono-oxygenase reaction (Zanger et al. 1988a). By kinetic analysis of microsomes from liver biopsies of in vivo phenotyped extensive- and poor-metabolizing subjects, a striking selectivity of the CuOOH-mediated activity of P450db1 in identifying the poor-metabolizing condition was achieved, namely a drastically reduced V_{max} paralleled by an increased K_m and a loss of stereoselectivity in poor-metabolizer microsomes.

Immunoquantitation of P450db1. Different types of antibodies, all specifically recognizing P450db1, have been developed or discovered in our laboratory. These include rabbit polyclonal antibodies and mouse monoclonal antibodies specifically recognizing P450db1. Moreover, in collaboration with L. Kiffel and J.-C. Homberg (Hôpital Necker and Hôpital St. Antoine, Paris), we have discovered that circulating antibodies which occur in some children with chronic active hepatitis (anti-LKM1 antibodies) uniquely recognize P450db1-type activity, as demonstrated by complete inhibition and immunoprecipitation of CuOOH-mediated microsomal bufuralol-1'-hydroxylation. We used anti-LKM1 IgG to immunoisolate the microsomal LKM1 antigen. The eluted

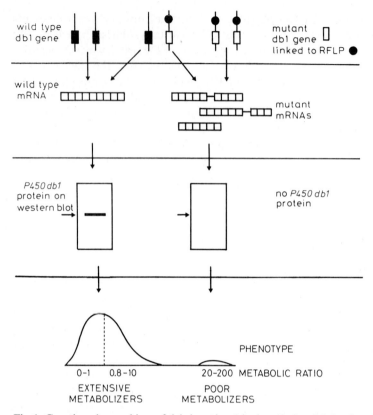

Fig. 1. Genetic polymorphism of debrisoquine-4-hydroxylation. Molecular characterization of the human cytochrome *P450db1* gene. The scheme should give an idea about how splicing defects may cause mutant mRNAs which yield no detectable *P450db1* protein and result in the debrisoquine poor metabolizer phenotype

protein was identical to P450db1 in its M_r of 50 000 and its N-terminal amino acid sequence (Zanger et al. 1988 b). By the same procedure the anti-LKM1 antigen was isolated from solubilized microsomes of human livers, including liver biopsies from in vivo phenotyped extensive- and poor-metabolizing subjects. The amount of P450db1 immunoisolated or immunoquantitated on Western blots correlated closely with the V_{max} of CuOOH mediated bufuralol-1'-hydroxylation. No protein could be demonstrated in poor metabolizers' livers (Zanger et al. 1988 a).

Collectively, our immunological data provide convincing evidence for the specific absence rather than a functional alteration of P450db1 in most poor metabolizers as the cause of debrisoquine polymorphism.

Studies at the DNA Level. A full-length human cDNA (db1-cDNA) was cloned by screening cDNA expression libraries derived from livers of extensive metabolizers with anti-P450db1 antibodies (Gonzalez et al. 1988). The relationship of the db1-cDNA to P450db1 was convincingly demonstrated by identical N-terminal sequence and functional expression in COS-1 cells. The db1 gene was localized on human chromosome 22, in agreement with linkage studies in poor-metabolizer families by Eichelbaum et al. (1987). In livers with markedly decreased bufuralol-1′-hydroxylase activity, different aberrant pre-mRNA splicing defects were discovered which could explain the absence of the P450db1 protein in the livers of poor metabolizers (Gonzalez et al. 1988).

We have also used the db1-cDNA to analyse leucocyte DNA from in vivo phenotyped extensive- and poor-metabolizing subjects in order to identify mutant alleles of the db1 gene locus (Skoda et al. 1988). Restriction fragment length polymorphisms (RFLPs) generated by several endonucleases were found to be associated with the poor metabolizer phenotype when DNA from unrelated poor metabolizers and unrelated extensive metabolizers was compared. The segregation of these RFLPs was studied in families of poor metabolizer propositi in which obligate heterozygote carriers of the recessive gene could be identified. These studies revealed that each of two polymorphic fragments is allelic with a fragment present in all extensive metabolizers and suggests that these two RFLPs identify two independent mutated alleles of the db1 gene. Among poor metabolizers, 75% had at least one of these mutated alleles (Skoda et al. 1988). Our studies thus suggest that a third (or probably several additional) mutated allele not detected by these methods must be present in the population and associated with decreased metabolism of debrisoquine. The mutations leading to the RFLPs and their relationship to the aberrant splicing defects observed in poor metabolizers' livers are presently being investigated. A scheme of these recent findings is presented in Fig. 1.

4.2 Mephenytoin Polymorphism

Studies at the Microsomal Level. The inherited deficiency of mephenytoin metabolism affects one of the two major metabolic pathways of mephenytoin, namely stereoselective 4-hydroxylation of S-mephenytoin. The other main reaction, N demethylation to nirvanol, remains unaffected. Our initial studies in microsomes of liver biopsies of in vivo phenotyped extensive- and poor-metabolizing subjects suggested the deficiency of a P450 isozyme different from P450db1. Poor metabolizer microsomes could be distinguished from those of extensive metabolizers by a decreased V_{max} and increased K_m for S-mephenytoin hydroxylation and a loss in stereoselectivity for the S enantiomer (Meier et al. 1985). P450 isozyme fractions (P450meph) which catalyse mephenytoin hydroxylation have been purified and characterized from human livers (Gut et al. 1986b). The only other substrate known to be subject to this polymorphism is mephobarbital (Jacqz et al. 1986).

Immunoquantitation of Cytochrome P450meph. In sera of patients suffering from tienilic acid induced hepatitis, high titres of anti-liver kidney microsome (anti-LKM2) antibodies have been detected (Beaune et al. 1987). These autoimmune antibodies strongly inhibit the microsomal oxidation of tienilic acid and recognize the P450 responsible for microsomal S-mephenytoin hydroxylation (Meier and Meyer 1987). They potently inhibited S-mephenytoin 4-hydroxylation and immunoprecipitated the same single protein as rabbit anti-P450meph antibodies. The same amount of protein was immunopurified from solubilized liver microsomes of extensive metabolizers and one in vivo phenotyped poor metabolizer subject. Comparison of the extensive metabolizer type of P450 with that isolated from poor metabolizer liver revealed no difference in regard to M_r, isoelectric point, relative content in microsomes, peptide maps, amino acid composition, or N-terminal protein sequence (Meier and Meyer 1987). However, our recent studies also suggest that different but immunologically indistinguishable P450 isozymes may catalyse the metabolism of tolbutamide, tienilic acid and mephenytoin. If these are recognized and inhibited by the same antibodies, one may fail to detect a decrease in enzyme protein such as the P450meph because other unaffected proteins are recognized. Thus, the mechanism of the mephenytoin polymorphism remains unresolved, and studies at the DNA level have not yet been possible.

4.3 N-Acetyltransferase Polymorphism

We have studied the human defect at the level of enzyme expression by developing sensitive enzyme assays and by raising antibodies against N-acetyltransferase purified from the cytosol of several human livers. So far our results suggest that the large variations in cytosolic enzyme activity are accompanied by parallel differences in the quantity of at least two distinct but closely related isozymes of N-acetyltransferase, NAT-1 and NAT-2. In livers with low N-acetyltransferase activity no protein could be detected by the anti-N-acetyltransferase serum in either of the isozyme fractions (Grant and Meyer, submitted). We are unable to say at the present time whether this results from genetic variation in regulatory elements controlling synthesis of these acetylating isozymes, or whether gene mutations in coding sequences lead to the production of unstable structurally variant enzymes which are rapidly degraded. Nonetheless, our studies provide yet another example of an enzyme system which seems to display unexpected complexity at the molecular level when considered in the context of its phenotypic expression in vivo. Molecular studies currently in progress should allow us to clarify the precise nature of the interindividual differences which we have detected at the protein level.

5 Conclusions

Studies at the protein and gene level of the enzymes affected by common genetic polymorphisms will ultimately allow the development of clinical tests to predict poor metabolizers and improve the efficacy and safety of drug therapy.

References

Beaune P, Dansette PM, Mansuy D, Kiffel L, Finck M, Amar C, Leroux JP, Homberg JC (1987) Human anti-endoplasmic reticulum autoantibodies appearing in a drug-induced hepatitis are directed against a human liver cytochrome P450 that hydroxylates the drug. Proc Natl Acad Sci USA 84:551–555

Dayer P, Kronbach T, Eichelbaum M, Meyer UA (1987) Enzymatic basis of the debrisoquine/sparteine-type genetic polymorphism of drug oxidation. Biochem Pharmacol 36:4145–4152

Eichelbaum M (1984) Polymorphic drug oxidation in humans. Fed Proc 43:2298–2302

Eichelbaum M, Baur MP, Dengler HJ, Osikowska-Evers BO, Tieves G, Zekorn C, Rittner C (1987) Chromosomal assignment of human cytochrome P-450 (debrisoquine/sparteine type) to chromosome 22. Br J Clin Pharmacol 23:455

Gonzalez FJ, Skoda RC, Kimura S, Umeno M, Zanger UM, Nebert DW, Gelboin HV, et al. (1988) Characterization of the common genetic defect in humans deficient in debrisoquine metabolism. Nature 331:442–446

Grant DM, Tang BK, Kalow W (1984) A simple test for acetylator phenotype using caffeine. Br J Clin Pharmacol 17:459–464

Gut J, Catin T, Dayer P, Kronbach T, Zanger U, Meyer UA (1986a) Debrisoquine/sparteine-type polymorphism of drug oxidation: purification and characterization of two functionally different human liver cytochrome P450 isozymes involved in impaired hydroxylation of the prototype substrate bufuralol. J Biol Chem 261:11734

Gut J, Meier UT, Catin T, Mayer UA (1986b) Mephenytoin-type polymorphism of drug oxidation: purification and characterization of a human liver cytochrome P-450 isozyme catalyzing microsomal mephenytoin hydroxylation. Biochim Biophys Acta 884:435–447

Jacqz E, Hall SD, Branch RA, Wilkinson GR (1986) Polymorphic metabolism of mephenytoin in man. Pharmacokinetic interaction with a co-regulated substrate, mephobarbital. Clin Pharmacol Ther 39:646–653

Kronbach T, Mathys D, Gut J, Catin T, Meyer UA (1987) High performance liquid chromatographic assays for bufuralol 1'-hydroxylase, debrisoquine 4-hydroxylase, and dextromethorphan O-demethylase in microsomes and purified cytochrome P-450 isozymes of human liver. Anal Biochem 162:24–32

Küpfer A, Preisig R (1983) Inherited defects of hepatic drug metabolism. Semin Liver Dis 3:341–354

Meier UT, Meyer UA (1987) Genetic polymorphism of human cytochrome P450 S-mephenytoin-4-hydroxylase. Biochemistry 26:8466–8474

Meier UT, Kronbach T, Meyer UA (1985) Assay of mephenytoin metabolism in human liver microsomes by high-performance liquid chromatography. Anal Biochem 151:286–291

Meier UT, Dayer P, Male PJ, Kronbach T, Meyer UA (1986) Mephenytoin hydroxylation polymorphism: characterization of the enzymatic deficiency in liver microsomes of poor metabolizers phenotyped in vivo. Clin Pharmacol Ther 38:488–494

Meyer UA (1987) Polymorphisms of human drug metabolising enzymes. In: Benford DJ, Bridges JW, Gibson GG (eds) Drug metabolism – from molecules to man. Taylor and Francis, London, pp 95–105

Skoda RC, Gonzalez FJ, Demierre A, Meyer UA (1988) Two mutant alleles of the human cytochrome *P450db1*-gene associated with genetically deficient metabolism of debrisoquine and other drugs. Proc Natl Acad Sci USA 85:5240–5243

Weber WW, Hein DW (1985) N-acetylation pharmacogenetics. Pharmacol Rev 37:25–79

Zanger UM, Vilbois F, Hardwick JP, Meyer UA (1988a) Absence of hepatic cytochrome P450bufI causes genetically deficient debrisoquine oxidation in man. Biochemistry 27:5447–5454

Zanger UM, Hauri HP, Loeper J, Homberg JC, Meyer UA (1988b) Antibodies against human cytochrome P450db1 in autoimmune hepatitis type II. Proc Natl Acad Sci USA 85:8256–8260

Genetic Polymorphism in Drug Oxidation

W. Kalow [1]

1 Introduction

As discussed by Meyer et al. (this volume), recent studies of drug-metabolizing enzymes at the molecular level have led to remarkable advances. We can expect that the rapid progress will continue. By contrast, studying the clinical consequences of the molecular discoveries will remain a slow process.

Polymorphism is a word of many meanings. In genetics, polymorphism refers to the simultaneous occurrence in a population of variant forms of a gene product. However, the occurrence of a variant is counted as polymorphic only if it has a frequency greater than can be accounted for by the mutation rate. In practice, a variant is called polymorphic only if its gene frequency in a population exceeds 2%. In other words, the term excludes rare variants. This definition fits only two variants, which have been referred to as debrisoquine polymorphism and mephenytoin polymorphism. Meyer et al. (this volume) have outlined the current knowledge of these polymorphisms at the molecular level. Some particular aspects of these polymorphisms will be emphasized in subsequent chapters. I will try to provide an overview mainly from a pharmacokinetic and clinical perspective.

I will use the term debrisoquine hydroxylase for the human enzyme which has been characterized genetically, and which is homologous to the rat enzyme db1 (Gonzales et al. 1988). I will use the term mephenytoin hydroxylase, realizing that this may represent one, or two closely related enzymes which act only on the S enantiomer of mephenytoin (Guengerich et al. 1986).

2 Debrisoquine Polymorphism

There are two kinds of interactions of drugs with debrisoquine hydroxylase. The drug may either be metabolized by debrisoquine hydroxylase or bind to the enzyme without being metabolized; the latter are inhibitors. For in vitro screening, we are reminded that all drug substrates are inhibitors by competing with other substrates, but a drug which is not a competitive inhibitor can also not be a substrate. Drugs with extremely high affinity are also not good substrates, since high affinity implies a slow release of enzyme from the enzyme-substrate complex.

[1] Department of Pharmacology, University of Toronto, Toronto, Canada

Clinical Pharmacology in Psychiatry
Editors: S. G. Dahl and L. F. Gram
(Psychopharmacology Series 7)
© Springer-Verlag Berlin Heidelberg 1989

2.1 Substrates of Debrisoquine Hydroxylase

Table 1 lists the substrates of debrisoquine hydroxylase in terms of a pharmacological classification. With three exceptions (discussed below), inclusion of a drug into this list is based on in vivo studies in patients, volunteers or both. The metabolism by debrisoquine hydroxylase of some drugs,

Table 1. Drugs metabolized by debrisoquine hydroxylase

Drugs	Consequences for poor metabolizers	References
β-Blockers		
Metoprolol	Loss of selectivity, side effects	13, 18, 20, 34
Bufuralol	Increased side effects	7, 15, 20, 37
Timolol	Moderate pharmacokinetic alteration	19, 20
Bopindolol	Minimal pharmacokinetic alteration	13
Propranolol	No clinical change	19, 20
Other cardiovascular drugs		
Debrisoquine	Hypotension, collapse	10, 33,37
Guanoxan	Hypotension	31
Sparteine	Uterine rupture	8, 10, 34
N-Propylajmaline	Overdose effects	39
Propafenone	CNS and neurological side effects	29, 34
Encainide	Reduced effect (only after single dose)	21, 25, 35
Perhexiline	Neuropathy, hepatotoxicity, myopathy	11, 14, 28
Diltiazem	Cardiac failure (given with metoprolol)	34
Indoramin	Dizziness, hypotension	24
Antidepressants		
Nortriptyline	Slow elimination, cumulation	3, 22, 30
Desipramine	Slow elimination, cumulation	4, 8, 9, 30
Amitriptyline	Minor change	5
Imipramine	Minor change	3, 8, 9, 30
Clomipramine	Minor change	6
Miscellaneous drugs		
Dextromethorphan	Slight drowsiness if anything	17, 27, 38
Phenformin	Lactic acidosis	16, 23, 36
Codeine	Metabolism demonstrated in vitro	12
Amiflamine	Overdose effects expected	1, 2
Methoxyphenamine	Experimental administration	26
Methoxyamphetamine	Prolonged hallucinations	32
Lasiocarpine	In vitro demonstration	37
Monocrotaline	In vitro demonstration	37

1. Alvan et al. (1986); 2. Alvan et al. (1984); 3. van Bahr et al. (1986); 4. van Bahr et al. (1985); 5. Balant-Gorgia et al. (1982); 6. Balant-Gorgia et al. (1986); 7. Boobis et al. (1985); 8. Brøsen (1988); 9. Brøsen and Gram (1988); 10. Cooper and Evans (1984); 11. Cooper et al. (1984); 12. Dayer et al. (1988); 13. Dayer et al. (1986); 14. Gould et al. (1986); 15. Gut et al. (1984); 16. Idle et al. (1981); 17. Kupfer et al. (1986); 18. Lennard et al. (1986b); 22. Mellstrom et al. (1981); 23. Oates et al. (1983); 24. Pierce et al. (1987); 25. Roden and Woosley (1988); 26. Roy et al. (1985); 27. Schmid et al. (1985); 28. Shah et al. (1982); 29. Siddoway et al. (1987); 30. Sjoqvist and Wagner et al. (1987); 35. Wang et al. (1984); 36. Wiholm et al. (1981); 37. Wolff et al. (1987); 38. Woodworth et al. (1987); 39. Zekorn et al. (1985).

Table 2. Drugs not metabolized by debrisoquine hydroxylase as determined in vivo

Acetanilid	Wakile et al. (1979)
Aminorex	Saner et al. (1986)
Amobarbital	Inaba et al. (1980)
Antipyrine	Eichelbaum et al. (1983)
Benzodiazepine	Syvalahti et al. (1986)
Caffeine	Unpublished observation
Ethanol	Male et al. (1982)
Maprotiline	Gabris et al. (1985)
Methaqualone	Oram et al. (1982)
Midazolam	Klotz et al. (1986)
Phenytoin	Kadar et al. (1983)
Prazosin	Lennard et al. (1988)
Theophylline	Dahlqvist et al. (1984)
Tolbutamide	Peart et al. (1987

prominently bufurarol, debrisoquine, sparteine, nortriptyline and desipramine, has been investigated both in vivo and in vitro. Table 2 lists drugs which have been shown not to be metabolized by debrisoquine hydroxylase in vivo.

For most of the drugs listed in Table 1, the metabolic dependence on debrisoquine hydroxylase has been known for some years, and there are sufficient published comments to allow me to be brief regarding them. Most drugs with serious toxicities for poor metabolizers are no longer on the market. These include debrisoquine, sparteine and phenformin. It is my understanding that perhexiline can still be used by patients in the United Kingdom if prior testing has shown them to be extensive metabolizers of debrisoquine.

Studies with db1 antibodies suggest that the debrisoquine hydroxylase participates in the metabolism of the pyrrhol derivatives lasiocarpine and monocrotaline.

Of considerable interest is a newcomer to this list, codeine. Probably every medical student has learned that the analgesic action of codeine depends on its demethylation to morphine. This conversion has recently been shown by Dayer et al. (1988) in isolated human liver to be catalysed by debrisoquine hydroxylase. Metabolism studies in vivo are still to be done, and it remains to be shown in clinical studies whether poor metabolizers of debrisoquine derive the expected pain relief from codeine. Another question that remains to be answered is based on the observation that debrisoquine hydroxylase occurs in brain cells (Fonne-Pfister et al. 1987). It is thus a possibility that conversion of codeine into morphine may take place in the brain.

In this context, we should remember that numerous studies of cytochromes P450 in the brain have been conducted during recent years. The cytochromes in brain represent a variety of enzymes and isozymes, many with specific distributions (Warner et al. 1988), some prominently in the globus pallidus (Kapitulnik et al. 1987). The P450 concentration in brain is generally much lower than in the liver, often in the order of 1% of that found in liver. However, some cells, or particular cells groups, seem to have rather high concentrations of inducible cytochromes (Volk et al. 1988). This could mean that the occurrence of genetic variants in the liver reflects variation in the brain, with direct implications for some cerebral functions. In any case, this is an area of investigation which will require much attention in the future.

2.2 Inhibitors of Debrisoquine Hydroxylase

Otton et al. in Toronto (1983, 1984; Inaba et al. 1985), used human liver preparations to screen drugs for their capacity to bind to debrisoquine hydroxylase, using competitive inhibition of sparteine metabolism as the criterion for binding (Table 3). Our selection of drugs was influenced by the fact that sparteine – a prominent substrate of debrisoquine hydroxylase – was a natural alkaloid. We asked ourselves whether it could be that the debrisoquine polymorphism represents genetic adaptation against alkaloids or other toxic food constituents. At our request, Boehringer Ingelheim in the Federal Republic of Germany kindly supplied us with a series of the natural alkaloids which they had in their chemical storeroom. It thus happened that Otton found the very high affinity of quinidine for debrisoquine hydroxylase. Also yohimbine showed substantial binding. (These binding studies were called useless and misleading by the first reviewers of the manuscripts, which lead to rejection of the papers by one of the publications.) In the meantime, the clinical importance of inhibition of debrisoquine hydroxylase has been well established. Table 4 is based on in vivo evidence of such inhibition. Quinidine

Table 3. Strong inhibitors of debrisoquine hydroxylase in vitro ($K_i < \mu M$)

Quinidine	Otton et al. (1984)
Cinchonidine	Otton et al. (1984)
Desipramine	Otton et al. (1983)
Nortriptyline	Otton et al. (1983)
Chlorpromazine	Otton et al. (1983)
Thioridazine	van Bahr et al. (1985)
Haloperidol	Inaba et al. (1985)
Domperidone	Inaba et al. (1985)
Pipamperone	Inaba et al. (1985)
Labetalol	Inaba et al. (1985)
Ajmaline	Inaba et al. (1985)
Lobeline	Inaba et al. (1985)
Yohimbine	Inaba et al. (1985)
Corynantheine	Inaba et al. (1984)
MPTP	Fonne-Pfister et al. (1987)

Table 4. Inhibition of debrisoquine hydroxylase observed in vivo

Quinidine	Brøsen et al. (1987); Inaba et al. (1986); Leemann et al. (1986); Steiner and Spina (1987)
Thioridazine	Syvalahti et al. (1986)
Levomepromazine	Syvalahti et al. (1986)
Diphenhydramine	Poirier et al. (1987)
Orphenadrine	Poirier et al. (1987)
Diltiazem	Bottorff et al. (1988)
Propafenone	Siddoway et al. (1985)
Cimetidine	Steiner and Spina (1987)
Carbamazepine (?)	Roots et al. (1985)

has been shown to affect the metabolism of various substrates of debrisoquine hydroxylase, causing an extensive metabolizer to appear as a poor metabolizer (e.g. Inaba et al. 1986; Brøsen et al. 1987).

Among the drugs tested by Otton, chlorpromazine showed a high affinity for the enzyme. In vivo studies have shown in the meantime that levomepromazine and thioridazine are also potent inhibitors of the enzyme (Table 4). Since these neuroleptics tend to produce extrapyramidal symptoms such as parkinsonism, it was not surprising that the investigation of patients with parkinsonism in a psychiatric hospital revealed many to have a reduced capacity for metabolizing debrisoquine. This gave rise to the idea of an association between the debrisoquine polymorphism and parkinsonism (Barbeau et al. 1985). Barbeau, who first developed this idea, died shortly after publication of this paper. His collaborators have shown in a recent publication that the antihistaminics diphenhydramine and orphenadrine increase the metabolic ratio in patients with parkinsonism (Poirier et al. 1987). In the meantime, Meyer and his collaborators have shown through in vitro studies that N-methyl-4-phenyl-1,2,3,6-tetrahydropyridine, the neurotoxic substance referred to as MPTP, was in vitro a potent inhibitor of debrisoquine hydroxylase (Fonne-Pfister et al. 1987); they also demonstrated the presence of the enzyme in human and in rat brain. Since the illicit recreational use of MPTP has given rise to severe parkinsonism, Meyer has reopened the question of any special connection between susceptibility to parkinsonism and debrisoquine polymorphism.

2.3 Variation Between Extensive Metabolizers of Debrisoquine

It is part of the lore of human genetics that there is often less person-to-person variation between homozygotes for a monogenic trait than between heterozygotes. This is likely to be true also for the debrisoquine polymorphism. This aspect of its population distribution has been neglected in the computer simulations of both Jackson et al. (1986) and Steiner (1987).

Table 5. Kinetics of sparteine oxidation by the microsomal enzyme component of human liver susceptible to inhibition by quinidine (from Tyndale 1988)

Liver no.	n	K_m (μM)	$\pm$ SE of K_m	V_{max} (pmol mg^{-1} 0.5 h^{-1})
K18	2	167.8	1.3	7019
AL9	3	101.3	20.6	1687
K14	1	101.3		3768
K12	1	95.4		5700
K15	8	94.2	4.1	4138
K10	1	44.4		5738
K20	3	38.0	9.1	14413
AL10	1	37.0		718
K21	8	33.6	3.8	1137
K16	6	18.8	1.7	735

Nevertheless, one cannot distinguish phenotypically between homozygous and heterozygous extensive metabolizers (Brøsen 1988). A potential reason became apparent in recent studies by Tyndale (1988). Tyndale reinvestigated sparteine oxidation in a series of human livers using an exceptionally wide range of substrate concentrations. In most livers, she could identify two enzyme components, one susceptible to inhibition by quinidine and one not susceptible. The nonsusceptible component had the lower affinities for sparteine. The Michaelis constant (K_m) in the quinidine-susceptible component of the sparteine-oxidizing enzyme varied over a ten-fold range within the livers investigated (Table 5). This variability far exceeds the limits of experimental error. It seems likely that this variability of K_m values indicates structural variations within the wild-type debrisoquine hydroxylase. This could well be the main factor obscuring the phenotypic distinctions between the two extensive metabolizer genotypes. It could also be this factor which is responsible for the peculiar association between bronchial carcinoma and the subgroup of extensive metabolizers with very high metabolic ratios (Ayesh and Idle 1985).

2.4 Clinical Consequences of a Drug-Metabolizing Failure: Principle Questions

Let us ask as a general question: What can happen to a drug if a particular drug-metabolizing activity is absent, as for instance, in a poor metabolizer of debrisoquine or sparteine (Kalow 1987)?

As a rule, the mammalian body has several means of getting rid of a drug. Not only is there renal and biliary excretion besides metabolism, but there are often two or three competing reactions leading to different metabolites of a given drug. In that case, if one reaction fails, it may not much alter the metabolic clearance of a drug. An example is propranolol: only one of its three metabolic pathways depend on debrisoquine hydroxylase. Propanolol can be, and has been, used to detect poor metabolizers of debrisoquine, although their metabolic failure does not make the slightest difference for the pharmacological action of propranolol (Lennard et al. 1986a). If the person has two defects, knocking out two of the metabolic pathways, the clinical consequence could be drug toxicity. A variant of this kind of protective multimetabolism is represented by cases in which the same reaction is produced by two different enzymes. The classical example is alcohol oxidation by both alcohol dehydrogenase and a cytochrome P450 formerly referred to as MEOS; the enzyme molecule is now known and is designated P450IIE1 (Nebert and Gonzalez 1987).

More frequent are the cases in which a given reaction of a given substrate can be produced by more than one cytochrome. Reilly et al. (1983) in Toronto found many years ago that the side-chain hydroxylation of amobarbital, the main elimination pathway of that drug, was catalysed by two cytochromes. We concluded at that time that an inability to hydroxylate amobarbital should be a rare event, in spite of the fact that the rate of metabolism was predominently under genetic control and highly variable between persons (Endrenyi et al. 1976). In the meantime, this kind of metabolic safeguard has been found for a number of drugs, among which are some drug substrates whose first biotransforming enzyme is debrisoquine hydroxylase. For instance, debrisoquine hydroxylase is under most circumstances the main enzymemetabolizing sparteine. The enzyme is easily identified by its genetic variability and by its susceptability to inhibition by quinidine. The "back-up enzyme" has a somewhat lower affinity for sparteine and is not inhibited by quinidine (Tyndale 1988).

Metoprolol and other β-blockers are racemates. Debrisoquine hydroxylase oxidizes one of the enantiomers more effectively than the other, while the back-up enzyme produces the same action but without distinction between the enantiomers (Lennard et al. 1986b). The enantiomers also differ in potency for β-blockade. It thus happens that the increased plasma concentration in poor metabolizers is composed to a large extent of the less active enantiomer.

Similarity of pharmacological action of drug and metabolite is another major reason for a lack of clinical consequences of a drug-metabolizing deficiency. A classical example, revealed during studies of N-acetyltransferase, is procainamide and acetylprocainamide (Uetrecht et al. 1984). Both have similar pharmacological actions although the toxic effects are different; the parent drug tends to produce antinuclear antibodies, in contrast to the acetylated metabolite. There are equivalent examples pertaining to the debrisoquine polymorphism. Bufuralol has served as a model substrate for in vitro investigations of debrisoquine hydroxylase (Dayer et al. 1986). However, since hydroxybufuralol is about as effective in producing β-blockade as is the parent drug, the metabolic difference is clinically hardly noticeable, at least in respect to β-blockade.

The consequences of a metabolic deficiency may be shaped by pharmacokinetic factors. Thus, one can distinguish between an alteration in first-pass metabolism and a deficiency in metabolic clearance which translates into a prolonged half-life. Usually both factors are apparent (Kalow 1987).

A good example of modification of a first-pass effect in poor metabolizers is represented by the pharmacokinetics of debrisoquine itself. The now classical illustration by Sloan et al. (1983) shows that the oral intake of a single dose of debrisoquine leads to an approximately four-fold higher plasma level in a poor than in an extensive metabolizer. The decline of the plasma level in a semilogarithmic plot is the same for the poor metabolizer and the extensive metabolizer. This means that the normal debrisoquine hydroxylase is acting very fast upon debrisoquine, so that about 80% of the drug is destroyed in the liver as it enters via the portal blood, and before it can leave via the hepatic vein. In other words, only about 20% of the absorbed drug gets into the general circulation. After completion of the absorption phase, the rate of metabolism of debrisoquine must be determined by access to the enzyme, probably by the rate at which it is carried by the hepatic artery into the liver, in other words, by hepatic blood flow.

Good examples of half-life modulation by the debrisoquine polymorphism are sparteine (Eichelbaum 1982) and propylajmaline (Zekorn et al. 1985). A standard oral dose of these drugs leads to similar initial blood levels in poor and extensive metabolizers. In extensive metabolizers, debrisoquine hydroxylase activity is rate limiting and determines the half-life; other, less efficient elimination mechanisms determine the half-life of the drug in poor metabolizers.

This pharmacokinetic distinction between first-pass metabolism and half-life prolongation is important particularly during chronic administration of a drug. Thus, in chronic administration of sparteine to extensive metabolizers there is no particular tendency for cumulation of the drug within the body. On the other hand, sparteine tends to accumulate on repeated doses in a poor metabolizer over a considerable period of time (Eichelbaum 1982). Mathematically speaking, it takes 3.5 times the half-life of the drug in order practically to reach steady-state concentrations during chronic drug administration. Thus, even if the half-life is only moderately prolonged, it takes much longer to reach the steady-state levels, and these will be elevated.

3 Mephenytoin Polymorphism

It is now almost 10 years since the hereditary metabolic defect of mephenytoin hydroxylation was discovered by Kupfer et al. (1979) at Vanderbilt University. In spite of many efforts by various investigators, there are still not many drugs known to be affected by this polymorphism (see reviews by Kalow 1986; Wilkinson 1986). It is of course possible that future discoveries will reveal many drugs to be metabolized by mephenytoin hydroxylase without us currently suspecting it. However, at the present time we must accept at face value that mephenytoin hydroxylase is a cytochrome P450 with more restricted functions than is debrisoquine hydroxylase.

The mephenytoin polymorphism represents a structural alteration which affects enzyme activity (Meier and Meyer 1987). There is a complicating aspect of this alteration: not all of its substrates are affected by the structural change. There is in vitro evidence that tolbutamide can be hydroxylated by mephenytoin hydroxylase, but not with the same person-to-person variation of activity as with mephenytoin (Knodell et al. 1987). The distribution curves in a population must be different for tolbutamide and for mephenytoin. Analogous situations are known for other enzymes: paraoxonase activity is bimodally distributed in a population while the hydrolysis of phenylacetate by the same enzyme is unimodally distributed (Eckerson et al. 1983). Also, organophosphates do not discriminate between the genetic variants of plasma cholinesterase while inhibitors of the amine type do (Kalow and Davies 1958). In any case, the mephenytoin hydroxylase appears to have two classes of substrates. Since we have looked at only one class, because it was revealed by genetic variation, we may be underestimating the overall importance of this enzyme. Meehan et al. (1988) showed mephenytoin hydroxylase to belong to a cytochrome P450 family with members involved in steroid oxidations.

The enantiomeric selectivity of the enzyme has received much attention, and the clinical importance of the genetic defect for the therapeutic use of mephenytoin is well documented (Kalow 1986; Wilkinson 1986). Mephenytoin is a valuable but rarely used antiepileptic. More widely used is mephobarbital; its primary metabolism also depends on mephenytoin hydroxylase (Kupfer and Branch 1985). It is very likely that mephobarbital would tend to show overdose toxicity in poor metabolizers of mephenytoin. In addition, one route of hexobarbital metabolism depends on this enzyme.

Several groups of investigators have tested drugs for their capacity to inhibit mephenytoin hydroxylase in the hope of identifying further substrates of this enzyme. In the large random screening test of Inaba et al. (1985) tranylcypromine was the only competitive inhibitor with a micromolar value of K_i. Weaker but consistent inhibition was shown by diazepam and other benzodiazepines; the observation was confirmed by Hall et al. (1987), but a relationship between mephenytoin hydroxylation and 3-hydroxylation of diazepam could be excluded (Tait 1987). According to the inhibition data by Hall et al. (1987), potential substrates are also methsuximide and ethytoin. The antifungal agent ketoconazole also inhibited mephenytoin hydroxylation in vivo (Atiba et al. 1988). From among a series of steroids, only norethindrone proved a fairly potent ($K_i = 20 \mu M$) inhibitor (Jurima et al. 1985). We recently excluded inhibition by glutethimide and by aminoglutethimide (unpublished observation).

The frequency of the mephenytoin polymorphism is roughly 5% in Caucasian and 20% in Japanese populations (Kalow 1986; Wilkinson 1986). No poor metabolizer was found among 90 Cuna Indians in Panama (Inaba et al. 1988).

4 Summary and Conclusions

Of the two clearly established drug oxidation polymorphisms, only the one referred to as debrisoquine polymorphism affects many drugs. The only known polymorphic substrates of mephenytoin hydroxylase are mephenytoin and mephobarbital. Relatively recently discovered drug substrates of debrisoquine hydroxylase are propafenone, diltiazem, and codeine. The list of substrates contains 28 items. The fate of slightly less than half of these is clinically affected in poor metabolizers, and several of the latter drugs are no longer marketted. There are many reasons why a failure of metabolism may not alter the fate of a drug sufficiently to affect its clinical use.

Of interest and clinical importance is the inhibition of debrisoquine hydroxylase by inhibitors such as quinidine and by some neuroleptics; also the simultaneous use of two substrates has led to serious toxicity by mutual metabolic inhibition.

The study of these oxidation polymorphisms has been instructive not only for formal pharmacogenetics but also for the understanding of problems of therapy in patients without genetic defects.

References

Alvan G, Grind M, Graffner C, Sjoqvist F (1984) Relationship of N-demethylation of amiflamine and its metabolite to debrisoquine hydroxylation polymorphism. Clin Pharmacol Ther 36:515–519

Alvan G, Graffner C, Grind M, Gustafsson LL, Lindgren JE, Nordin C, Ross S et al. (1986) Tolerance and pilot pharmacokinetics of amiflamine after increasing single oral doses in healthy subjects. Clin Pharmacol Ther 40:81–85

Atiba JO, Blaschke TF, Wilkinson GR (1988) Effect of ketoconazole on polymorphic 4-hydroxylation of S-mephenytoin and debrisoquine. Clin Pharmacol Ther 43:136

Ayesh R, Idle JR (1985) Evaluation of drug oxidation phenotypes in the biochemical epidemiology of lung cancer risk. In: Boobis AR, Caldwell J, de Metteis F, Elcombe CR (eds) Microsomes and drug oxidation. Taylor and Francis, London, pp 340–346

Balant-Gorgia AE, Schulz P, Dayer P, Balant L, Kubli A, Gertsch C, Garrone G (1982) Role of oxidation polymorphism on blood and urine concentrations of amitriptyline and its metabolites in man. Arch Psychiatr Nervenkr 232:215–222

Balant-Gorgia AE, Balant LP, Genet C, Dayer P, Aeschlimann JM, Garrone G (1986) Importance of oxidative polymorphism and levomepromazine treatment on the steady-state blood concentrations of clomipramine and its major metabolites. Eur J Clin Pharmacol 31:449–455

Barbeau A, Roy M, Paris S, Cloutier T, Plasse L, Poirier J (1985) Ecogenetics of Parkinson's disease: 4-hydroxylation of debrisoquine. Lancet 2:1213–1216

Boobis AR, Murray S, Hampden CE, Davies DS (1985) Genetic polymorphism in drug oxidation: in vitro studies of human debrisoquine 4-hydroxylase and bufuralol 1'-hydroxylase activities. Biochem Pharmacol 34:65–71

Bottorff MB, Hoon TJ, Lalonde RL, Kazierad DJ, Mirvis DM (1988) Effects of diltiazem (D) on the disposition of encainide (E) and its active metabolites. Clin Pharmacol Ther 43:195

Brøsen K (1988) The relationship between imipramine metabolism and the sparteine oxidation polymorphism. Laegeforeningens, Copenhagen

Brøsen K, Gram LF (1988) First-pass metabolism of imipramine and desipramine: impact of the sparteine oxidation phenotype. Clin Pharmacol Ther 43:400–406

Brøsen K, Gram LF, Haghfelt T, Bertilsson L (1987) Extensive metabolizers of debrisoquine become poor metabolizers during quinidine treatment. Pharmacol Toxicol 60:312–314

Cooper M, Idle JR, Kong I, Sloan TP, Smith RL (1983) The quantitative contribution of debrisoquine oxidation capacity to variation in the metabolism of other substrates. Br J Clin Pharmacol 15:585P–586P

Cooper RG, Evans DAP (1984) Oxidation polymorphism has clinical relevance. Lancet 2:227

Cooper RG, Evans DAP, Whibley EJ (1984) Polymorphic hydroxylation of perhexiline maleate in man. J Med Genet 21:27–33

Dahlqvist R, Bertilsson L, Birkett DJ, Eichelbaum M, Sawe J, Sjoqvist F (1984) Theophylline metabolism in relation to antipyrine, debrisoquine, and sparteine metabolism. Clin Pharmacol Ther 35:815–821

Davies DS, Kahn GC, Murray S, Brodie MJ, Boobis AR (1981) Evidence for an enzymatic defect in the 4-hydroxylation of debrisoquine by human liver. Br J Clin Pharmacol 11:89–91

Dayer P, Merier G, Perrenoud JJ, Marmy A, Leemann T (1986) Interindividual pharmacokinetic and pharmacodynamic variability of different beta blockers. J Cardiovasc Pharmacol [Suppl 16] 8:S20–S24

Dayer P, Desmeules J, Leemann T, Striberni R (1988) Bioactivation of the narcotic drug codeine in human liver is mediated by the polymorphic monooxygenase catalyzing debrisoquine 4-hydroxylation. Biochem Biophys Res Commun 152:411–416

Eckerson HW, Wyte CM, La Du BN (1983) The human serum paraoxonase/arylesterase polymorphism. Am J Hum Genet 35:1126–1138

Eichelbaum M (1982) Defective oxidation of drugs: pharmacokinetic and therapeutic implications. Clin Pharmacokinet 7:1–22

Eichelbaum M, Bertilsson L, Sawe J (1983) Antipyrine metabolism in relation to polymorphic oxidations of sparteine and debrisoquine. Br J Clin Pharmacol 15:317–321

Endrenyi L, Inaba T, Kalow W (1976) Genetic study of amobarbital elimination based on its kinetics in twins. Clin Pharmacol Ther 20:701–714

Fonne-Pfister R, Bargetzi MJ, Meyer UA (1987) MPTP, the neurotoxin inducing Parkinson's disease, is a potent competitive inhibitor of human and rat cytochrome P450 isozymes (P450bufI, P450dbl) catalyzing debrisoquine 4-hydroxylation. Biochem Biophys Res Commun 148:1144–1150

Gabris G, Baumann P, Jonzier-Perey M, Bosshart P, Woggon B, Kupfer A (1985) N-methylation of maprotiline in debrisoquine/mephenitoin-phenotyped depressive patients. Biochem Pharmacol 34:409–410

Gonzalez FJ, Skoda RC, Kimura S, Umeno M, Zanger UM, Nebert DW, Gelboin HY et al. (1988) Characterization of the common genetic defect in humans deficient in debrisoquine metabolism. Nature 331:442–446

Gould BJ, Amoah AGB, Parke DV (1986) Stereoselective pharmacokinetics of perhexiline. Xenobiotica 16:491–502

Guengerich FP, Distlerath LM, Reilly PEB, Wolff T, Shimada T, Umbenhauer DR, Martin MV (1986) Human-liver cytochromes P-450 involved in polymorphisms of drug oxidation. Xenobiotica 16:367–378

Gut J, Gasser R, Dayer P, Kronbach T, Catin T, Meyer UA (1984) Debrisoquine-type polymorphism of drug oxidation: purification from human liver of a cytochrome P450 isozyme with high activity for bufuralol hydroxylation. FEBS Lett 173:287–290

Hall SD, Guengerich FP, Branch RA, Wilkinson GR (1987) Characterization and inhibition of mephenytoin 4-hydroxylase activity in human liver microsomes. J Pharmacol Exp Ther 240:216–222

Idle JR, Sloan TP, Smith RL, Wakile LA (1979) Application of the phenotyped panel approach to the detection of polymorphism of drug oxidation in man. Br J Pharmacol 66:430P

Idle JR, Oates NS, Shah RR, Smith RL (1981) Is there a genetic predisposition to phenformin-induced lactic acidosis? Br J Clin Pharmacol 11:418P–419P

Inaba T, Otton SV, Kalow W (1980) Deficient metabolism of debrisoquine and sparteine. Clin Pharmacol Ther 27:547–549

Inaba T, Nakano M, Otton SV, Mahon WA, Kalow W (1984) A human cytochrome P-450 characterized by inhibition studies as the sparteine-debrisoquine monooxygenase. Can J Physiol Pharmacol 62:860–862

Inaba T, Jurima M, Mahon WA, Kalow W (1985) In vitro inhibition studies of two isozymes of human liver cytochrome P-450. Drug Metab Dispos 13:443–448

Inaba T, Tyndale RE, Mahon WA (1986) Quinidine: potent inhibition of sparteine and debrisoquine oxidation in vivo. Br J Clin Pharmacol 22:199–200

Inaba T, Jorge LF, Arias TD (1988) Mephenytoin hydroxylation in the Cuna Amerindians of Panama. Br J Clin Pharmacol 25:75–79

Jackson PR, Tucker GT, Lennard MS, Woods HF (1986) Polymorphic drug oxidation: pharmacokinetic basis and comparison of experimental indices. Br J Clin Pharmacol 22:541–550

Jacqz E, Hall SD, Branch RA (1986) Genetically determined polymorphisms in drug oxidation. Hepatology 6:1020–1032

Jurima M, Inaba T, Kalow W (1985) Mephenytoin hydroxylase activity in human liver: inhibition by steroids. Drug Metab Dispos 13:746–749

Kadar D, Fecycz TD, Kalow W (1983) The fate of orally administered [4-^{14}C]phenytoin in two healthy male volunteers. Can J Physiol Pharmacol 61:403–407

Kahn GC, Boobis AR, Davies DS (1984) Interindividual differences in monooxygenase activities of human liver. In: de Serres FJ, Pero RW (eds) Individual susceptibility to genotoxic agents in the human population. Plenum, New York, pp 109–153

Kahn GC, Boobis AR, Brodie MJ, Toverud EL, Murray S, Davies DS (1985) Phenacetin O-deethylase: an activity of a cytochrome P-450 showing genetic linkage with that catalysing the 4-hydroxylation of debrisoquine? Br J Clin Pharmacol 20:67–76

Kalow W (1986) The genetic defect of mephenytoin hydroxylation. Xenobiotica 16:379–389

Kalow W (1987) Genetic variation in the human hepatic cytochrome P-450 system. Eur J Clin Pharmacol 31:633–641

Kalow W, Davies RO (1958) The activity of various esterase inhibitors towards atypical human serum cholinesterase. Biochem Pharmacol 1:183–192

Kapitulnik J, Gelboin HV, Guengerich FP, Jacobowitz DM (1987) Immunohistochemical localization of cytochrome P-450 in rat brain. Neuroscience 20:829–833

Klotz U, Mikus G, Zekorn C, Eichelbaum M (1986) Pharmacokinetics of midazolam in relation to polymorphic sparteine oxidation. Br J Clin Pharmacol 22:618–620

Knodell RG, Hall SD, Wilkinson GR, Guengerich FP (1987) Hepatic metabolism of tolbutamide: characterization of the form of cytochrome P-450 involved in methyl hydroxylation and relationship to in vivo disposition. J Pharmacol Exp Ther 241:1112–1119

Kupfer A, Branch RA (1985) Stereoselective mephobarbital hydroxylation cosegregates with mephenytoin hydroxylation. Clin Pharmacol Ther 38:414–418

Kupfer A, Desmond P, Schenker S, Branch R (1979) Family study of a genetically determined deficiency of mephenytoin hydroxylation in man. Pharmacologist 21:173

Kupfer A, Schmid B, Pfaff G (1986) Pharmacogenetics of dextromethorphan O-demethylation in man. Xenobiotica 16:421–433

Leemann T, Dayer P, Meyer UA (1986) Single-dose quinidine treatment inhibits metoprolol oxidation in extensive metabolizers. Eur J Clin Pharmacol 29:739–741

Lennard MS, Ramsay LE, Silas JH, Tucker GT, Woods HF (1983) Protecting the poor metabolizer: clinical consequences of genetic polymorphism of drug oxidation. Pharm Int 4:61–65

Lennard MS, Tucker GT, Silas JH, Woods HF (1986a) Debrisoquine polymorphism and the metabolism and action of metoprolol, timolol, propranolol and atenolol. Xenobiotica 16:435–447

Lennard MS, Tucker GT, Woods HF (1986b) The polymorphic oxidation of beta-adrenoceptor antagonists. Clin Pharmacokinet 11:1–17

Lennard MS, McGourty JC, Silas JH (1988) Lack of relationship between debrisoquine oxidation phenotype and the pharmacokinetics and first dose effect of prazosin. Br J Clin Pharmacol 25:276–278

Male PJ, Dayer P, Deom A, Pometta D, Fabre J (1982) Elimination de l'alcool et profil lipidique chez les bons et mauvais oxydateurs du bufuralol et de la débrisoquine. Schweiz Med Wochenschr 114:1860

McAllister CB, Wolfenden HT, Aslanian WS, Woosley RL, Wilkinson GR (1986) Oxidative metabolism of encainide: polymorphism, pharmacokinetics and clinical considerations. Xenobiotica 16:483–490

Meehan RR, Gosden JR, Rout D, Hastie ND, Friedberg T, Adesnik M, Buckland R et al. (1988) Human cytochrome P-450 PB-1: a multigene family involved in mephenytoin and steroid oxidations that maps to chromosome 10. Am J Hum Genet 42:026–037

Meier UT, Meyer UA (1987) Genetic polymorphism of human cytochrome P-450 (S)-mephenytoin 4-hydroxylase. Studies with human autoantibodies suggest a functionally altered cytochrome P-450 isozyme as cause of the genetic deficiency. Biochemistry 26:8466–8474

Mellstrom B, Bertilsson L, Sawe J, Schulz H-U, Sjoqvist F (1981) E- and Z-10-hydroxylation of nortriptyline: relationship to polymorphic debrisoquine hydroxylation. Clin Pharmacol Ther 30:189–193

Nebert DW, Gonzales FJ (1987) P450 genes: structure, evolution, and regulation. Annu Rev Biochem 56:945–993

Oates NS, Shah RR, Drury PL, Idle JE, Smith RL (1982) Captopril-induced agranulocytosis associated with an impairment of debrisoquine hydroxylation. Br J Clin Pharmacol 14:601P

Oates NS, Shah RR, Idle JR, Smith RL (1983) Influence of oxidation polymorphism on phenformin kinetics and dynamics. Clin Pharmacol Ther 34:827–834

Oram M, Wilson K, Burnett D, Al-Dabbagh SG, Idle JR, Smith RL (1982) Metabolic oxidation of methaqualone in extensive and poor metabolisers of debrisoquine. Eur J Clin Pharmacol 23:147–150

Otton SV, Inaba T, Kalow W (1983) Inhibition of sparteine oxidation in human liver by tricyclic antidepressants and other drugs. Life Sci 32:795–800

Otton SV, Inaba T, Kalow W (1984) Competitive inhibition of sparteine oxidation in human liver by beta-adrenoceptor antagonists and other cardiovascular drugs. Life Sci 34:73–80

Otton SV, Brinn RU, Gram LF (1988) In vitro evidence against the oxidation of quinidine by the sparteine/debrisoquine monooxygenase of human liver. Drug Metab Dispos 16:15–17

Peart GF, Boutagy J, Shenfield GM (1987) Lack of relationship between tolbutamide and debrisoquine oxidation phenotype. Eur J Clin Pharmacol 33:397–402

Pierce DM, Smith SE, Franklin RA (1987) The pharmacokinetics of indoramin and 6-hydroxyindoramin in poor and extensive hydroxylators of debrisoquine. Eur J Clin Pharmacol 33:59–65

Poirier J, Roy M, Campanella G, Cloutier T, Paris S (1987) Debrisoquine metabolism in parkinsonian patients treated with antihistamine drugs. Lancet 2:386

Reilly PA, Tang BK, Stewart DJ, Kalow W (1983) The occurrence of two hepatic microsomal sites for amobarbital hydroxylation. Can J Physiol Pharmacol 61:67–71

Roden DM, Woosley RL (1988) Clinical pharmacokinetics of encainide. Clin Pharmacokinet 14:141–147

Roots I, Otte F, Berchtold C, Heinemeyer G, Schmidt D, Cornaggia C (1985) Debrisoquine phenotyping in epileptic patients treated with phenytoin and carbamazepine. Biochem Pharmacol 34:447–448

Roy SD, Hawes EM, McKay G, Korchinski ED, Midha KK (1985) Metabolism of methoxyphenamine in extensive and poor metabolizers of debrisoquin. Clin Pharmacol Ther 38:128–133

Saner H, Gurtner HP, Preising R, Kupfer A (1986) Polymorphic debrisoquine and mephenytoin hydroxylation in patients with pulmonary hypertension of vascular origin after aminorex fumarate. Eur J Clin Pharmacol 31:437–442

Schmid B, Bircher J, Preising R, Kupfer A (1985) Polymorphic dextromethorphan metabolism: co-segregation of oxidative O-demethylation with debrisoquin hydroxylation. Clin Pharmacol Ther 38:618–624

Shah RR, Oates NS, Idle JR, Smith RL, Lockhart JDF (1982) Impaired oxidation of debrisoquine in patients with perhexiline neuropathy. Br Med J 284:295–298

Siddoway LA, Thompson KA, McAllister CB, Wang T, Wilkinson GR, Roden DM, Woosley RL (1987) Polymorphism of propafenone metabolism and disposition in man: clinical and pharmacokinetic consequences. Circulation 75:785–791

Sjoqvist F, Bertilsson L (1986) Slow hydroxylation of tricyclic antidepressants – relationship to polymorphic drug oxidation. In: Kalow W, Goedde HW, Agarwal DP (eds) Ethnic differences in reactions to drugs and xenobiotics. Liss, New York, pp 169–188

Sloan TP, Mahgoub A, Lancaster R, Idle JR, Smith RL (1978) Polymorphism of carbon oxidation of drugs and clinical implications. Br Med J 2:655–657

Sloan TP, Lancaster R, Shah RR, Idle JR, Smith RL (1983) Genetically determined oxidation capacity and the disposition of debrisoquine. Br J Clin Pharmacol 15:443–450

Smith RL (1986a) Polymorphism in drug metabolism – implications for drug toxicity. Arch Toxicol [Suppl] 9:138–146

Smith RL (1986b) Introduction. Xenobiotica 16:361–365

Steiner E (1987) Polymorphic debrisoquine hydroxylation. Thesis, Karolinska Institute, Huddinge Hospital

Steiner E, Spina E (1987) Differences in the inhibitory effect of cimetidine on desipramine metabolism between rapid and slow debrisoquin hydroxylators. Clin Pharmacol Ther 42:278–282

Steiner E, Alvan G, Garle M, Maguire JH, Lind M, Nilson SO, Thomson T et al. (1987a) The debrisoquin hydroxylation phenotype does not predict the metabolism of phenytoin. Clin Pharmacol Ther 42:326–333

Steiner E, Dumont E, Spina E, Dahlqvist R (1987b) Inhibition of desipramine 2-hydroxylation by quinidine and quinine. Clin Pharmacol Ther 43:577–581

Syvalahti EKG, Lindberg R, Kallio J, de Vocht M (1986) Inhibitory effects of neuroleptics on debrisoquine oxidation in man. Br J Clin Pharmacol 22:89–92

Tait A (1987) In vitro metabolism of diazepam by human liver. Thesis, University of Toronto

Tyndale RF (1988) In vitro research into the genetic polymorphism of sparteine metbolism. Thesis, University of Toronto

Uetrecht JP, Sweetman B, Woosley R, Oates J (1984) Metabolism of procainamide to a hydroxylamine by rat and human hepatic microsomes. Drug Metab Dispos 12:77–81

Volk B, Amelizad Z, Anagnostopoulos J, Knoth R, Oesch F (1988) First evidence of cytochrome P-450 induction in the mouse brain by phenytoin. Neurosci Lett 84:219–224

Von Bahr C, Spina E, Birgersson C, Ericsson O, Goransson M, Henthorn T, Sjoqvist F (1985) Inhibition of desmethylimipramine 2-hydroxylation by drugs in human liver microsomes. Biochem Pharmacol 34:2501–2505

Von Bahr C, Birgersson C, Morgan ET, Eriksson O, Goransson M, Spina E, Woodhouse K (1986) Oxidation of tricyclic antidepressant drugs, debrisoquine and 7-ethoxyresorufin, by human liver preparations. Xenobiotica 16:391–400

Wagner F, Jahnchen E, Trenk D, Eichelbaum M, Harnasch P, Hauf G, Roskamm H (1987) Severe complications of antianginal drug therapy in a patient identified as a poor metabolizer of metoprolol, propafenone, diltiazem, and sparteine. Klin Wochenschr 65:1164–1168

Wakile LA, Sloan TP, Idle JR, Smith RL (1979) Genetic evidence for the involvement of different oxidative mechanisms in drug oxidation. J Pharm Pharmacol 31:350–352

Wang T, Roden DM, Wolfenden HT, Woosley RL, Wood AJJ, Wilkinson GR (1984) Influence of genetic polymorphism on the metabolism and disposition of encainide in man. J Pharmacol Exp Ther 228:605–611

Warner M, Kohler C, Hansson T, Gustafsson J-A (1988) Regional distribution of cytochrome P-450 in the rat brain: spectral quantitation and contribution of P-450b,e and P-450c,d. J Neurochem 50:1057–1065

Wiholm B-E, Alvan G, Bertilsson L, Sawe J, Sjoqvist F (1981) Hydroxylation of debrisoquine in patients with lacticacidosis after phenformin. Lancet 1:1098–1099

Wilkinson GR (1986) Genetic polymorphism of mephenytoin hydroxylation in man. In: Gorrod (ed) Development of drugs and modern medicines. Horwood, Chichester, pp 474–493

Wolff T, Strecker M (1985) Lack of relationship between debrisoquine 4-hydroxylation and other cytochrome P-450 dependent reactions in rat and human liver. Biochem Pharmacol 34:2593–2598

Wolff T, Distlerath LM, Worthington MT, Guengerich FP (1987) Human liver debrisoquine 4-hydroxylase: test for specifity toward various monooxygenase substrates and model of the active site. Arch Toxicol 60:89–90

Woodworth JR, Dennis SRK, Moore L, Rotenberg KS (1987) The polymorphic metabolism of dextromethorphan. J Clin Pharmacol 27:139–143

Zekorn C, Achtert G, Hausleiter HJ, Moon CH, Eichelbaum M (1985) Pharmacokinetics of N-propylajmaline in relation to polymorphic sparteine oxidation. Klin Wochenschr 63:1180–1186

The Use of Human Liver Banks in Pharmacogenetic Research *

C. VON BAHR, F. P. GUENGERICH, G. MOVIN, and C. NORDIN [1]

1 Introduction

The plasma concentrations of certain drugs have been shown to exhibit very large differences following similar standard doses, leading to different effects of, for example, tricyclic antidepressant drugs. This report will attempt to show how simple in vitro experiments may give valuable information as to the in vivo interindividual variability in drug metabolism kinetics in man, which enzymes are involved in the metabolism of a drug, and clinically important metabolic interaction potentials.

2 Methods

Livers from our human liver bank were used, microsomes prepared (von Bahr et al. 1980), and the formation of desipramine from imipramine and 2-hydroxydesipramine from desipramine in microsomal incubations were measured (Spina et al. 1984).

3 Results and Discussion

3.1 Plasma Levels of Desipramine in Patients

After a standard dose of desipramine the steady-state plasma levels vary markedly between subjects (Hammer and Sjöqvist 1967). Some patients show very high levels and are more prone to side effects. Such subjects have been shown to be slow hydroxylators of the antihypertensive drug debrisoquine (Sjöqvist 1988). About 10% of Caucasian subjects have a poor ability to

* This study was supported by grants from the Swedish Natural Science Research Council (B-TF 9202-100) and by funds from the Karolinska Institute.
[1] Department of Clinical Pharmacology, Astra Research Centre, S-15185 Södertälje, and Departments of Clinical Pharmacology and Psychiatry at Huddinge Hospital, Karolinska Institute, 14186 Huddinge, Sweden

Clinical Pharmacology in Psychiatry
Editors: S. G. Dahl and L. F. Gram
(Psychopharmacology Series 7)
© Springer-Verlag Berlin Heidelberg 1989

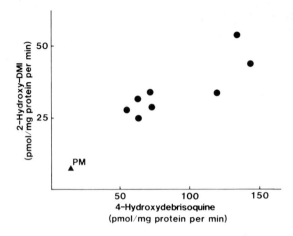

Fig. 1. Relationship between debrisoquine 4-hydroxylation and desipramine (*DMI*) 2-hydroxylation in microsomes from nine different human livers. *PM*, Poor in vivo metabolizer of debrisoquine, having a debrisoquine/4-hydroxydebrisoquine urinary ratio of 50. (From von Bahr et al. 1986)

hydroxylate this drug (Mahgoub et al. 1977), due to an inherited recessive trait (Price-Evans et al. 1980). We have shown that the hydroxylation of desipramine follows the debrisoquine phenotype in vivo (Spina et al. 1984). Desmethylimipramine and debrisoquine are probably hydroxylated by the same cytochrome P-450 isoenzyme.

3.2 Correlation Between Desipramine and Debrisoquine Hydroxylation in Human Liver Microsomes

We have incubated debrisoquine and desipramine with liver microsomes from several human subjects. The rates of 4-hydroxylation of debrisoquine and 2-hydroxylation of desipramine varied markedly among the livers. This variation in enzyme activity is probably the main determinant of the large variation in plasma levels of desipramine in vivo. The two metabolic activities correlated with each other (Fig. 1). A liver from a "poor" in vivo hydroxylator of debrisoquine had an unusually low capacity to hydroxylate both drugs in vitro.

A good correlation between two reactions indicates that they may be catalysed by the same enzyme, but this is not proof, as two enzymes regulated in common may be involved. Inhibition and antibody studies can clarify this further (see below).

The *N*-demethylation of imipramine in different human liver microsomes does not correlate well with the hydroxylation of debrisoquine and desipramine hydroxylation (von Bahr et al. 1986). However, microsomes from a slow in vivo hydroxylator of debrisoquine had a low capacity to demethylate imipramine. A poor correlation does not exclude the possibility that the drugs are metabolized by the same enzyme, but in this case it is likely that at least one additional enzyme is involved.

3.3 Inhibition Studies with "Genetic Marker Drugs"

When a drug, at defined in vitro conditions, is metabolized almost exclusively by one enzyme, inhibition studies may provide a useful indication of whether other compounds are metabolized by that enzyme. Drugs that can be regarded as "marker drugs" for the enzyme debrisoquine hydroxylase, also known as cytochrome P-450db1 (Gonzales et al. 1988), include debrisoquine (Boobis et al. 1983), sparteine (Inaba et al. 1985) and bufuralol (Gut et al. 1986). We have used desipramine as a marker drug (von Bahr et al. 1985). Debrisoquine competitively inhibited the 2-hydroxylation of desipramine (Fig. 2). Conversely, desipramine inhibited the 4-hydroxylation of debrisoquine with an IC_{50} value of $35\ \mu M$. This indicates that the two reactions are catalysed by the same cytochrome P-450 isoenzyme. The combination of (a) a good correlation between the hydroxylations of desipramine and debrisoquine in various livers and (b) these inhibition data strongly indicates that debrisoquine hydroxylase is of major importance for the hydroxylation of desipramine. The fact that the hydroxylation of desipramine co-varies with the debrisoquine hydroxylation in vivo in man supports this (Spina et al. 1984).

Interestingly, imipramine inhibited the desipramine hydroxylation competitively (not shown). Debrisoquine inhibits the demethylation of imipramine (von Bahr et al. 1986). These data indicate that imipramine interacts with debrisoquine or desipramine hydroxylase. The fairly poor correlation between imipramine N-demethylation, on the one hand, and the hydroxylation of debrisoquine and desipramine on the other (von Bahr et al. 1986) indicates, however, that this N-demethylation is mainly catalysed by at least one other enzyme. Recent in vivo data in man showed that this seems to be the case (Brøsen et al. 1986). We have shown that purified debrisoquine or "desipramine hydroxylase" can catalyse the N-demethylation of imipramine, but at a slow rate (Birgersson et al. 1986). Also the 2-hydroxylation of imipramine seems to be influenced by the slow phenotype of sparteine (and thereby debrisoquine) metabolism (Brøsen et al. 1986). This example il-

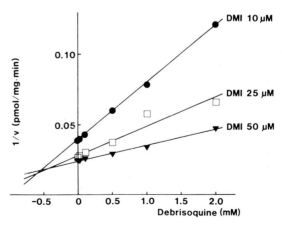

Fig. 2. Effect of different concentrations of debrisoquine on the rate (v) of 2-hydroxylation from different concentrations of desipramine (*DMI*) in human liver microsomes. Dixon plot. (From von Bahr et al. 1986)

Table 1. Effect of neuroleptic drugs on 2-hydroxylation of desipramine in human liver microsomes

Compound (10 µM)	% of control[a]
Haloperidol	69
Perphenazine	18
Chlorpromazine	54
Thioridazine	12

[a] Microsomes were incubated with 25 µM desipramine.

lustrates that a drug can inhibit a marker reaction even if it is metabolized mainly by other enzymes.

The antiarrhythmic drug quinidine markedly inhibits the hydroxylation of desipramine in vitro (von Bahr et al. 1985). Steiner et al. (1987) showed later that this was also true in vivo. Quinine also inhibited desipramine hydroxylation in vitro and in vivo, but less efficiently than quinidine. Quinidine is not itself metabolized to any detectable degree by the enzyme (Guengerich et al. 1986). This shows that in vitro experiments with human liver can predict important clinical interactions with an enzyme, even if the compound itself is not metabolized by the enzyme.

Table 1 shows that the neuroleptic drugs haloperidol, perphenazine, chlorpromazine and thioridazine inhibit the hydroxylation of desipramine in

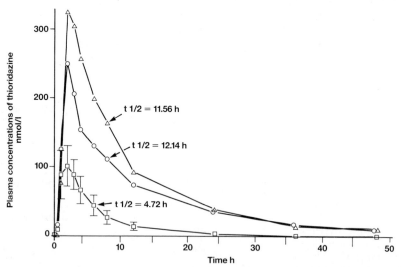

Fig. 3. Plasma concentrations of thioridazine following a single oral dose of thioridazine (25-mg tablet) in 13 rapid (mean ± SD) and 2 slow hydroxylators of debrisoquine. Apparent plasma half-lives ($t\,\frac{1}{2}$) are depicted

human livers in vitro. Gram and Overø (1972) have shown that perphenazine inhibits the in vivo hydroxylation of nortriptyline in man. Nortriptyline is 10-hydroxylated by debrisoquine hydroxylase (von Bahr et al. 1983). Haloperidol also inhibits the oxidation of sparteine in man (Gram and Brøsen, this volume). Thioridazine markedly increases the plasma levels of desipramine in man, probably by inhibiting the metabolism of desipramine (Hirschowitz et al. 1983). Thioridazine also increases the ratio between debrisoquine and 4-hydroxydebrisoquine in the urine, indicating inhibition of the enzyme (Syvälahti et al. 1986). These data are not sufficient to predict whether or not thioridazine itself is metabolized to any quantitatively important degree by the debrisoquine or desipramine hydroxylase. Therefore we included to slow hydroxylators of debrisoquine in a pharmacokinetic study on thioridazine. Figure 3 shows that the two poor hydroxylators of debrisoquine had much higher plasma levels of thioridazine than the rapid hydroxylators. The active metabolite, thioridazine side-chain sulphoxide (mesoridazine), appeared in blood more slowly and had a longer half-life in slow hydroxylators of debrisoquine (not shown). In this case in vitro inhibition studies were able to predict in vivo drug metabolic inhibition. Complementary in vivo studies in man showed that the metabolism of thioridazine was markedly influenced by the debrisoquine hydroxylation phenotype.

3.4 Inhibition Studies with Antibodies

Distlerath and Guengerich (1984) and Wolff et al. (1985) have used an antibody against the rat debrisoquine hydroxylase that specifically inhibits the human liver debrisoquine hydroxylase but not other cytochrome P-450 forms. This antibody almost completely (>75%) inhibited the in vitro oxidation of

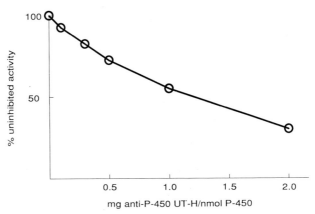

Fig. 4. Anti-rat P-450 antibody inhibition of 2-hydroxylation of desipramine by human liver microsomes. The antibody against rat debrisoquine hydroxylase (*UT-H*) was added to human liver microsomes in increasing concentrations. Pre-immune IgG fractions did not inhibit the desipramine hydroxylation. The antibodies were the same as those used by Distlerath and Guengerich (1984)

debrisoquine and sparteine in human liver, only partly inhibited (30%–70%) the oxidation of propranolol and encainide, and did not significantly inhibit (<15%) the o-deethylation of phenacetin or the 4-hydroxylation of S-mephenytoin. These two latter reactions are catalysed by other cytochrome P-450 isozymes (Distlerath et al. 1985; Meier and Meyer 1987). Figure 4 shows that this antibody against debrisoquine hydroxylase inhibited the 2-hydroxylation of desipramine (about 70%) in human liver microsomes, indicating that debrisoquine hydroxylase is of major importance for desipramine metabolism.

These data show that such antibodies can give information on how much an individual cytochrome P-450 form contributes to the overall microsomal metabolism of a compound. Such information is of value for quantitative predictions of the role of a certain cytochrome P-450 for the kinetics of a drug in vivo in man. If it is known that the metabolism of a drug is almost completely inhibited by an antibody that is monospecific to one enzyme, and if it already is known how the activity of this enzyme varies among patients, reliable predictions of the variability in the kinetics of a new drug can be made from in vitro experiments.

3.5 Metabolism by Purified Enzyme

Debrisoquine hydroxylase has been purified from human liver. The purified cytochrome can hydroxylate debrisoquine and bufuralol (Distlerath et al. 1985; Gut et al. 1986). We have also purified this enzyme and have found that it hydroxylates desipramine (Birgersson et al. 1986). The purified enzyme could also N-demethylate imipramine, but at a slow rate. The fact that a purified enzyme can metabolize a certain compound is proof that an enzyme can catalyse a specified reaction. However, this approach could be cumbersome since it is very difficult to purify cytochrome P-450 from human liver. A large amount of liver is needed, which is not readily available to most investigators.

3.6 Combined Use of Inhibition Studies and Antibodies

There are four in vitro approaches that can be used for the evaluation of whether a drug is metabolized by a known enzyme:

– Correlation between a new reaction and a "marker reaction" for an enzyme
– Inhibition of a "marker reaction" by a new compound
– Inhibition of a new reaction by a monospecific antibody
– Metabolism by a purified enzyme

The "correlation approach" with incubation of two drugs in many livers is useful and seems to predict correlations occurring in vivo. By including livers from subjects who have been phenotyped in vivo, the approach proves even stronger, especially if livers lacking a polymorphically regulated enzyme are included. Tissue from subjects exposed to environmental chemicals are also of value. This approach may be difficult for most investigators, since tissue from many donors are needed.

Inhibition studies in human liver microsomes with marker drugs are very useful for screening if a compound can interact with a certain enzyme. They also seem to have good predictive value for drug metabolic interactions occurring in vivo. The approach is simple, and material from only a few livers is needed. Furthermore, only one analytical method for screening several compounds is needed.

Inhibition studies in intact human liver microsomes with monospecific antibodies are very useful for evaluation if an enzyme catalyses a reaction. With knowledge of how this enzyme behaves in vivo, many predictions of kinetics in vivo can be made. The drawback is that it may be hard to produce monospecific inhibitory antibodies in enough quantities in a standardized way. In a few years monoclonal inhibitory antibodies will probably be available for more general use.

Work with purified human enzymes is useful, but difficult and costly. This approach enables the making of antibodies and synthesizing of oligonucleotide probes deduced from amino acid sequences. These are useful for evaluating the genetic mechanism regulating the enzymes (see below).

We recommend the combined use of inhibition studies with marker drugs and inhibitory antibody studies with human liver microsomes as a simple approach to determine whether compounds are metabolized by a certain enzyme. Many compounds can be screened easily. Only one method for analyses of a metabolite and only a few livers are needed to obtain substantial information that is predictive for the in vivo situation.

4 Future Possibilities

As shown above, the human liver bank can easily be used to identify whether a compound is metabolized by a known enzyme, e.g. debrisoquine hydroxylase.

By examination of several livers one may occasionally find "outliers" with unusually low or high activity. The latter may be due to metabolism by an induced enzyme. A very low activity may be due to an abnormal or lacking enzyme that is polymorphically regulated. The debrisoquine hydroxylation polymorphism could probably be identified in this way.

We have identified a new human liver glutathione S-transferase (μ) and have found it to be present in only some livers (Warholm et al. 1980). Board (1981) has shown that this is due to a genetic polymorphism of the enzyme (GST_1). Similarly, by performing in vitro experiments with several human livers, Price-Evans and White (1964) showed that the in vivo polymorphic acetylation of sulphamethazine and isonidazide was due to a polymorphism in the activity of acetyltransferase in the liver.

Modern enzyme-characterizing and molecular biology techniques simplify the analyses of hereditary traits responsible for abnormal drug metabolism.

By purifying the enzymes antibodies can be made, amino acid sequences determined, and oligonucleotide probes deduced from these and synthesized. With these techniques, cDNA and expression libraries can be screened and cDNA for the enzyme cloned. Gonzalez et al. (1988) have used such approaches and characterized the molecular mechanisms behind debrisoquine hydroxylation. Such approaches can be used to clarify the relationship between phenotype and genotype and to elucidate whether a deficient enzyme activity is due to a lacking or an abnormal enzyme. Further work is needed to elucidate whether probes against DNA isolated from peripheral blood cells can be used as a simple diagnostic test for poor hydroxylation of debrisoquine. If this is possible, patients at risk for dose-dependent adverse reactions could easily be identified prior to therapy and given lower drug doses.

Acknowledgement. We wish to thank Dr Anders Lidén for analysing the thioridazine plasma levels.

References

Birgersson C, Morgan ET, Jörnvall H, von Bahr C (1986) Purification of a demethylimipramine and debrisoquine hydroxylating cytochrome P-450 from human liver. Biochem Pharmacol 35:3165–3166

Board PG (1981) Biochemical genetics of glutathione-S-transferase in man. Am J Human Genet 33:36–43

Boobis AR, Murray S, Kahn GC, Robertz G-M, Davies DS (1983) Substrate specificity of the form of cytochrome P-450 catalyzing the 4-hydroxylation of debrisoquine in man. Mol Pharmacol 23:474–481

Brøsen K, Otton V, Gram L (1986) Imipramine demethylation and hydroxylation: impact of the sparteine oxidation phenotype. Clin Pharmacol Ther 40:543–549

Distlerath LM, Guengerich FP (1984) Characterization of a human liver cytochrome P-450 involved in the oxidation of debrisoquine and other drugs by using antibodies raised to the analogous rat enzyme. Proc Natl Acad Sci USA 81:7348–7352

Distlerath LM, Reilly PEB, Martin MV, Davies GG, Wilkinson GR, Guengerich FP (1985) Purification and characterization of the human liver cytochromes P-450 involved in debrisoquine prototypes for genetic polymorphism in oxidative drug metabolism. J Biol Chem 260:9057–9067

Gonzalez FJ, Skoda RC, Kimura S, Umeno M, Zanger UM, Nebert DW, Gelboin HV et al. (1988) Characterization of the common genetic defect in humans deficient in debrisoquine metabolism. Nature 331:442–446

Gram LF, Overø FK (1972) Drug interaction: inhibitory effect of neuroleptics on metabolism of tricyclic antidepressants in man. Br Med J 1:463–465

Guengerich FP, Müller-Enoch D, Blair IA (1986) Oxidation of quinidine by human liver cytochrome P-450. Mol Pharmacol 30:287–295

Gut J, Catin T, Dager P, Kronbach T, Zanger U, Meyer UA (1986) Debrisoquine/sparteine-type polymorphism of drug oxidation. J Biol Chem 261:11734–11743

Hammer W, Sjöqvist F (1967) Plasma levels of monomethylated tricyclic antidepressants during treatment with imipramine-like compounds. Life Sci 6:1895–1903

Hirschowitz J, Bennett JA, Zemlan FP, Garrer DL (1983) Thioridazine effect on desipramine plasma levels. J Clin Psychopharmacol 3:376–379

Inaba T, Jurima M, Mahon WA, Kalow W (1985) In vitro inhibition studies of two isozymes of human liver cytochrome P-450. Mephenytoin p-hydroxylase and sparteine monooxygenase. Drug Metab Dispos 13:443–448

Mahgoub A, Idle JR, Dring LG, Lancaster R, Smith RL (1977) Polymorphic hydroxylation of debrisoquine in man. Lancet 2:584–586

Meier UT, Meyer VA (1987) Genetic polymorphism of human cytochrome P-450 (S)-mephenytoin 4-hydroxylase. Studies with human antibodies suggest a functionally altered cytochrome P-450 isozyme as a cause of the genetic deficiency. Biochemistry 26:8466–8474

Price-Evans DA, White TA (1964) Human acetylation polymorphism. J Lab Clin Med 63:394–403

Price-Evans DA, Mahgoub A, Sloan TP, Idle JR, Smith RL (1980) A family and population study of the genetic polymorphism of debrisoquine oxidation in a white British population. J Med Genet 17:102–105

Sjöqvist F (1988) Slow drug hydroxylation – implications for patient management and drug utilization. 2nd International ISSX Meeting, Kobe

Spina E, Birgersson C, von Bahr C, Ericsson Ö, Mellström B, Steiner E, Sjöqvist F (1984) Phenotypic consistency in hydroxylation of demethylimipramine and debrisoquine in healthy subjects and in human liver microsomes. Clin Pharmacol Ther 36:677–682

Steiner E, Dumont E, Spina E, Dahlqvist R (1987) Inhibition of desipramine 2-hydroxylation by quinidine and quinine. Clin Pharmacol Ther 43:577–581

Syvählahti EKG, Lindberg R, Kallio J, de Vocht M (1986) Inhibitory effects of neuroleptics on debrisoquine oxidation in man. Br J Clin Pharmacol 22:89–92

Von Bahr C, Groth C-G, Jansson H, Lundgren H, Lind M, Glaumann H (1980) Drug metabolism in human liver in vitro: establishment of a human liver bank. Clin Pharmacol Ther 27:711–725

Von Bahr C, Birgersson C, Blanck A, Göransson M, Mellström B, Nilsell K (1983) Correlation between nortriptyline and debrisoquine hydroxylation in the human liver. Life Sci 33:631–636

Von Bahr C, Spina E, Birgersson C, Göransson M, Henthorn T, Sjöqvist F (1985) Inhibition of desmethylimipramine 2-hydroxylation by drugs in human liver microsomes. Biochem Pharmacol 34:2501–2505

Von Bahr C, Birgersson C, Morgan ET, Eriksson Ö, Göransson M, Spina E, Woodhouse K (1986) Oxidation of tricyclic antidepressant drugs, debrisoquine and 7-ethoxyresorufin by human liver preparations. Xenobiotica 16:391–400

Warholm M, Gutenberg C, Mannervik B, von Bahr C, Glaumann H (1980) Identification of a new glutathione S-transferase in human liver. Acta Chem Scand [B] 34:607–610

Wolff T, Distlerath LM, Worthington MT, Groopman JP, Hammons GJ, Kadlubar FF, Prough RA, et al. (1985) Substrate specificity of human liver cytochrome P-450 debrisoquine 4-hydroxylase probed using immunochemical inhibitor and chemical modeling. Cancer Res 45:2116–2122

Inhibitors of the Microsomal Oxidation of Psychotropic Drugs: Selectivity and Clinical Significance

L. F. GRAM and K. BRØSEN [1]

1 Introduction

The use of human liver microsomal preparations as a tool in drug metabolism research has potentials in a number of areas, not least in pharmacogenetics. The testing of different compounds for their ability competitively to inhibit the oxidation of model compounds such as sparteine/debrisoquine or mephenytoin is a particularly useful primary screening procedure (Otton et al. 1983, 1984; Boobis et al. 1983; von Bahr et al. 1985; Inaba et al. 1984, 1985; see Table 1). Substances not acting as inhibitors of the sparteine/debrisoquine

Table 1. The sparteine/debrisoquine oxygenase: in vitro competitive inhibitors and co-segregation in phenotyped subjects

In vitro inhibition	In vivo co-segregation	Drug examples
−	−	Antipyrine Mephenytoin Sulphamethazine
−	+	?
+	+	Tricyclics Metoprolol Timolol
+	−	Quinidine? Haloperidol?

oxygenase can safely be excluded as substrates of this P450 isozyme and will, accordingly, not exhibit the corresponding monogenetic polymorphism in metabolism in vivo. There appear to be no false negatives contradicting this assumption. However, if a compound is extensively bound to tissue components in the in vitro preparation, apparent high K_i values may lead to the erroneous conclusion that the compound is a weak in vitro inhibitor. Among the substances that act as competitive inhibitors of this oxygenase (Table 1), several different tricyclic antidepressants and β-blockers are notable substrates of this oxygenase and show in vivo the corresponding oxidation

[1] Department of Clinical Pharmacology, School of Medicine, Odense University, J. B. Winsløws Vej 19, 5000 Odense C, Denmark

Clinical Pharmacology in Psychiatry
Editors: S. G. Dahl and L. F. Gram
(Psychopharmacology Series 7)
© Springer-Verlag Berlin Heidelberg 1989

polymorphism, at least for one metabolic pathway. The in vitro inhibition is also reflected in vivo: imipramine treatment caused a moderate increase in sparteine and debrisoquine metabolic ratio (MR) in patients, without changing their phenotype (Brøsen et al. 1986).

Cimetidine is a nonspecific, potent in vivo inhibitor of the oxidation of many drugs (Somogyi and Gugler 1982), including some psychotropic drugs such as diazepam (Klotz and Reimann 1980) and imipramine (Wells et al. 1986). Cimetidine is not a potent in vitro inhibitor of the sparteine/debrisoquine oxygenase or the mephenytoin oxygenase (Inaba et al. 1985) and appears to act by non-substrate binding to the heme moiety of different P450 isozymes. Cimetidine is not discussed further in this chapter.

2 Quinidine

As shown in Table 2, some drugs, in particular quinidine, are extremely potent inhibitors of the sparteine/debrisoquine oxygenase. This inhibitor potency was reflected in vivo in patients on therapeutic quinidine doses (600–800 mg/day) with quinidine plasma concentrations of 2–7 μM, who were transformed into phenotypically poor metabolizers with practically abolished oxidation of sparteine or debrisoquine (Fig. 1; Brinn et al. 1986; Brøsen et al. 1987). Data from volunteer studies (Boobis et al. 1988) indicate that quinidine doses as low as 5 mg can cause an increase in the sparteine or debrisoquine MR by a factor of 2–6. It can be inferred from these studies that quinidine

Table 2. Potency of various drugs acting as competitive inhibitors of the sparteine/debrisoquine oxygenase

Drug	Apparent K_i (μM)	Substrate[a]	Reference
Amitriptyline	50	SP	Otton et al. (1983)
Nortriptyline	15	SP	Otton et al. (1983)
Imipramine	40	SP	Otton et al. (1983)
Desipramine	8	SP	Otton et al. (1983)
Chlorpromazine	7	SP	Inaba et al. (1985)
Chlorpromazine	6	DMI	v. Bahr et al. (1985)
Thioridazine	0.75	DMI	v. Bahr et al. (1985)
Haloperidol	1	SP	Inaba et al. (1985)
Metoprolol	18	SP	Otton et al. (1984)
Propranolol	15	SP	Otton et al. (1984)
Timolol	18	SP	Otton et al. (1984)
Bufarolol	7	DB	Boobis et al. (1983)
Quinidine	0.06	SP	Otton et al. (1984)
Quinidine	0.07	DB	Inaba et al. (1984)

[a] Substrate: SP, sparteine; DMI, desipramine; DB, debrisoquine.

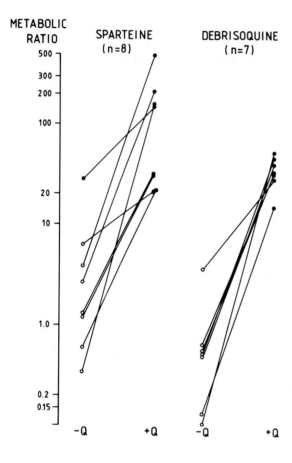

Fig. 1. Patients' metabolic ratio of sparteine and debrisoquine before ($-Q$) and during ($+Q$) treatment with quinidine (600–800 mg/day). *Open circles,* before quinidine ($-Q$); *filled circles,* during quinidine ($+Q$). (Data from Brinn et al. 1986, for sparteine; Brøsen et al. 1987, for debrisoquine)

Table 3. Studies on the role of the sparteine/debrisoquine oxygenase for the oxidation of quinidine

Human liver microsomal preparations:	No effect of sparteine on the formation of 3-OH-quinidine or the overall disappearance rate of quinidine (Otton et al. 1988)
Panel study in sparteine extensive ($n=3$) and poor metabolizers ($n=3$)	No difference in total clearance after single intravenous dose of quinidine (Mikus et al. 1986)
Panel study in sparteine extensive ($n=4$) and poor metabolizers ($n=4$)	No difference in total clearance but 20% lower 3-OH-clearance in poor metabolizers after single oral dose of quinidine (Brøsen et al. (1989)
Steady-state levels in quinidine-treated patients phenotyped prior to treatment	3-OH-Quinidine/quinidine ratio lower in a poor metabolizers (0.09; $n=1$) than in any of the extensive metabolizers (0.10–0.53; $n=7$) (Brinn et al. 1986)

doses of 100–200 mg/day are sufficient to increase the MR by a factor of about 50. To what extent quinidine is a substrate of the sparteine/ debrisoquine oxygenase has been examined in several studies (Table 3). Generally, these studies suggest that quinidine is eliminated via other routes, but it appears possible that 3-OH-quinidine formation may be mediated via the sparteine/debrisoquine oxygenase, at least partly.

Since quinidine acts as an inhibitor at very low concentrations, it may be expected that a selective blockade of the sparteine/debrisoquine oxygenase can be obtained at these low concentrations. So far only few studies have addressed the question of selectivity in inhibitory action. The metabolism of antipyrine, which is an established non-substrate of the sparteine/ debrisoquine oxygenase (Inaba et al. 1985; Bertilsson et al. 1980) has been shown not to be influenced by quinidine (Boobis, personal communication). In a recent volunteer study with single doses of imipramine and desipramine (Brøsen and Gnam 1989), we found that co-administration of quinidine (200 mg/day) to extensive metabolizers of sparteine leads to a quite precise mimicking of the pattern of metabolism seen in poor metabolizers, i.e. a drastically reduced rate of 2-hydroxylation and an unchanged or slightly reduced imipramine demethylation. Quinidine at low doses thus appears to be a promising tool for testing oxidation of a drug via the sparteine/debrisoquine oxygenase, but a wider testing of its selectivity is required (Speirs et al. 1986; Brøsen and Gnam).

3 Neuroleptics

As shown in Table 2, several neuroleptics are potent in vitro inhibitors of the sparteine/debrisoquine oxygenase. In the following, the questions of in vivo potency, inhibitor selectivity, and the extent to which the neuroleptics are a substrate of the sparteine/debrisoquine oxygenase will be discussed.

Sylvälahti et al. (1986) carried out debrisoquine tests in a large sample of psychiatric patients and compared the results for groups on different psychotropic medication. A striking finding was that patients on levo- mepromazine or thioridazine had a much higher MR with about 40% of the patients appearing as phenotypically poor metabolizers. Patients on other drugs (antidepressants, benzodiazepines, antiepileptics) showed normal MR values.

In a recent study at the University of Caen in France (Gram et al. 1989), this problem was addressed by carrying out sparteine tests before (MR_c) and during (MR_d) haloperidol administration, given in an initial fixed dose (10 mg/day) for 1 week and then at a dose two to four times higher. A linear relationship between the haloperidol plasma level and the log MR_d/MR_c was found. At the highest haloperidol levels (60–80 nM) the MR increased by a factor of about 50. No extensive metabolizers were transformed to poor metabolizers in this study.

Table 4. Inhibition of the sparteine oxygenase: inhibitor concentrations in vitro and in vivo

	In vitro	In vivo	
	(human liver) K_i (nM)	Free plasma concentration (nM)	Degree of inhibition (MR_d/MR_c)
Quinidine	60[a]	100[b]	50[b]
Haloperidol	1 000[a]	8[c]	50[c]

[a] Inaba et al. (1985).
[b] Brinn et al. (1986); Boobis et al. (1988).
[c] Gram et al. (1989).
Free plasma concentrations have been estimated on the basis of data reported in the literature on protein binding: free fraction of quinidine $\sim 20\%$ (Ochs et al. 1980), free fraction of haloperidol $\sim 10\%$ (Jørgensen 1986). MR, Metabolic ratio = (excretion of sparteine)/(excretion of dehydrosparteines) before drug treatment (control, MR_c) and during drug treatment (drug, MR_d).

As shown in Table 4, the in vivo potency assessed from the free plasma concentration appeared to be much higher for haloperidol than for quinidine. This is in marked contrast to the in vitro data, which suggest that quinidine is by far the more potent inhibitor. We can not readily explain these results, which illustrate the general problems in transferring in vitro experimental concentrations to clinically effective concentrations (Gram et al. 1987). The lack of direct concentration measurements in the in vitro setting and the unknown ratio between free blood concentration and intrahepatocyte concentration are some of the factors to be accounted for.

The haloperidol steady-state level on the initial fixed dose was about the same in one poor metabolizer and in nine extensive metabolizers (all phenotyped before treatment). This could indicate that haloperidol is not metabolized to any extent by the sparteine/debrisoquine oxygenase, but larger patient samples or panels will be required to settle this issue definitely. As reported recently (von Bahr et al., this volume; Dahl-Puustinen et al. 1988), data on thioridazine and perphenazine suggest a co-segregation with the sparteine/debrisoquine oxidation.

4 Neuroleptics as Inhibitors of the Metabolism of Antidepressants

The dominant role of the sparteine/debrisoquine oxygenase in the hydroxylation of tricyclic antidepressants and the inhibitory effect of neuroleptics on this P450 isozyme points back to the observations we made in the early 1970s, that neuroleptics are potent inhibitors of the metabolism of tricyclic antidepressants (Gram et al. 1971; Gram and Overø 1972; Gram 1975). These findings have subsequently been confirmed by several groups (Olivier-Martin et al. 1975; Vandel et al. 1979; Nelson and Jatlow 1980; Siris et al.

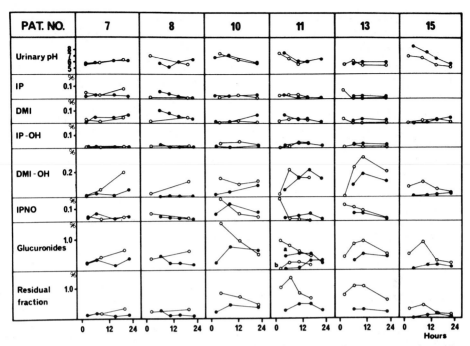

Fig. 2. Urinary excretion of imipramine/desipramine, the primary non-conjugated metabolites and the glucuronide fraction after single doses of [^{14}C]imipramine or [^{14}C]desipramine in patients 1 h before (o—o) and during treatment with perphenazine (•—•). *IP*, Imipramine; *DMI*, desipramine; *IP-OH*, 2-OH-imipramine; *DMI-OH*, 2-OH-desipramine; *IPNO*, imipramine-neoxide. (From Gram 1975)

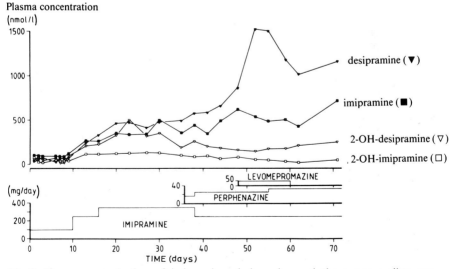

Fig. 3. Plasma concentration of imipramine, desipramine and the corresponding non-conjugated 2-hydroxymetabolites during imipramine treatment before and during concomitant treatment with perphenazine and levopromazine. (From Brøsen et al. 1986)

1982). Several neuroleptics, both phenothiazines, thioxanthenes, and butyrophenones appear to be potent inhibitors of the metabolism of typical tricyclic antidepressants, such as imipramine, desipramine, amitriptyline and nortriptyline. These neuroleptics include chlorpromazine, perphenazine, thioridazine, levomepromazine, fluphenazine, chlorprothixene and haloperidol. Studies on the effect of perphenazine on formation and excretion of metabolites of imipramine and desipramine suggested that the major effect was an inhibition of the 2-hydroxylation of imipramine and, in particular, desipramine (Fig. 2; Gram 1975). This has been confirmed in studies on imipramine metabolite levels in plasma (Brøsen et al. 1986). These studies also showed that the demethylation of imipramine, leading to formation of desipramine, was unaffected by the co-administration of neuroleptics (Fig. 3). These findings are compatible with the view that the neuroleptics act as relatively selective inhibitors of the sparteine/debrisoquine oxygenase. Since the earliest report on this interaction using steady-state plasma level measurements (Gram 1977; Nelson and Jatlow 1980), it has become clear that this effect of neuroleptics is often quite pronounced. In elderly depressed patients given additional treatment with perphenazine 8–16 mg/day, a 50%–200% increase in steady-state levels of imipramine plus desipramine or nortriptyline was seen (Gram et al. 1984).

In conclusion, neuroleptics cause a pharmacokinetically well documented and clinically significant inhibition of the metabolism of tricyclic antidepressants. In light of the frequent use of this drug combination, particularly in delusional depressions (Gram et al. 1984), it is strange that this interaction is not generally acknowledged. Even in recent issues or leading textbooks on pharmacotherapy (Gilman et al. 1985; Speight 1987), no mention of this interaction may be found.

References

Bertilsson L, Eichelbaum M, Mellström B, Säwe J, Schulz H-U, Sjöqvist F (1980) Nortriptyline and antipyrine clearance in relation to the debrisoquine hydroxylation in man. Life Sci 27:1673–1677

Boobis AR, Murray S, Kahn GC, Robertz G-M, Davies DS (1983) Substrate specificity of the form of cytochrome P-450 catalysing the 4-hydroxylation of debrisoquine in man. Mol Pharmacol 23:474–481

Boobis A, Edwards RJ, Singleton A, Sesardic D, Murray B, Speirs CJ, Murray S, et al. (1988) The contribution of polymorphic isozymes of cytochrome P-450 to the pharmacokinetics and toxicity of foreign compounds in man. In: Miners J, Birkett DJ, Drew R, McManus M (eds) Microsomes and drug oxidation. Taylor and Francis, London, pp 216–223

Brinn R, Brøsen K, Gram LF, Haghfelt T, Otton SV (1986) Sparteine oxidation is practically abolished in quinidine-treated patients. Br J Clin Pharmacol 22:194–197

Brøsen K, Gram LF, (1989) Quinidine potently inhibits the 2-hydroxylation of imipramine and desipramine, but not the demethylation of imipramine. Eur J Clin Pharmacol (in press)

Brøsen K, Gram LF, Klysner R, Bech P (1986) Steady-state levels of imipramine and its metabolites: significance of dose-dependent kinetics. Eur J Clin Pharmacol 30:43–49

Brøsen K, Gram LF, Haghfelt T, Bertilsson L (1987) Extensive metabolizers of debrisoquine become poor metabolizers during quinidine treatment. Pharmacol Toxicol 60:312–314

Brøsen K, Davidsen F, Gram LF (1989) Quinidine kinetics after a single oral dose in relation to the sparteine oxidation polymorphism in man. (submitted)

Dahl-Puustinen M-L, Lidén A, Bertilsson L (1988) Disposition of perphenazine in man – relationship to polymorphic debrisoquine hydroxylation (Poster). 5th International Meeting on Clinical Pharmacology in Psychiatry, Tromsø

Gilman AG, Goodman LS, Rall TW, Murad F (eds) (1987) The pharmacological basis of therapeutics, 7th edn. Macmillan, New York

Gram LF (1975) Effects of perphenazine on imipramine metabolism in man. Psychopharmacol Commun 1:165–175

Gram LF (1977) Effect of neuroleptics on the metabolism of tricyclic antidepressants. In: Deniker P, Radouco-Thomas C, Villeneuve A (eds) Neuropsychopharmacology. Pergamon, New York, pp 1061–1062

Gram LF, Overø FK (1972) Drug interaction: inhibitory effect of neuroleptics on the metabolism of tricyclic antidepressants in man. Br Med J 1:165–175

Gram LF, Kofod B, Christiansen J, Rafaelsen OJ (1971) Drug interaction: inhibitory effect of neuroleptics on metabolism of tricyclic antidepressants in man. In: Vinar O, Votava Z, Bradley PB (eds) Advances in neuropsychopharmacology. North-Holland, Amsterdam, pp 447–452

Gram LF, Kragh-Sørensen P, Kristensen CB, Møller M, Pedersen OL, Thayssen P (1984) Plasma level monitoring of antidepressants: theoretical basis and clinical application. In: Usdin E, Åsberg M, Bertilsson L, Sjöqvist F (eds) Frontiers in biochemical and pharmacological research in depression. Raven, New York, pp 399–411

Gram LF, Brøsen K, Christensen P, Kragh-Sørensen P (1987) Pharmacokinetic considerations relevant to the pharmacodynamics of antidepressants. In: Dahl SG, Gram LF, Paul SM, Potter WZ (eds) Clinical pharmacology in psychiatry: selectivity in drug action, promises or problems? Springer, Berlin Heidelberg New York, pp 184–192

Gram LF, Debruyne D, Caillard V, Boulenger JP, Lacotte J, Moulin M, Zarifian E (1989) Substanial rise in Sparteine metabolic ratio during haloperidol treatment. Br J Pharmacol 27:272–275

Inaba T, Nakano M, Otton SV, Mahon WA, Kalow W (1984) A human cytochrome P450 characterized by inhibition studies as the sparteine-debrisoquine monooxygenase. Can J Physiol Pharmacol 62:860–862

Inaba T, Jurima M, Mahon WA, Kalow W (1985) In vitro inhibition studies of two isozymes of human liver cytochrome P-450. Mephenytoine p-hydroxylase and sparteine monooxygenase. Drug Metab Dispos 13:443–448

Jørgensen A (1986) Metabolism and pharmacokinetics of antipsychotic drugs. Prog Drug Metab 9:111–174

Klotz U, Reimann I (1980) Delayed clearance of diazepam due to cimetidine. N Engl J Med 302:1012–1014

Mikus G, Ha HR, Vozeh S, Zekorn C, Follath F, Eichelbaum M (1986) Pharmacokinetics and metabolism of quinidine in extensive and poor metabolizers of sparteine. Eur J Clin Pharmacol 31:69–72

Nelson JC, Jatlow PI (1980) Neuroleptic effect on desipramine steady-state plasma concentrations. Am J Psychiatry 137:1232–1234

Ochs HR, Greenblatt DJ, Woo E (1980) Clinical pharmacokinetics of quinidine. Clin Pharmacokinet 5:150–168

Olivier-Martin R, Marzin D, Buschenschutz E, Pichot P, Boissier J (1975) Concentration plasmatique de l'imipramine et de la desmethylimipramine et effet anti-depresseur au cours d'un traitement contrôlé. Psychopharmacologie 41:187–195

Otton SV, Inaba T, Kalow W (1983) Inhibition of sparteine oxidation in human liver by tricyclic antidepressants and other drugs. Life Sci 32:795–800

Otton SV, Inaba T, Kalow W (1984) Competitive inhibition of sparteine oxidation in human liver by beta-adrenoceptor antagonists and other cardiovascular drugs. Life Sci 34:73–80

Otton SV, Brinn R, Gram LF (1988) In vitro evidence against the oxidation of quinidine by the sparteine/debrisoquine monooxygenase of the human liver. Drug Metab Dispos 16:15–17

Siris SG, Cooper TB, Rifbein AE, Brenner R, Lieberman JA (1982) Plasma imipramine concentration in patients receiving concomitant fluphenazine decanoate. Am J Psychiatry 139:104–106

Somogyi A, Gugler R (1982) Drug interactions with cimetidine. Clin Pharmacokinet 7:23–41

Speight TM (ed) (1987) Avery's drug treatment, 3rd edn. ADIS, Auckland

Speirs CJ, Murray S, Boobis AR, Seddon CE, Davies DS (1986) Quinidine and the identification of drugs whose elimination is impaired in subjects classified as poor metabolizers of debrisoquine. Br J Clin Pharmacol 22:739–743

Sylvälahti EKG, Lindberg R, Kallio J, de Vocht M (1986) Inhibitory effects of neuroleptics on debrisoquine oxidation in man. Br J Clin Pharmacol 22:89–92

Vandel B, Vandel S, Allers G, Bechtel P, Volmat R (1979) Interaction between amitriptyline and phenothiazine in man: effect on plasma concentration of amitriptyline and its metabolite nortriptyline and the correlation with clinical response. Psychopharmacology (Berlin) 65:185–190

Von Bahr C, Spina E, Birgersson C, Ericsson O, Göransson M, Henthorn T, Sjöqvist F (1985) Inhibition of desmethylimipramine 2-hydroxylation by drugs in human liver microsomes. Biochem Pharmacol 34:2501–2505

Wells BG, Pieper, Self TH, Stewart CF, Waldon SL, Bobo L, Warner C (1986) The effect of ranitidine and cimetidine on imipramine disposition. Eur J Clin Pharmacol 31:285–290

Pharmacogenetics of Antidepressants *

F. SJÖQVIST [1]

1 Introduction

The metabolism of tricyclic antidepressants is catalysed by the cytochrome P-450 family of isozymes. The tertiary amines amitriptyline, imipramine and chlorimipramine are all demethylated to active secondary amines. Des-methylimipramine and nortriptyline, on the other hand, are hydroxylated in aromatic and benzylic positions, respectively. The latter involves the formation of two isomers, E and Z, each of which occurs in the R and in the S form. These metabolic changes modify the effects of the drugs on monoaminergic neurons.

It has now been confirmed in independent studies from different countries that the clinical effects of many tricyclic antidepressants are concentration dependent, and that the best therapeutic outcome in endogenous depression is obtained within relatively well-defined ranges of plasma concentrations (Sjöqvist et al. 1980; Åsberg 1983; Gram et al. 1984; Perry et al. 1987). Serious toxicity usually occurs at concentrations well above the therapeutic ranges (Gram 1977). Monitoring of drug plasma levels is particularly important in patients with extreme rates of drug oxidation. It would therefore be of interest to find means to diagnose individuals who might fall outside the "therapeutic window" when treated with commonly recommended doses. Here, we report our attempts to find such predictors using a pharmacogenetic research strategy.

2 Early Pharmacogenetic Observations

Our early studies of the pharmacokinetics of tricyclic antidepressants revealed a pronounced inter-individual variability in the steady-state plasma concentrations obtained on fixed dosage schedules. Already in the first study we found two outliers with markedly higher plasma concentrations than among the other subjects. We therefore speculated that pharmacogenetic factors governed the hydroxylation of these drugs (Hammer and Sjöqvist 1967). Twin and family studies clearly established that the steady-state plasma concentra-

* This study was supported by a grant from the Swedish Medical Research Council (3902).
[1] Department of Clinical Pharmacology of the Karolinska Institute, Huddinge University Hospital, 141 86 Huddinge, Sweden

Clinical Pharmacology in Psychiatry
Editors: S. G. Dahl and L. F. Gram
(Psychopharmacology Series 7)
© Springer-Verlag Berlin Heidelberg 1989

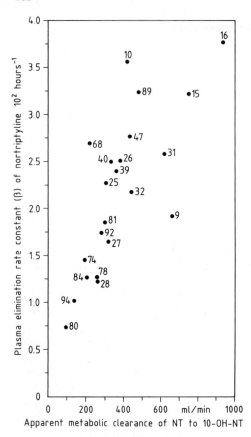

Fig. 1. Correlation between the β-slope elimination rate constant (β) of nortriptyline (NT) in plasma and the corresponding apparent metabolic clearance of nortriptyline to 10-hydroxy-nortriptyline (10-OH-NT) – unconjugated and conjugated – in 22 healthy twins (five monozygotic and six dizygotic pairs) given a single oral dose of nortriptyline (1 mg/kg). The subject code numbers for monozygotic twins were: 15/16, 25/26, 39/40, 47/89, 78/84; for dizygotic twins: 9/10, 27/28, 31/32, 68/81, 78/80, 92/94. (From Alexanderson 1972a, 1973)

tion is under genetic control but suggested polygenic rather than monogenic mechanisms (Alexanderson et al. 1969; Åsberg et al. 1971). This would be in keeping with the fact that the steady-state plasma concentration is dependent on several kinetic and metabolic factors. Alexanderson (1972a, b, 1973) was the first to study the clearance of a drug by hydroxylation in a pharmacogenetic perspective. He demonstrated a ten-fold difference between healthy twin volunteers in their capacity to hydroxylate nortriptyline, which is the rate-limiting step in its elimination. Significant intra-pair similarities were found in the ability of non-drug-exposed identical twins to dispose of nortriptyline, compared to non-identical twins (Fig. 1).

An early observation in this work was that the different tricyclic antidepressants behaved similarly within an individual (Hammer et al. 1969). Thus the plasma clearance and the steady-state plasma concentration of the two secondary amines desmethylimipramine and nortriptyline, which are hydroxylated, covaried within individuals. The same was true for the reciprocal plasma levels of the tertiary amines amitriptyline and chlorimipramine, which reflect their rates of demethylation (Table 1). These studies clearly indicated that the hydroxylating and demethylating enzymes involved in these reactions could not distinguish between the pair of substrates used.

Table 1. Intra-individual correlations between the kinetics of tricyclic antidepressants. (From Sjöqvist and Bertilsson 1984)

Variable	Drug 1	Drug 2	No. of individuals	r	p
Plasma half-life (single dose)	DMI	NT	8	0.88	<0.005
Plasma clearance	DMI	NT	8	0.90	<0.005
Observed mean steady-state concentrations	DMI	NT	11	0.94	<0.001
Reciprocal plasma levels	AT	CI	15	0.87	<0.001
Reciprocal plasma levels of demethylated metabolites formed from AT and CI	NT	DMCI	15	0.77	<0.001

DMI, Desmethylimipramine; NT, nortriptyline; AT, amitriptyline; CI, chlorimipramine; DMCI, desmethylchlorimipramine.

3 The New Pharmacogenetics

After the independent discoveries of the debrisoquine and sparteine oxidation polymorphisms (Mahgoub et al. 1977; Eichelbaum et al. 1979) we decided to explore further the mechanisms involved in the oxidation of tricyclic antidepressants by using individuals whose oxidation phenotype had been determined with debrisoquine. This was of particular interest in view of the

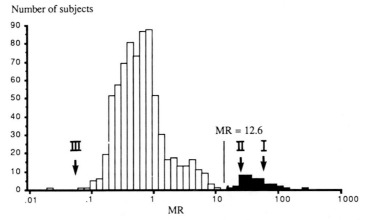

Fig. 2. Distribution of the metabolic ratios (*MR*) between the urinary concentrations of debrisoquine and 4-hydroxydebrisoquine in the urine of 757 Swedish healthy volunteers. An antimode at metabolic ratio 12.6 distinguishes rapid and slow hydroxylators. Patients I, II and III are described in the text. (Modified from Steiner et al. 1988a)

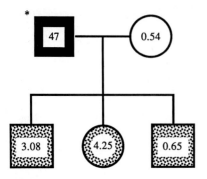

Fig. 3. Pedigree of the adult members of the author's family (*asterisk,* propositus); ■, slow hydroxylator; ○, rapid hydroxylator of unknown genotype; ⊠ ⊕, obligate heterozygote rapid hydroxylator of debrisoquine. *Numbers* indicate the ratio between debrisoquine and 4-hydroxydebrisoquine in urine after a single oral dose of 10 mg

fact that both debrisoquine and nortriptyline are hydroxylated in benzylic positions. Up to now we have phenotyped 757 healthy Swedish volunteers (Fig. 2). Approximately 6%–9% of Caucasian populations are slow hydroxylators of debrisoquine (Steiner et al. 1988 a). Family studies in Great Britain (Evans et al. 1980) and Sweden (Steiner et al. 1985) have shown that the hydroxylation of debrisoquine is controlled by two alleles at a single gene locus, and that slow hydroxylators are homozygous recessives. It is not possible to distinguish homo- and heterozygotic rapid hydroxylators with a debrisoquine test. As shown in Fig. 3 the debrisoquine hydroxylation ratio varies markedly between obligate heterozygote rapid hydroxylators.

We now have unequivocal evidence that individuals belonging to the slow phenotype are identical to those who are slow in hydroxylating nortriptyline and desmethylimipramine (see Sjöqvist and Bertilsson 1984, 1986). As an example, we found a significant association between the debrisoquine hydroxylation index and the 10-hydroxylation of nortriptyline both in Swedish and Ghanaian human volunteers (Fig. 4). It was also possible to

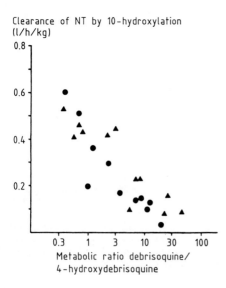

Clearance of NT by 10-hydroxylation (l/h/kg)

Metabolic ratio debrisoquine/ 4-hydroxydebrisoquine

Fig. 4. Relationship between the debrisoquine hydroxylation index and the plasma clearance of nortriptyline (*NT*) by formation of 10-hydroxynortriptyline (*10-OH-NT;* sum of levels of *E* and *Z* isomers). ●, Ghanaians; ▲, Swedes. (From Woolhouse et al. 1984)

demonstrate this association in vitro using human liver microsomes as the enzymatic source (von Bahr et al. 1982). Interestingly, only the plasma clearance of nortriptyline by E-10-hydroxylation correlated with the debrisoquine hydroxylation index while Z-10-hydroxylation did not (Mellström et al. 1981).

In an unstratified series of human volunteers we found no apparent relationship between the clearance of amitriptyline by demethylation and the debrisoquine hydroxylation phenotype (Mellström et al. 1983), but there was a significant correlation in non-smokers, suggesting that smokers have an induced demethylase that operates in addition to the debrisoquine hydroxylase (Mellström et al. 1983, 1985). Previous studies have shown that the hydroxylation of amitriptyline depends on the debrisoquine hydroxylation phenotype (Balant-Gorgia et al. 1982).

These studies therefore strongly suggest an association between the debrisoquine hydroxylation phenotype and the benzylic hydroxylation of nortriptyline in the E position, but also that additional hydroxylases might be involved in the oxidation of nortriptyline. We therefore decided to perform similar studies with desmethylimipramine, the main metabolite of which is hydroxylated in the phenolic position. We found the ratio between desmethylimipramine and 2-OH-desmethylimipramine in 24-h urinary specimens to correlate strongly with the debrisoquine hydroxylation index (Spina et al. 1987b). Both the total plasma clearance of desmethylimipramine and the clearance by 2-hydroxylation were found to covary with the debrisoquine hydroxylation index (Fig. 5). These observations have been confirmed in independent studies by Brøsen et al. (1986a, b), who used subjects phenotyped with sparteine. These authors have also demonstrated that the first-pass hydroxylation of desmethylimipramine is saturable in rapid but not in slow

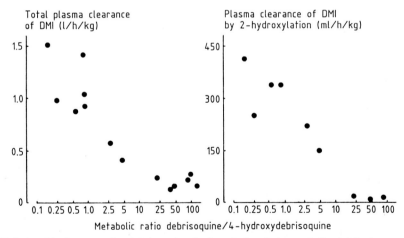

Fig. 5. Relationship between the debrisoquine hydroxylation index and the total plasma clearance of desmethylimipramine (*DMI*) and clearance by 2-hydroxylation, respectively. (From Spina et al. 1987b)

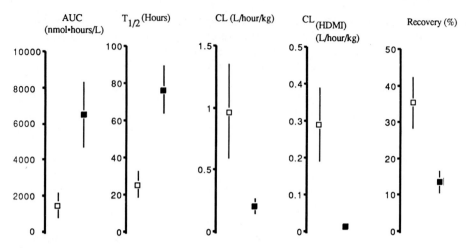

Fig. 6. Summary of the differences in the kinetics of desmethylimipramine (*DMI*) and 2-hydroxydesmethylimipramine (*HDMI*) between rapid (□) and slow (■) hydroxylators (mean ±SD). (From Steiner 1987)

hydroxylators (Brøsen and Gram 1988). The overall differences in des-methylimipramine kinetics between the two phenotypes are shown in Fig. 6.

In vitro data also show that the rates of hydroxylation of des-methylimipramine and debrisoquine correlate strongly within each individual liver (Spina et al. 1984). Competitive inhibition of the 2-hydroxylation of des-methylimipramine is obtained with substrates that have been shown or sug-gested to be oxidized by the debrisoquine hydroxylase (debrisoquine, nortrip-tyline, metoprolol, thioridazine) but not with other drugs (von Bahr et al.

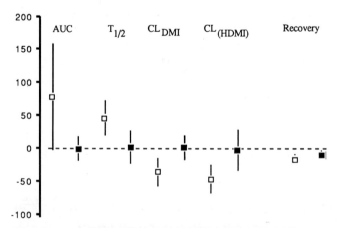

Fig. 7. Desmethylimipramine (*DMI*) kinetics before and during treatment with cimetidine in rapid (□) and slow (■) hydroxylators (mean ±SD). While cimetidine inhibits the hydroxyla-tion of desmethylimipramine in rapid hydroxylators, there is no discernible effect in slow hydroxylators. (Data from Steiner and Spina 1987)

1985). This is in keeping with the preliminary physical characteristics of purified human desmethylimipramine-2-hydroxylase (Birgersson et al. 1986; Ingelman Sundberg, personal communication), which seem to agree with those described for debrisoquine hydroxylase (Gut et al. 1986).

Using inhibitors of drug metabolism we were able to demonstrate another clinically important difference between the two phenotypes. Thus, cimetidine (Fig. 7) and quinidine markedly decreased the hydroxylation of des-methylimipramine in rapid but not in slow hydroxylators (Steiner and Spina 1987; Steiner et al. 1988b). Quinidine is a potent inhibitor of both desmethylimipramine-2-hydroxylation and debrisoquine-4-hydroxylation in vitro (for references see von Bahr et al. 1985).

4 Discussion

Tricyclic antidepressants fulfil two criteria: (a) their metabolism depends on the debrisoquine/sparteine type of polymorphism and (b) their clinical effects correlate with plasma drug levels (Åsberg 1983; Perry et al. 1987). With the use of nortriptyline, approximately 65% of patients with endogenous depression achieve plasma concentrations within the so-called therapeutic window (50–150 ng/ml) on a dosage of 50 mg t.i.d. while very rapid and very slow hydroxylators fall outside this range (Fig. 8). It would be of considerable value if these patients could be identified before selecting the initial dosage schedule. Since the majority of patients respond to a commonly recommended dose, therapeutic drug monitoring could be reserved for patients with extreme rates of drug oxidation. Such patients might be diagnosed by measuring the ratio between desmethylimipramine and 2-OH-desmethylimipramine in urine (after a single oral dose). Spina et al. (1987a) have shown that this ratio varies almost 100-fold between patients, and that it correlates significantly with steady-state plasma concentrations of desmethylimipramine in patients treated with either desmethylimipramine or the parent drug imipramine (Fig. 9). The desmethylimipramine/2-OH-desmethylimipramine ratio should

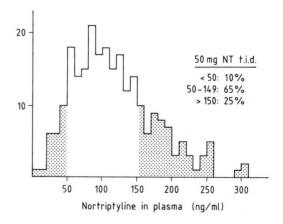

Fig. 8. Distribution of nortriptyline plasma concentrations in depressed patients treated with 50 mg t.i.d. The therapeutic effect is usually obtained within a therapeutic window of 50–150 ng/ml, since the concentration-effect curve is curvilinear (see Åsberg 1983)

50 mg NT t.i.d.

< 50: 10%
50–149: 65%
> 150: 25%

Nortriptyline in plasma (ng/ml)

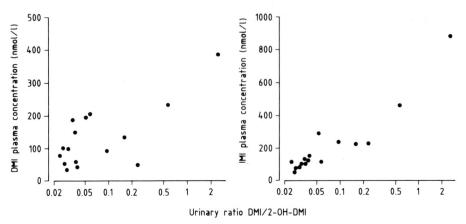

Fig. 9. Relationship between the desmethylimipramine hydroxylation index (*DMI/2-OH-DMI*) and the steady-state plasma levels of imipramine (*IMI*; $r_s = 0.41$; $n = 16$; NS; *left panel*) and desmethylimipramine (*DMI*; $r_s = 0.85$; $n = 16$; $p < 0.01$; *right panel*) in 16 patients on chronic treatment with imipramine, 75 mg daily by mouth. (From Spina et al. 1987 b)

also predict steady-state plasma concentrations of nortriptyline, the metabolism of which cosegregates with that of desmethylimipramine (Sjöqvist and Bertilsson 1984).

The potential strength offered by the approach of prophylactically determining the oxidation phenotype before long-term treatment with tricyclic antidepressants is illustrated with three cases whose debrisoquine ratios are indicated in Fig. 2. Patient I was the first subject to exhibit signs of slow hydroxylation of desmethylimipramine by developing excessive plasma concentrations and side effects on a dose of 25 mg t.i.d. She was reexamined 15 years later with a debrisoquine test and found to be a slow hydroxylator (patient GD in Hammer and Sjöqvist 1967). During these years she had had several prescriptions of psychotropic drugs and had often experienced marked side effects at common doses. Case II represents a similar association between slow hydroxylation and serious side effects (confusion, vertigo) on nortriptyline 25 mg t.i.d. (Bertilsson et al. 1981). This patient needed only 20 mg per day to maintain plasma levels within the therapeutic window. Our third case represents the other extreme. It concerns a middle-aged woman who was treated with various antidepressants, most notably nortriptyline and amitriptyline, with poor results. Very high doses had to be given in order to achieve an apparent therapeutic range, and it turned out that the patient was an extremely rapid hydroxylator of debrisoquine. The patient had plasma concentrations of the 10-OH metabolite that were ten times higher than those obtained in 30 control subjects (Bertilsson et al. 1985).

The clinical implications of the occurrence of extreme rates of drug hydroxylation in the population will depend largely on the shape of the concentration-effect relationships for each drug. Drug-metabolic phenotyping tests might be successfully combined with conventional monitoring of plasma drug levels to optimize the management of patients treated with drugs having concentration-dependent effects and side effects that are difficult to evaluate solely on clinical grounds. Tricyclic antidepressants represent a good example of such drugs. Phenotyping tests may also be used to predict whether or not drug metabolic interactions will occur in an individual. Possibly, phenotyping tests and, in the future, genotyping tests may be applied systematically to optimize the treatment with potentially toxic but useful drugs and thus save them from being withdrawn from the market due to inappropriate utilization. An important aspect of pharmacogenetics is that inter-ethnic differences have been demonstrated in the occurrence of slow hydroxylators of debrisoquine and mephenytoin. This may turn out to be of importance for the therapeutic "reputation" of a drug in different parts of the world.

References

Alexanderson B (1972a) On interindividual variability in plasma levels of nortriptyline and desmethylimipramine in man: a pharmacokinetic and genetic study. Medical Dissertation, Linköping University, Linköping

Alexanderson B (1972b) Pharmacokinetics of desmethylimipramine and nortriptyline in man after single and oral doses – a crossover study. Eur J Clin Pharmacol 5:7–10

Alexanderson B (1973) Prediction of steady-state plasma levels of nortriptyline from single oral dose kinetics: a study in twins. Eur J Clin Pharmacol 6:44–53

Alexanderson B, Price-Evans DA, Sjöqvist F (1969) Steady-state plasma levels of nortriptyline in twins: influence of genetic factors and drug therapy. Br Med J 2:764–768

Åsberg M (1983) On the relationship between plasma concentrations of tricyclic antidepressant drugs and therapeutic response. In: Clayton PJ, Barrett JE (eds) Treatment of depression: old controversies and new approaches. Raven, New York, pp 85–104

Åsberg M, Price-Evans D, Sjöqvist F (1971) Genetic control of nortriptyline kinetics in man – a study of relatives of propositi with high plasma concentrations. J Med Genet 8:129–135

Balant-Gorgia AE, Schulz P, Dayer P, Balant L, Kubli A, Gertsch C, Garrone G (1982) Role of oxidation polymorphism on blood and urine concentrations of amitriptyline and its metabolites in man. Arch Psychiatr Nervenkr 232:215–222

Bertilsson L, Mellström B, Sjöqvist F, Mårtenson B, Åsberg M (1981) Slow hydroxylation of nortriptyline and concomitant poor debrisoquine hydroxylation: clinical implications. Lancet 1:560–561

Bertilsson L, Åsberg-Wistedt A, Gustafsson LL, Nordin C (1985) Extremely rapid hydroxylation of debrisoquine – a case report with implication for treatment with nortriptyline and other tricyclic antidepressants. Ther Drug Monit 7:242–243

Birgersson C, Morgan ET, Jörnvall H, von Bahr C (1986) Purification of a desmethylimipramine and debrisoquine hydroxylation cytochrome P-450 from human liver. Biochem Pharmacol 35:3165–3166

Brøsen K, Gram LF (1988) First-pass metabolism of imipramine and desipramine: impact of the sparteine oxidation phenotype. Clin Pharmacol Ther 43:400–406

Brøsen K, Otton V, Gram LF (1986a) Imipramine demethylation and hydroxylation: impact of the sparteine oxidation phenotype. Clin Pharmacol Ther 40:543–549

Brøsen K, Klysner R, Gram LF, Otton SV, Bech P, Bertilsson L (1986b) Steady-state concentrations of imipramine and its metabolites in relation to the sparteine/debrisoquine polymorphism. Eur J Clin Pharmacol 30:679–684

Eichelbaum M, Spannbrucker N, Steinke B, Dengler HJ (1979) Defective N-oxidation of sparteine in man: a new pharmacogenetic defect. Eur J Clin Pharmacol 16:183–187

Evans DAP, Mahgoub A, Sloan TP, Idle JR, Smith RL (1980) A family and population study at the genetic polymorphism of debrisoquine in white British population. J Med Genet 17:102–105

Gram LF (1977) Plasma level monitoring of tricyclic antidepressant therapy. Clin Pharmacokinet 2:237–251

Gram LF, Kragh-Sørensen P, Kristensen CB, Møller M, Pedersen OL, Thayssen P (1984) Plasma level monitoring of antidepressants: theoretical basis and clinical applications. In: Usdin E, Åsberg M, Bertilsson L, Sjöqvist F (eds) Frontiers in biochemical and pharmacological research in depression. Advances in psychopharmacology. Raven, New York, pp 399–411

Gut J, Catin T, Dayer P, Kronbach T, Zanger U, Meyer UA (1986) Debrisoquine/sparteine-type polymorphism of drug oxidation. J Biol Chem 261:11734–11743

Hammer W, Sjöqvist F (1967) Plasma levels of monomethylated tricyclic antidepressants during treatment with imipramine-like compounds. Life Sci 6:1895–1903

Hammer W, Mårtens S, Sjöqvist F (1969) Comparative studies of the metabolism of desmethylimipramine, nortriptyline, and oxyphenylbutazone in man. Clin Pharmacol Ther 10:44–49

Mahgoub A, Idle JR, Dring LG, Lancaster R, Smith RL (1977) Polymorphic hydroxylation of debrisoquine in man. Lancet 2:584–586

Mellström B, Bertilsson L, Säwe J, Schulz H-U, Sjöqvist F (1981) E- and Z-hydroxylation of nortriptyline – relationship to polymorphic debrisoquine hydroxylation. Clin Pharmacol Ther 30:189–193

Mellström B, Säwe J, Bertilsson L, Sjöqvist F (1983) Metabolism of amitriptyline – relationship to polymorphic debrisoquine hydroxylation. Clin Pharmacol Ther 24:516–520

Mellström B, Säwe J, Bertilsson L, Sjöqvist F (1985) Amitriptyline metabolism: relation with debrisoquine hydroxylation in nonsmokers. Clin Pharmacol Ther 39:369–371

Perry PJ, Pfohl BM, Holstad SG (1987) The relationship between antidepressant response and tricyclic antidepressant plasma concentrations. A retrospective analysis of the literature using logistic regression analysis. Clin Pharmacokinet 13:381–392

Sjöqvist F, Bertilsson L (1984) Clinical pharmacology of antidepressant drugs. In: Usdin E, Åsberg M, Bertilsson L, Sjöqvist F (eds) Frontiers in biochemical and pharmacological research in depression. Advances in biochemical psychopharmacology. Raven, New York, pp 359–372

Sjöqvist F, Bertilsson L (1986) Slow hydroxylation of tricyclic antidepressants – relationship to polymorphic drug oxidation. In: Kalow W (ed) Ethnic differences in reactions to drugs and xenobiotics. Liss, New York, pp 169–188

Sjöqvist F, Bertilsson L, Åsberg M (1980) Monitoring tricyclic antidepressants. Ther Drug Monit 25:85–93

Spina E, Birgersson C, von Bahr C, Ericsson Ö, Mellström B, Steiner E, Sjöqvist F (1984) Phenotypic consistency in the hydroxylation of desmethylimipramine and debrisoquine in healthy subjects and in human liver microsomes. Clin Pharmacol Ther 36:677–682

Spina E, Arena A, Pisani F (1987a) Urinary desipramine hydroxylation index and steady-state plasma concentrations of imipramine and desipramine. Ther Drug Monit 9:129–133

Spina E, Steiner E, Ericsson Ö, Sjöqvist F (1987b) Hydroxylation of desmethylimipramine: dependence on the debrisoquine hydroxylation phenotype. Clin Pharmacol Ther 41:457–461

Steiner E (1987) Polymorphic debrisoquine hydroxylation. Thesis, Karolinska Institute, Stockholm

Steiner E, Spina E (1987) Differences in the inhibitory effect of cimetidine on desipramine metabolism between rapid and slow debrisoquine hydroxylators. Clin Pharmacol Ther 42:272–282

Steiner E, Iselius L, Alván G, Lindsten J, Sjöqvist F (1985) A family study of genetic and environmental factors determining polymorphic hydroxylation of debrisoquine. Clin Pharmacol Ther 38:394–401

Steiner E, Bertilsson L, Säwe J, Bertling I, Sjöqvist F (1988a) Polymorphic debrisoquine hydroxylation in 757 Swedish subjects. Clin Pharmacol Ther 44:431–435

Steiner E, Dumont E, Spina E, Dahlqvist R (1988b) Inhibition of desipramine 2-hydroxylations by quinidine and quinine in rapid and slow hydroxylators. Clin Pharmacol Ther 43:577–581

Von Bahr C, Birgersson C, Bertilsson L, Göransson M, Mellström B, Nilsell K, Sjöqvist F (1982) Drug metabolism in human liver microsomes: towards marker substrates for different enzymes. Br J Clin Pharmacol 14:603P–604P

Von Bahr C, Spina E, Birgersson C, Ericsson Ö, Göransson M, Henthorn T, Sjöqvist F (1985) Inhibition of desmethylimipramine 2-hydroxylation by drugs in human liver microsomes. Biochem Pharmacol 34:2501–2505

Woolhouse N, Adjepon-Yamoah KK, Mellström B, Hedman A, Bertilsson L, Sjöqvist F (1984) Nortriptyline and debrisoquine hydroxylations in Ghanaian and Swedish subjects. Clin Pharmacol Ther 36:374–378

Pharmacokinetic and Clinical Significance of Genetic Variability in Psychotropic Drug Metabolism *

K. Brøsen and L. F. Gram [1]

1 Introduction

The discovery of a common genetic polymorphism in the oxidation of sparteine and debrisoquine (Mahgoub et al. 1977; Eichelbaum et al. 1979) has created new interest in the role of genetic factors for individual variations in the oxidation of psychotropic drugs, notably tricyclic antidepressants.

In Caucasians, two phenotypes are clearly distinguished: poor metabolizers, who make up about 7% of the population, and extensive metabolizers, who make up more than 90%. The sparteine/debrisoquine oxidation polymorphism expresses the activity of a distinctive isozyme of cytochrome P450, the socalled P450dbl, and poor metabolizers have negligible amounts of this isozyme (Gonzalez et al. 1988). The elimination of several drugs depends on P450dbl, and in poor metabolizers these drugs are either excreted slowly via the kidneys or oxidized very slowly by alternative P450s.

The discovery of the sparteine/debrisoquine oxidation polymorphism has had a tremendous impact on biochemical drug metabolism research, but the consequences of this research for the practical use of psychotropic as well as other drugs are still limited.

2 Clinical Significance of the Sparteine/Debrisoquine Oxidation Polymorphism

Individual variations in the oxidation of psychotropic drugs are often inconvenient from a clinical point of view. A genetic polymorphism is a special case in which the extreme variability is due to genetic inheritance. This is not a particular disadvantage, since the optimal treatment or dosage can be predicted from determination of the patient's phenotype. The clinical significance of the sparteine/debrisoquine oxidation polymorphism may thus be

---

* This paper has in part been draftet within the aims of the European concerted action, the COST B1 programme "Criteria for the Choice and Definition of Healthy, Volunteers and/or Patients for Phase I and II studies in Drug Development".

[1] Department of Clinical Pharmacology, Odense University, School of Medicine, J.B. Winsløws Vej 19, 5000 Odense C, Denmark

Clinical Pharmacology in Psychiatry
Editors: S. G. Dahl and L. F. Gram
(Psychopharmacology Series 7)
© Springer-Verlag Berlin Heidelberg 1989

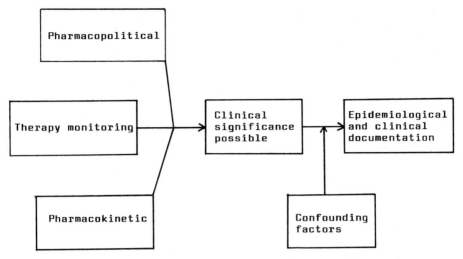

Fig. 1. Factors and mechanisms that determine the clinical significance of the sparteine/ debrisoquine oxidation polymorphism

defined according to the usefulness of phenotyping patients prior to the treatment with a particular drug.

The elimination of more than 20 different drugs depends on P450dbl, but several of these are either unimportant or obsolete. The pharmacopolitical aspects of the discussion (see Fig. 1) involve the restriction of psychotropic drugs to those that are essential and universally available for the treatment of particular psychiatric disorders. The clinical significance in relation to a particular drug should be analysed in three steps. Firstly, are the elimination kinetics of the drug significantly dependent on P450dbl? If so, is the resulting variability in plasma concentrations important to the safety and efficacy of the drug? And, finally, is it possible to carry out dose adjustments according to the clinical or paraclinical effects of the drug?

3 Drug Elimination Kinetics and P450dbl

Sparteine, debrisoquine, dextromethorphan or another test drug of choice may be used for phenotyping. The poor-metabolizer phenotype is defined by a metabolic ratio (ratio of amount of parent compound to that of metabolite) in an 8- to 12-h urine sample of >20 for sparteine, >12.6 for debrisoquine and >0.3 for dextromethorphan (antimodes). The phenotype can predict the total elimination of a drug only if the drug and/or its active metabolite is a substrate for P450dbl and elimination via alternative P450s; non-oxidative metabolism or excretion of unchanged drug does not take place in extensive metabolizers. These criteria are approximately met by tricyclic antidepressants (Table 1), as

Table 1. Elimination psychotropic drugs in relation to the sparteine/debrisoquine oxidation polymorphism

Biotrans-formation	Consequence for poor metabolizers	Drug	Reference

$D \overset{*}{\Rightarrow} M_a$
 $\downarrow$
 M_b
	Accumulation of drug	Nortriptyline
		 Desipramine
		
		 Clomipramine
		 Perphenazine
		 Thioridazine
			Bertilsson et al. (1980)
			 Bertilsson and
			    Åberg-Wistedt (1983)
			 Balant-Gorgia et al. (1986)
			 Dahl-Puustinen et al. (1989)
			 von Bahr et al.
			    (this volume)

$D \Rightarrow M_a$ $*\downarrow \quad \Downarrow*$ $M_b \quad M_c$	Accumulation of active metabolite	Imipramine (active metabolite: desipramine)	Brøsen et al. (1986 a, b)
$D \overset{*}{\Rightarrow} M_a$ $*\downarrow \quad \Downarrow*$ $M_b \quad M_c$	Accumulation of drug and active metabolite	Amitriptyline (active metabolite: nortriptyline)	Mellström et al. (1983)

D, Drug; M_a, active metabolite; M_b, M_c, other oxidative metabolites
$\Rightarrow$, important pathways; $\blacktriangleright$, less important pathway; *, pathway catalysed by the P450 which oxidizes sparteine and debrisoquine (P450dbl).

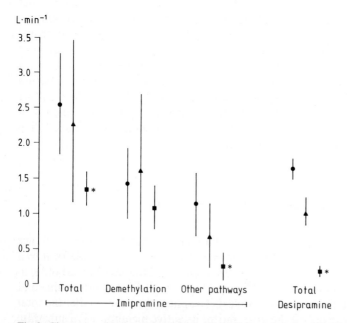

Fig. 2. Clearance of imipramine (total and partial) and desipramine after single oral doses. Mean $\pm$SD in six rapid extensive metabolizers ($\bullet$), six slow extensive metabolizers ($\blacktriangle$) and six poor metabolizers ($\blacksquare$). *Asterisk*, $p < 0.05$ Mann-Whitney U test, extensive versus poor metabolizers. (Data from Brøsen et al. 1986a; figure published in Brøsen 1988)

Table 2. Clinical significance of P450dbl

- Genetic polymorphism (sparteine/debrisoquine type)
- Stereoselective metabolism
- Site of interaction by inhibition (e.g. tricyclic antidepressants, neuroleptic and quinidine)
- Saturated by therapeutic doses (e.g. imipramine and desipramine)
- Almost uninducible

well as by thioridazine (von Bahr et al., this volume) and perphenazine (Dahl-Puustinen et al. 1989).

Ideally, the impact of the sparteine/debrisoquine oxidation polymorphism for the elimination of a given psychotropic drug should be established on the basis of cross-over population and family studies, but no such study has been performed.

Tricyclic antidepressants and several neuroleptics are competitive inhibitors of sparteine and debrisoquine oxidation in human liver microsome preparations in vitro (Inaba et al. 1985), thereby raising the possibility that the drugs themselves are substrates for P450dbl (Gram and Brøsen, this volume). As mentioned, this has been confirmed in vivo for the tricyclic antidepressants. In the typical case (e.g. desipramine; Brøsen et al. 1986a) the total clearance is on the average five times lower (Fig. 2) and hence the steady-state concentration five times higher in poor than in extensive metabolizers after the same dose. With the neuroleptic haloperidol there appeared to be no phenotype differences in the steady-state concentrations (Gram et al. 1989), and it was therefore concluded that haloperidol is oxidized by other P450s than P450dbl. An intermediate result (e.g. imipramine; Brøsen et al. 1986a) is obtained if the drug is only in part oxidized by P450dbl (Fig. 2).

The pharmacokinetic picture is complicated by a number of confounding factors that may alter the relative importance of P450dbl in the individual patient, with the result that the predictive value of the metabolic ratio for elimination of a drug is reduced or even lost. The phenotype difference is increased by selective induction in extensive metabolizers, but the effect is negligible (Eichelbaum et al. 1986; Table 2). Conversely, P450dbl becomes less important by induction of alternative P450s, as suggested for amitriptyline demethylation in smokers (Mellström et al. 1983). A reduced or non-existent phenotype difference may also be a consequence of the functional impairment of P450dbl. Thus, the phenotype difference in oxidation is completely lost during treatment with a very potent inhibitor such as quinidine (Gram and Brøsen, this volume).

Another functional characteristic of P450dbl is non-linear kinetics at therapeutic doses with some substrates. On oral administration the saturation probably takes place during the first pass through the liver (Brøsen and Gram 1988). The consequences are illustrated in a clinical study with imipramine (Brøsen et al. 1986c; Fig. 3). The steady-state concentration of imipramine plus desipramine ranged from 89 to 1437 nM in 16 extensive metabolizers

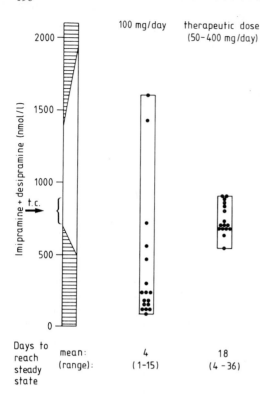

Fig. 3. Distribution of steady-state concentration of imipramine plus desipramine and distribution of therapeutic doses in 17 depressed patients during treatment with imipramine. (Data from Brøsen et al. 1986c)

patients and was 1603 nM in one poor metabolizer treated with 100 mg imipramine per day. However, due to non-linear kinetics in most extensive metabolizers, but linear kinetics in one poor metabolizer, the 18-fold difference in steady-state concentrations was corrected by an eight-fold difference in therapeutic dose (Fig. 3; Brøsen et al. 1986c).

4 Therapeutic Aspects of the Sparteine/Debrisoquine Oxidation Polymorphism

Until now, pharmacokinetics has been the main area of research, but before genetic polymorphism can be said to be of possible clinical significance, a number of criteria related to therapeutic drug monitoring must also be met.

Some drugs have a wide therapeutic plasma concentration range whereas others are easily dose-titrated according to their clinical effects (e.g. benzodiazepines). Even in the case of genetic polymorphism, phenotyping or direct assessment of the pharmacokinetic variability is unnecessary for either class of drugs. The sparteine/debrisoquine oxidation polymorphism is of possible clinical significance only if the drug has a narrow plasma concentration

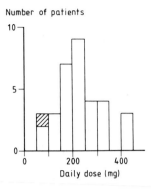

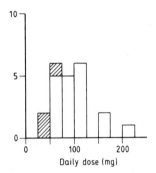

Fig. 4. *Upper panel*, distribution of the imipramine dose (mg/dg) necessary to obtain a mean (±SD) steady-state concentration of 713 ± 132 nmol/l for imipramine plus desipramine in 33 depressed patients (data from Brøsen et al. 1986b). *Lower panel*, distribution of the nortriptyline dose necessary to obtain a mean (±SD) steady-state concentration of 349 ± 121 nmol/l in 22 patients (Gram et al. 1989b). *Hatched bars*, poor metabolizers; *open bars*, extensive metabolizers

range, and clinical dose titration is not possible. Thus, if there is no rationale for plasma concentration monitoring, there is also no rationale for phenotyping. This applies to tricyclic antidepressants where the onset of action is slow, and where adverse reactions are unpleasant but difficult to distinguish from symptoms of persistent depression (dry mouth, sedation, constipation).

With tricyclic antidepressants there appear to be two patient groups at risk. One group consists of poor and of slow extensive metabolizers who show toxic plasma concentrations when treated with textbook-recommended doses. These patients often become non-compliant or drop-outs due to unpleasant adverse reactions. The other group consists of rapid extensive metabolizers who suffer from therapeutic failure due to plasma concentrations that are too low. The former group requires a low dose and the latter group a high dose in order to reach a therapeutic plasma concentration level (Fig. 4). The clinical picture in the two risk groups is very similar: recurrent depressions that do not respond to treatment, simply because appropriate dose adjustments are not carried out.

The distribution of therapeutic imipramine and nortriptyline doses did not exhibit bimodality, but poor metabolizers represented the lower extreme (Fig. 4). However, more than 90% of the patients are extensive metabolizers, and even within this phenotype there was a large variability in dose (Fig. 4).

The correlation between metabolic rate and imipramine dose in extensive metabolizers was poor although statistically significant (Brøsen et al. 1986 b), and phenotyping could not replace plasma concentration monitoring.

5 Conclusions and Perspectives

The presence and functional state of a particular isozyme, P450dbl, are major determinants of the overall elimination of tricyclic antidepressants (Table 1), some neuroleptics and other drugs. The impact on the oxidation of other psychotropic drugs such as benzodiazepines and most neuroleptics has been poorly investigated. Some of the most important characteristics of P450dbl have been summarized in Table 2.

A phenotyping test with sparteine, debrisoquine or dextromethorphan before treatment with a tricyclic antidepressant may serve as a simple and safe test to enable the clinician to select an appropriate initial dose. The test result (metabolic ratio) is not sufficiently precise to replace plasma concentration monitoring, but the optimal strategy for handling drug level monitoring (time to reach steady-state, dose-dependent kinetics and interactions with neuroleptics) is different in extensive metabolizers than in poor metabolizers. Thus, in most extensive metabolizers an appropriate initial dose of imipramine is 200 mg per day (Fig. 4). Steady-state is reached within a few days, but achievement of the therapeutic level is hampered by dose-dependent kinetics and inhibition by neuroleptics (Fig. 2; Gram and Brøsen, this volume). In poor metabolizers the appropriate initial dose is 50–75 mg per day. Due to the very long elimination half-life of desipramine (4–6 days; Brøsen et al. 1986 a) it may

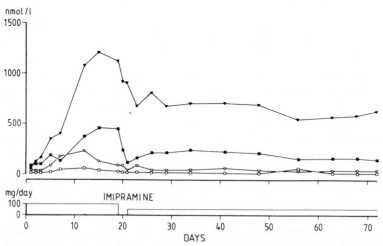

Fig. 5. Plasma concentrations of imipramine (■), desipramine (▼), 2-OH-imipramine (□) and 2-OH-desipramine (▽) during treatment with different imipramine doses in 66-year-old man, a poor metabolizer of sparteine. (Data from Brøsen et al. 1986 c)

take several weeks before steady-state is reached (Fig. 5). Final adjustments are carried out on the basis of linear kinetics. Poor metabolizers show, as expected, less inhibition by other drugs, such as cimetidine and quinidine (Steiner and Spina 1987; Steiner et al. 1988).

Since the rest result is valid for several tricyclic antidepressants and must only be performed once in a life time, the test appears to be of particular value for patients with recurrent depressions.

Recent studies have shown that the sparteine/debrisoquine oxidation polymorphism has an impact on the elimination of thioridazine and perphenazine, and analogous considerations may apply to treatment of psychotic patients.

However, the final epidemiological and clinical documentation for the usefulness of phenotyping is still lacking. As for any clinical test, its introduction into routine use should be implemented under continuous surveillance in a follow-up programme that will ultimately refine our understanding of its potentials and limitations.

References

Balant-Gorgia AE, Balant LP, Genet C, Dayer P, Aeschlimann JM, Garrone G (1986) Importance of oxidative polymorphism and levomepromazine treatment on the steady-state blood concentrations of clomipramine and its major metabolites. Eur J Clin Pharmacol 31:449–455

Bertilsson L, Åberg-Wistedt A (1983) The debrisoquine hydroxylation test predicts steady-state plasma levels of desipramine. Br J Clin Pharmacol 15:388–390

Bertilsson L, Eichelbaum M, Mellström B, Säwe J, Schulz H-U, Sjöqvist F (1980) Nortriptyline and antipyrine clearance in relation to debrisoquine hydroxylation in man. Life Sci 27:1673–1677

Brøsen K (1988) The relationship between imipramine metabolism and the sparteine oxidation polymorphism. Dan Med Bull 35:460–468

Brøsen K, Gram LF (1988) First-pass metabolism of imipramine and desipramine: impact of the sparteine oxidation phenotype. Clin Pharmacol Ther 43:400–406

Brøsen K, Otton SV, Gram LF (1986a) Imipramine demethylation and hydroxylation: impact of the sparteine oxidation phenotype. Clin Pharmacol Ther 40:543–549

Brøsen K, Klysner R, Gram LF, Otton SV, Bech P, Bertilsson L (1986b) Steady-state concentrations of imipramine and its metabolites in relation to the sparteine/debrisoquine polymorphism. Eur J Clin Pharmacol 30:679–684

Brøsen K, Gram LF, Klysner R, Bech P (1986c) Steady-state levels of imipramine and its metbolites: significance of dose-dependent kinetics. Eur J Clin Pharmacol 30:43–49

Dahl-Puustinen ML, Liden A, Bertilsson L (1989) Disposition of perphenazine in man related to polymorphic debrisoquine hydroxylation in man. Clin Pharmacol Ther (in press)

Eichelbaum M, Spannbrucker N, Steincke B, Dengler HJ (1979) Defective N-oxidation of sparteine in man: a new pharmacogenetic defect. Eur J Clin Pharmacol 16:183–187

Eichelbaum M, Mineshita S, Ohnhaus EE, Zekorn C (1986) The influence of enzyme induction on polymorphic sparteine oxidation. Br J Clin Pharmacol 22:49–53

Gonzalez FJ, Skoda R, Kimura S, Umeno M, Zanger UM, Nebert DW, Gelboin HV et al. (1988) Characterization of the common genetic defect in humans deficient in debrisoquine metabolism. Nature 331:442–446

Gram LF, Debruyne D, Caillard V, Boulenger JP, Lacotte J, Moulin M, Zarifian E (1989a)
    Substantial rise in sparteine metabolic ratio during haloperidol treatment. Br J Clin
    Pharmacol 27:272–275
Gram LF, Brøsen K, Kragh-Sorensen P, Christensen P (1989b) Steady-state levels of E- and
    Z-10-OH-nortriptyline in nortriptyline treated patients: significance of concurrent
    medication and the sparteine oxidation phenotype. Ther Drug Monit (in press)
Inaba T, Jurima M, Mahon WA, Kalow W (1985) In vitro inhibition studies of two isozymes
    of human liver cytochrome P-450. Mephenytoin p-hydroxylase and sparteine
    monooxygenase. Drug Metab Dispos 13:443–446
Mahgoub A, Idle JR, Dring LG, Lancaster R, Smith RL (1977) Polymorphic hydroxylation
    of debrisoquine in man. Lancet 2:584–586
Mellström B, Bertilsson L, Lou Y-C, Säwe J, Sjöqvist F (1983) Amitriptyline metabolism:
    relationship to polymorphic debrisoquine hydroxylation. Clin Pharmacol Ther
    34:516–520
Steiner E, Spina E (1987) Differences in the inhibitory effect of cimetidine on desipramine
    metabolism between rapid and slow debrisoquine hydroxylators. Clin Pharmacol Ther
    42:278–282
Steiner E, Dumont E, Spina E, Dahlqvist R (1988) Inhibition of desipramine 2-
    hydroxylation by quinidine and quinine. Clin Pharmacol Ther 43:577–581

Inhibition of Desipramine 2-Hydroxylation by Quinidine and Quinine in Rapid and Slow Debrisoquine Hydroxylators *

E. Spina [1], E. Steiner [2], E. Dumont [2], and R. Dahlqvist [2]

1 Polymorphic Debrisoquine Oxidation and Metabolism of Desipramine

Polymorphic oxidation has been described for debrisoquine (Mahgoub et al. 1977) and for sparteine (Eichelbaum et al. 1979). Reduced ability to oxidize these compounds is inherited as an autosomal recessive trait (Price-Evans et al. 1980), and the prevalence of the slow hydroxylator phenotype varies between 3% and 9%, depending on the country (Eichelbaum 1982). Biochemical studies indicate that this polymorphism is caused by an inherited absence or functional deficiency of a particular cytochrome P-450 isozyme, called debrisoquine hydroxylase (Boobies et al. 1983). The oxidative metabolism of several other drugs has been shown to cosegregate with the debrisoquine/sparteine oxidation polymorphism (Jacqz et al. 1986).

The tricyclic antidepressant desipramine is metabolized by hepatic microsomal mono-oxygenases, mainly by 2-hydroxylation. In vivo and in vitro studies (Spina 1987) have unequivocally demonstrated that the hydroxylation of desipramine is associated with the polymorphic debrisoquine oxidation. Urinary ratios between desipramine and its main metabolite, 2-hydroxydesipramine, after a single oral dose of desipramine can resolve rapid from slow hydroxylators (Spina et al. 1984) and significant differences in the pharmacokinetics of desipramine have been found between the two phenotypes (Spina et al. 1987). Moreover biochemical evidence supports the hypothesis that the hydroxylation of desipramine and debrisoquine are metabolized by the same enzyme (Spina et al. 1984).

2 Effect of Quinidine on the Metabolism of Drugs Associated with the Debrisoquine/Sparteine Oxidation Polymorphism

In order to investigate whether drugs interact with the debrisoquine hydroxylase, inhibition studies with human liver microsomes have been performed. Among several compounds submitted to such in vitro testing, the

* This study was supported by the Swedish Medical Research Council (grant 3902) and by funds from the Karolinska Institute.
[1] Institute of Pharmacology, University of Messina, 98100 Messina, Italy
[2] Department of Clinical Pharmacology, Karolinska Institute, Huddinge University Hospital, 14186 Huddinge, Sweden

antiarrhythmic drug quinidine was the most potent inhibitor of sparteine (Otton et al. 1984) and debrisoquine (Speirs et al. 1986) oxidation. This inhibition is highly selective since quinine, the diastereoisomer of quinidine, was much less potent as inhibitor of such oxidative reactions. Although quinidine binds avidly to the isozyme, it is not metabolized by the debrisoquine hydroxylase (Otton et al. 1986; Mikus et al. 1986). These observations were also confirmed in vivo. In fact, single and multiple oral doses of quinidine dramatically increased the metabolic ratios of sparteine (Inaba et al. 1986; Brinn et al. 1986) and debrisoquine (Inaba et al. 1986; Speirs et al. 1986; Brøsen et al. 1987), virtually transforming rapid into slow hydoxylators. Moreover, single doses of quinidine inhibited the oxidation of metoprolol, another substrate for the polymorphic enzyme (Leemann et al. 1986). Interestingly, the inhibitory effect was observed in rapid but not in slow hydroxylators.

3 Effect of Quinidine and Quinine on Desipramine Hydroxylation

3.1 In Vitro Studies

Using desipramine as probe drug for the polymorphic debrisoquine oxidation, von Bahr et al. (1985) investigated the effect of various compounds on desipramine hydroxylation in human liver microsomal preparations. Quinidine was the most potent competitive inhibitor of the reaction with an apparent inhibition constant (K_i) of 0.27 μM. Also quinine competitively inhibited the oxidation of desipramine, although to a lesser extent ($K_i = 12$ μM).

3.2 In Vivo Studies

We have recently studied the effect of quinidine and quinine on the urinary excretion of desipramine and 2-hydroxydesipramine in rapid and slow hydroxylators (Steiner et al. 1988). Ten healthy volunteers, seven rapid and three slow debrisoquine hydroxylators, received 25 mg desipramine as a single oral dose on three occasions: before treatment, after 2 days treatment with quinidine (800 mg daily) and after 2 days treatment with quinine (750 mg daily). Urine was collected for 24 h and urinary concentrations of desipramine and total 2-hydroxydesipramine (conjugated plus unconjugated) were determined by HPLC using a modification (Spina et al. 1984) of the method described by Sutfin and Jusko (1979). The results of this study are summarized in Table 1. In rapid hydroxylators treatment with quinidine and quinine decreased the urinary excretion of 2-hydroxydesipramine by 97% and 56%, respectively (Fig. 1, left panel). In slow hydroxylators the excretion of 2-hydroxydesipramine decreased significantly after treatment with quinidine (by 68%) but not with quinine (Fig. 1, right panel). Neither quinidine nor quinine modified the urinary excretion of desipramine in either phenotypic

Table 1. Urinary excretion of desipramine (DMI) and 2-hydroxy desipramine (2-OH-DMI) during the first 24 h after a single oral dose of 25 mg (82.50 μmol) desipramine in rapid and slow hydroxylators

	DMI (μmol)			2-OH-DMI (μmol)			DMI/2-OH-DMI ratio		
	Before treatment	Quinine	Quinidine	Before treatment	Quinine	Quinidine	Before treatment	Quinine	Quinidine
Rapid hydroxylators (n=7)									
Mean	0.78	1.02	0.92	20.86	9.19	0.69	0.04	0.14	1.65
SD	0.55	0.89	0.31	5.76	4.25	0.36	0.04	0.13	0.80
Slow hydroxylators (n=3)									
Mean	1.23	1.26	0.53	1.98	1.81	0.64	0.62	0.81	0.86
SD	0.15	0.50	0.31	0.25	0.60	0.43	0.06	0.60	0.08

group. Moreover, the urinary desipramine/2-hydroxydesipramine ratio of quinidine-treated rapid hydroxylators was even greater than that of (untreated) genetically slow hydroxylators.

The most likely explanation for our findings is an inhibition of desipramine metabolism by quinidine and quinine, as previously described in human liver microsomes (von Bahr et al. 1985). Also, in vivo quinidine was much more efficient as inhibitor than its diastereoisomer, virtually transforming rapid into slow hydroxylators. Interestingly, quinine decreased the excretion of 2-hydroxydesipramine in rapid but not in slow metabolizers. This is in

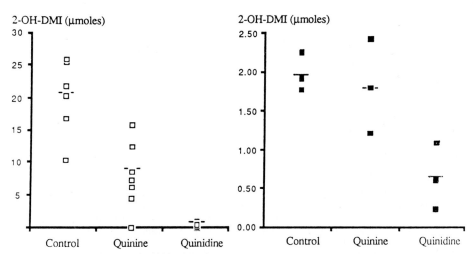

Fig. 1. Urinary recovery of 2-hydroxydesipramine (*2-OH-DMI*) before and during treatment with quinine and quinidine in seven rapid (*left panel*) and three slow (*right panel*) hydroxylators. (From Steiner et al. 1988)

agreement with the phenotypic differences reported in the interaction between quinidine and metoprolol (Leemann et al. 1986) and between cimetidine and desipramine (Steiner and Spina 1987). On the other hand, quinidine also modified the excretion of 2-hydroxydesipramine in the three slow hydroxylators.

From this and earlier studies we can conclude that quinidine is a strong inhibitor of the oxidative metabolism of drugs affected by the debrisoquine/sparteine polymorphism. This indicates that concomitant intake of other compounds may drastically alter drug metabolism even when it is mainly determined by genetic factors, causing errors in phenotype determination. Moreover quinidine treatment may be associated with clinically important drug interactions when combined with drugs that have a metabolism cosegregating with that of debrisoquine. Furthermore, as suggested by others (Leemann et al. 1986; Speirs et al. 1986), quinidine might be used as a tool to transform rapid into slow hydroxylators, providing a useful addition to panels of phenotyped subjects. New drugs under development might therefore be tested for this polymorphism without repeated exposure of slow hydroxylators.

References

Boobis AR, Murray S, Kahn GC, Robertz GM, Davies DS (1983) Substrate specificity of the form of cytochrome P-450 catalyzing the 4-hydroxylation of debrisoquine in man. Mol Pharmacol 23:474–481

Brinn R, Brøsen K, Gram LF, Haghfelt T, Otton V (1986) Sparteine oxidation is practically abolished in quinidine-treated patients. Br J Clin Pharmacol 22:194–197

Brøsen K, Gram LF, Haghfelt T, Bertilsson L (1987) Extensive metabolizers of debrisoquine become poor metabolizers during quinidine treatment. Pharmacol Toxicol 60:312–314

Eichelbaum M (1982) Defective oxidation of drugs: pharmacokinetic and therapeutic implications. Clin Pharmacokinet 7:1–22

Eichelbaum M, Spannbrucker N, Steincke B, Dengler HJ (1979) Defective N-oxidation of sparteine in man: a new pharmacogenetic defect. Eur J Clin Pharmacol 16:183–187

Inaba T, Tyndale RE, Mahon WA (1986) Quinidine: potent inhibition of sparteine and debrisoquine oxidation in vivo. Br J Clin Pharmacol 22:199–200

Jacqz E, Hall SD, Branch RA (1986) Genetically determined polymorphisms in drug oxidation. Hepatology 6:1020–1032

Leemann T, Dayer P, Meyer UA (1986) Single-dose quinidine treatment inhibits metoprolol oxidation in extensive metabolizers. Eur J Clin Pharmacol 29:739–741

Mahgoub A, Idle JR, Dring LG, Lancaster R, Smith RL (1977) Polymorphic hydroxylation of debrisoquine in man. Lancet 2:584–586

Mikus G, Ha HR, Vozeh S, Zekorn C, Follath F, Eichelbaum M (1986) Pharmacokinetics and metabolism of quinidine in extensive and poor metabolizers of sparteine. Eur J Clin Pharmacol 31:69–72

Otton SV, Inaba T, Kalow W (1984) Competitive inhibition of sparteine oxidation in human liver by β-adrenoceptor antagonists and other cardiovascular drugs. Life Sci 34:73–80

Otton SV, Brinn RU, Gram LF (1986) Quinidine 3-hydroxylase activity in human liver microsomes: effect of added debrisoquine, sparteine and desipramine (Abstr no 318). Acta Pharmacol Toxicol (Copenh) [Suppl 5] 59:113

Price-Evans DA, Mahgoub A, Sloan TP, Idle JR, Smith RL (1980) A family and population study of the genetic polymorphism of debrisoquine oxidation in a white British population. J Med Genet 17:102–105

Speirs CJ, Murray S, Boobis AR, Seddon CE, Davies DS (1986) Quinidine and the identification of drugs whose elimination is impaired in subjects classified as poor metabolizers of debrisoquine. Br J Clin Pharmacol 22:739–743

Spina E (1987) Hydroxylation of desmethylimipramine in man. Thesis, Karolinska Institute, Stockholm

Spina E, Birgersson C, von Bahr C, Ericsson O, Mellstrom B, Steiner E, Sjoqvist F (1984) Phenotypic consistency in hydroxylation of desmethylimipramine and debrisoquine in healthy subjects and in human liver microsomes. Clin Pharmacol Ther 36:677–682

Spina E, Steiner E, Ericsson O, Sjoqvist F (1987) Hydroxylation of desmethylimipramine: dependence on the debrisoquine hydroxylation phenotype. Clin Pharmacol Ther 41:314–319

Steiner E, Spina E (1987) Differences in the inhibitory effect of cimetidine on desipramine metabolism between rapid and slow debrisoquine hydroxylators. Clin Pharmacol Ther 42:278–282

Steiner E, Dumont E, Spina E, Dahlqvist R (1988) Inhibition of desipramine 2-hydroxylation by quinidine and quinine. Clin Pharmacol Ther 43:577–581

Sutfin TA, Jusko WJ (1979) High-performance liquid chromatographic assay for imipramine, desipramine and their 2-hydroxylated metabolites. J Pharm Sci 68:703–705

Von Bahr C, Spina E, Birgersson C, Ericsson O, Goransson M, Henthorn T, Sjöqvist F (1985) Inhibition of desmethylimipramine 2-hydroxylation by drugs in human liver microsomes. Biochem Pharmacol 34:2501–2505

Debrisoquine Oxidation Phenotype in Psychiatric Patients [*]

J. Benítez, B. Piñas, M. A. García, C. Martínez, A. Llerena, and J. Cobaleda [1]

1 Introduction

Between 5% and 10% of Caucasian populations exhibit poor metabolism of debrisoquine and sparteine (Clark 1985). Results obtained by our group indicate that among the Spanish population the percentage of poor metabolizers of debrisoquine is around 6% (Benítez et al. 1988). Generally the poor-metabolizer phenotype is at increased risk of toxicity when treated with drugs subjected to oxidative metabolism by the debrisoquine/sparteine type of pathway (Idle et al. 1983). A significant correlation between nortriptyline clearance and debrisoquine metabolic ratio has been demonstrated by Bertilsson et al. (1980). Steady-state concentrations of desipramine have also been shown to be highly correlated with the debrisoquine metabolic ratio (Bertilsson and Aberg-Wistedt 1983; Spina 1987).

It has been shown in biochemical studies that nortriptyline, desipramine, imipramine, amitriptyline and chlorpromazine inhibit the sparteine/debrisoquine mono-oxygenase in human liver preparations (Otton et al. 1983; Inaba et al. 1984). In another study by Inaba et al. (1985), several drugs used in the treatment of psychosis, such as chlorpromazine and haloperidol, were shown to inhibit the oxidation of sparteine in human liver preparations. A study by Syvälahti et al. (1986) comparing patients with and without neuroleptic treatment, suggested a competitive inhibition of oxidative metabolism by neuroleptics. The present study provides further in vivo evidence of such effects of neuroleptics on debrisoquine hydroxylation.

2 Methods

A total of 122 patients (95 men and 27 women) participated in the study. Their ages ranged from 19 to 72 years (mean 38.7 years). The study was conducted in accordance with the Helsinki Declaration. All patients were treated with neuroleptic drugs; the average number of drugs per patient was 1.6 (range,

[*] Supported in part by grants FISss 88/0898 from the Spanish Ministry of Health and CAICYT PB85-0154 from the Spanish Ministry of Education.
[1] Department of Pharmacology and Psychiatry, Medical School, University of Extremadura, 06071 Badajoz, Spain

Clinical Pharmacology in Psychiatry
Editors: S. G. Dahl and L. F. Gram
(Psychopharmacology Series 7)
© Springer-Verlag Berlin Heidelberg 1989

1–4). The control group consisted of 601 healthy volunteers, most of them students and staff at our Medical School. Their ages ranged from 18 to 83 years (mean 26 years). None of them had been taking any medication for at least 2 weeks before the study.

After an overnight fast, each patient or healthy volunteer emptied the bladder and was given a 10-mg tablet of debrisoquine (Dexlinax, Hoffman-La Roche). Thereafter, all urine was collected for 6 h. The volume of each specimen was measured, and an aliquot was stored at $-20\,^{\circ}$C until assayed.

The urine concentrations of debrisoquine and 4-hydroxydebrisoquine were determined by the flame ionization gas chromatographic method described by Lennard et al. (1977). Individual rates of metabolism were expressed as the ratios of parent drug and metabolite urinary concentrations.

3 Results

The debrisoquine metabolic ratio was 3.5 ± 0.5 (mean $\pm$ SE) in the control group of 601 healthy volunteers. Of these, 35 were poor metabolizers of debrisoquine (metabolic ratio ≥ 12.6).

Table 1. Poor metabolizers (PM) among patients on neuroleptic monotherapy plus other drugs

Neuroleptic	n	PM	%
Levomepromazine	11	5	45.5
Pericyazine	5	0	0
Thioridazine	16	10	65.5
Haloperidol	5	1	20.0
Clozapine	5	0	0
Clothiapine	5	0	0
Chlorpromazine	2	2	100
Fluphenazine	2	1	50
Thioproperazine	1	0	0
Trifluperazine	1	1	100
Sulpiride	1	0	0

Table 2. Poor metabolizers (PM) among patients on monotherapy

Neuroleptic	n	PM	%
Levomepromazine	4	2	50.0
Pericyazine	1	0	0
Thioridazine	6	5	83.3
Haloperidol	1	0	0
Clozapine	4	0	0
Clothiapine	2	0	0

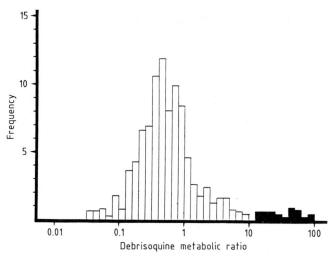

Fig. 1. Frequency distribution of log debrisoquine metabolic ratio in 601 healthy subjects. *Solid bars,* poor metabolizers, *open bars,* extensive metabolizers

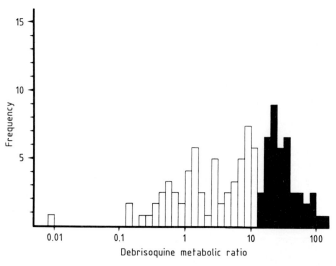

Fig. 2. Frequency distribution of log debrisoquine metabolic ratio in 122 psychiatric patients. *Solid bars,* poor metabolizers; *open bars,* extensive metabolizers

The patients receiving neuroleptics had a significantly higher mean metabolic ratio (19.1 ± 2.4; $p < 0.01$), 50 of them having a value of at least 12.6. The percentage of poor metabolizers was 65.7% for those receiving thioridazine ($n = 38$), 60% with fluphenazine ($n = 30$), 50% with levomepromazine ($n = 38$) and 24.2% with haloperidol ($n = 33$). The frequency of poor metabolizers among patients on neuroleptic monotherapy plus other drug and those on pure monotherapy with only one neuroleptic, are presented in Tables 1 and 2, respectively. The distribution of metabolic ratios among healthy subjects and patients are shown in Figs. 1 and 2, respectively.

Metabolic ratios were not higher in patients on monotherapy with clozapine or clothiapine than in the control group.

4 Discussion

The findings presented here show that the hydroxylation of debrisoquine is decreased in patients receiving common clinical doses of some neuroleptics.

The decreased oxidation of debrisoquine does not seem to be connected with the underlying disease, according to the results reported by Syvälahti et al. (1986). Their patients who were not receiving neuroleptic treatment, had normal low metabolic ratios. Inaba et al. (1984, 1985) have shown that chlorpromazine, haloperidol and some other neuroleptic drugs inhibit sparteine oxidation in vitro. Syvälahti et al. (1986) found a greater proportion of poor metabolizers among patients treated with thioridazine and levomepromazine than expected on the basis of results in healthy volunteers. This is confirmed by our results. Moreover, our study shows similar results for fluphenazine and, to a lesser extent, also for haloperidol. These effects are somewhat similar to, albeit more pronounced than, those found by Nordin et al. (1985) in depressed patients phenotyped with debrisoquine during and after nortriptyline treatment.

Nevertheless, we found no poor metabolizers among patients whose antipsychotic therapy was with clozapine or clothiapine only. Therefore, we could say that it is mainly the phenotiazines, and to a lesser extent haloperidol, among the neuroleptic drugs that interfere with debrisoquine oxidation. Neuroleptics of the dibenzodiazepine and dibenzothiazepine classes probably do not interfere, or at least not in a pronounced way. This would suggest that these two groups of drugs could be used instead of phenothiazines when dangerous interactions are expected, although more studies are needed before such a conclusion can be generalized. In addition, of course, side effects must be taken into account.

References

Benítez J, Llerena A, Cobaleda J (1988) Debrisoquine oxidation in a Spanish population. Clin Pharmacol Ther 44:74–77

Bertilsson L, Aberg-Wistedt A (1983) The debrisoquine hydroxylation test predicts steady-state plasma levels of desipramine. Br J Clin Pharmacol 15:388–389

Bertilsson L, Eichelbaum M, Mellström B, Säwe J, Schutz HV, Sjöqvist F (1980) Nortriptyline and antipyrine clearance in relation to debrisoquine hydroxylation in man. Life Sci 27:1673–1677

Clark DWJ (1985) Genetically determined variability in acetylation and oxidation. Therapeutic implications. Drugs 29:342–375

Idle JR, Oates NS, Shah RR, Smith RL (1983) Protecting poor metabolizers, a group at high risk of adverse drug reactions. Lancet 1:1388

Inaba T, Nakano M, Otton SV, Mahon WA, Kalow W (1984) A human cytochrome P-450 characterized by inhibition studies as the sparteine-debrisoquine monooxygenase. Can J Physiol Pharmacol 62:860–862

Inaba T, Jurima M, Mahon WA, Kalow W (1985) In vitro inhibition studies of two isozymes of human liver cytochrome P-450. Drug Metab Dispos 13:443–448

Lennard MS, Silas JH, Smith AJ, Tucker GT (1977) Determination of debrisoquine and its 4-hydroxy metabolites in biological fluids by gas chromatography with flame ionization and nitrogen-selective detection. J Chromatogr 133:161–166

Nordin C, Siwers B, Benítez J, Bertilsson L (1985) Plasma concentrations of nortriptyline and its 10-hydroxymetabolite in depressed patients – relationship to the debrisoquine hydroxylation metabolic ratio. Br J Clin Pharmacol 19:832–835

Otton SV, Inaba T, Kalow W (1983) Inhibition of sparteine oxidation in human liver by tricyclic antidepressants and other drugs. Life Sci 32:795–800

Spina E (1987) Hydroxylation of desmethylimipramine in man. Thesis, Karolinska Institute, Stockholm

Syvälahti EKG, Lindberg R, Kallio J, de Voch M (1986) Inhibitory effects of neuroleptics on debrisoquine oxidation in man. Br J Clin Pharmacol 22:89–92

Role of Pharmacogenetics in Drug Development

L. P. BALANT [1] and A. E. BALANT-GORGIA [2]

1 Introduction

Among the factors which hinder the introduction of a new drug onto the market, a narrow therapeutic range combined with large inter-individual variations in pharmacokinetics is of major concern. For a compound with these qualities, it may be expected that a proportion of the patient population receiving a standard dose will develop unwanted side effects related to higher than normal blood concentrations of the active substance, whereas other patients may show an apparent non-response due to unusually low concentrations.

It is now well recognized that drugs are eliminated by metabolic routes that are under genetic control. Some of these metabolic pathways show a distribution in their activity that allows patients and healthy volunteers to be classified into distinct subpopulations. Among the best studied routes showing genetic polymorphism are the sulphonamide type of acetylation and the debrisoquine type of hydroxylation. The latter is known as the debrisoquine/sparteine-type polymorphism of drug oxidation. It has a considerable incidence in the population, with 5% to 10% of investigated Caucasians falling into the category of poor hydroxylators (Alvan et al., in preparation; Eichelbaum 1982; Evans et al. 1980; Lennard et al. 1986). Other oxidative reactions seem to be independently polymorphically regulated; among these is mephenytoin hydroxylation.

The clinical relevance of such genetic variability depends strongly on the therapeutic class of the compound and on the concentration-effect relationships for the desired and the unwanted effects (Brøsen and Gram, this volume). Thus, β-blocking agents which display a large therapeutic margin can be used almost regardless of the patient's phenotype: large inter-individual variations of the steady-state blood concentrations are probably of minor clinical significance and certainly do not warrant blood concentration monitoring. In contrast, it is now generally recognized that for tricyclic antidepressants, blood level monitoring is important for the prevention of un-

[1] Clinical Research Unit, Department of Psychiatry, University of Geneva, P.O. Box 79, 1211 Geneva 8, Switzerland
[2] Therapeutic Drug Monitoring Unit, Department of Psychiatry, University Medical Center, 1211 Geneva 4, Switzerland

Clinical Pharmacology in Psychiatry
Editors: S. G. Dahl and L. F. Gram
(Psychopharmacology Series 7)
© Springer-Verlag Berlin Heidelberg 1989

wanted side effects and therapeutic failures, although this point of view is still not universally held.

In the present pharmaco-political context, the benefit to risk ratio for a new drug must be very stringently assessed. This may lead the pharmaceutical industry to stop the development of potentially important new chemical substances, for which early studies in man indicate the possibility of a higher than expected incidence of side effects or difficulties in managing the differences in dose requirements between different patients. The present paper discusses whether genetic polymorphism in drug metabolism represents an important factor in determining the overall benefit to risk ratio, and proposes suggestions as to how this problem may be handled during the development of a new drug. For practical reasons, examples will be limited to drugs associated with the debrisoquine/sparteine polymorphism of oxidative drug metabolism.

2 Inter-Individual Variability in Drug Response Linked to Genetic Polymorphism in Drug Metabolism

Any kind of genetic polymorphism in the disposition of a drug has the potential to enhance inter-individual variability in the pharmacokinetics of that drug. The dispersion on any relevant kinetic parameter is likely to be greater when the overall variation on the parameter is due to the existence of more than one discrete subpopulation than in the polygenic case, where there is a single population. As a rule, distributions in the former case tend to be highly skewed or bimodal, whereas in the latter case they tend towards normality. However, the likely extent and consistency of such variability are difficult to predict from published information.

Non-linear kinetics have been reported for the disposition of imipramine. Such dose-dependent behaviour contributes substantially to the variability of steady-state concentrations of imipramine and desipramine, although its relationship to the hydroxylation status of the patients has not been established (Brøsen et al. 1986). In other circumstances, non-linear kinetics could be related to the debrisoquine/sparteine phenotype. As an example, bufuralol (a β-blocking agent with an unusual, relatively small therapeutic index) may display non-linear disposition kinetics in poor metabolizers and linear kinetics in extensive metabolizers (Dayer et al. 1985). Case reports have also been published; one patient, phenotyped as a poor hydroxylator, showed non-linear kinetics of desmethylclomipramine disposition after co-administration of allopurinol (Balant-Gorgia et al. 1987). Depending on the values of V_{max} and K_m and on the drug concentration, it is conceivable that fast metabolizers could also exhibit non-linear kinetics as far as first-pass metabolism is concerned, as described for imipramine (Brøsen and Gram 1988). Further work in suitably planned studies is required before the practical relevance of these findings can be fully assessed. Nevertheless, the presently available information indicates that, under certain circumstances, genetic polymorphism may transform the kinetics of a compound from linear into non-linear. This could have important clinical implications.

3 Preclinical Investigations

Early in the development of a new drug, it is now customary to perform preliminary metabolic studies in animals. The data from such investigations, together with theoretical considerations, may help in determining whether a given compound is likely to be metabolized by pathways known to be under polymorphic genetic control in man. It must, however, be kept in mind that a given enzyme may metabolize a substrate in different positions. It is also possible, as demonstrated in the rabbit model of the acetylation polymorphism, that two drugs may be handled by the same enzyme, one in a polymorphic and the other in a non-polymorphic fashion. Accordingly, caution must be applied when extrapolating from in vitro or animal data to man.

At this stage it might be useful to extend further the predictability of such findings for man by using in vitro techniques with human hepatocytes or liver microsomes. The trend towards the establishment of human liver banks, comprising well characterized samples stored under defined conditions (Boobis et al. 1980; Meier et al. 1983; von Bahr et al. 1980; von Bahr et al., this volume) may prove invaluable in the application of such an approach. In the present situation, when neither pure cytochrome P-450 isoenzymes nor specific inhibitory antibodies against the isoenzymes are readily available, one must rely mainly on experiments with samples from subjects of defined phenotype or in which competitive inhibition of drug substrates is assessed. Thus, by using livers from subjects identified as poor metabolizers or by performing inhibition studies with marker drugs, valuable predictive information on the qualitative and quantitative importance of a polymorphic enzyme in the metabolism of a new compound should be obtained. Many clinically important drug-metabolic interactions could probably also be detected using such techniques.

If in vitro experiments provide an indication that polymorphic differences are indeed to be expected in man, it would be prudent to perform, as soon as possible, pharmacokinetic experiments in healthy volunteers, phenotyped as extensive and poor metabolizers for the metabolic pathway under consideration. This is presently quite feasible by using relatively simple methodology for the debrisoquine/sparteine type of polymorphism and also for the mephenytoin type. One may even use a combination of probes to phenotype volunteers for different polymorphisms in one session (Breimer et al. 1988). In addition, studies with specific inhibitors of a polymorphic enzyme such as quinidine, might be performed in extensive metabolizers (Inaba et al. 1986; Speirs et al. 1986). Such single-dose studies can be performed at a time when only minimal animal toxicological data are available (e.g. mutagenic potential, 1- or 2-week toxicity studies in two animal species and safety pharmacology).

The aim of such an investigation would be to confirm the findings in animals and in vitro and to determine the contribution of the polymorphic metabolic pathway to the overall elimination of the drug. Indeed, if the metabolic route represents only a small fraction of the overall disposition of the new compound, it is very unlikely that genetic polymorphism would be of clinical relevance as far as efficacy is concerned, since it would not lead to an increased variability in the elimination of the drug. However, a drug that is only slightly metabolized by a polymorphically regulated enzyme will still interact with it and may therefore inhibit the metabolism of other compounds, as in the case of quinidine, and this may be of clinical importance. As described above, such drug-drug interactions should be detectable at an early stage of drug development. Finally, such a drug could be metabolized to toxic products from which poor metabolizers would be relatively protected. The relevance of this last situation cannot be assessed with the data presently available.

On the other hand, if preliminary metabolic studies in man confirm the potential importance of genetically determined pharmacokinetic variability, it will be necessary to consider the magnitude of the therapeutic margin. Only if the therapeutic margin is small, should a "no-go" decision be considered. Such information can usually be inferred from the animal data available at this stage of the pharmacology, toxicology and safety pharmacology programmes.

If it is decided to proceed with the development of the new chemical entity, the design of the investigations to be performed during phase I, II and III studies should be tailored to the potential problem represented by genetic polymorphism in the metabolism of the drug. As an alternative, chemical analogues which retain the pharmacological properties of the drug, but which are metabolized by other routes, should be considered. It should, however, be emphasized that if a large proportion of the metabolism of a compound is subject to genetic polymorphism, this is not in itself an indication to stop development of the drug; the final decision should be made taking into account drug alternatives and the potential therapeutic progress offered by the new drug.

4 Clinical Pharmacology Investigations

In the context of genetic polymorphism, phase I studies in healthy volunteers should be aimed, among other things, at confirming the preliminary findings obtained in vitro and in animals. Parameters that should be evaluated are: the importance of the different disposition pathways in vivo, the pharmacokinetic variability of presystemic and systemic clearances, the consequence of such variability on steady-state blood concentrations, and possible non-linearity of elimination. At the same time, such studies should be aimed at the development of the phase II clinical trials in patients. Again, in the context of genetic polymorphism, it would be particularly useful to obtain information from the first patients in the phase II programme on the relationship between blood concentrations of the drug and pharmacodynamics, efficacy and side effects. This should enable an initial estimation of the therapeutic margin in the target population.

5 Clinical Investigations

If the results of the clinical pharmacology programme justify the continuation of the project, two extreme possible situations may be considered. (a) The drug has a wide therapeutic margin, no toxic metabolites are formed in any patient subgroup and the pharmacokinetic variability is almost negligible. Such a drug would then be developed as any other compound. Propranolol is a typical example. (b) The drug has a narrow therapeutic margin and the metabolic variability is a potential concern. In the case where the drug exhibits genetic polymorphism, one could envisage monitoring the blood concentrations of the drug during phase III clinical trials according to the "pharmacokinetic screen" concept (Temple 1983). The patients potentially at risk could then be identified using, for example, the "population kinetics" approach (Sheiner and Benet 1985). Although there are certainly many ways of coping with this problem, their discussion exceeds the scope of the present paper.

Finally, if a drug falls into this category, but it is felt that it represents a true therapeutic innovation, it would be useful to develop a drug-monitoring strategy, even before the drug is marketed. This should help to keep the drug free from an excessively high incidence of unwanted side effects which could otherwise lead to its early withdrawal.

6 Conclusions

The fact that the metabolism of a new drug is under substantial polymorphic genetic control, resulting in considerable pharmacokinetic variability, should not be a reason a priori for stopping its development. If exclusion of compounds had taken place on these grounds, valuable drugs such as the β-blocking agents and tricyclic antidepressants would not be available today or would have encountered additional difficulty in reaching the market.

For the pharmaceutical industry it is important to make the "go/no-go" decisions as soon as possible in the experimental life of a new drug. In vitro studies with human liver tissue and clinical pharmacological panel studies performed during phase I and phase II of drug development appear, at present, to represent the most suitable way of providing the necessary information on polymorphic drug metabolism at an early stage.

Acknowledgements. The authors wish to thank the members of the Management Committee of the European Concerted Action COST B1 (Criteria for the Choice and Definition of Healthy Volunteers and/or Patients for Phase I and II Studies in Drug Development) for their help during the preparation of the manuscript.

References

Balant-Gorgia AE, Balant L, Zysset T (1987) High plasma concentrations of desmethyl-clomipramine after chronic administration of clomipramine to a poor metabolizer. Eur J Clin Pharmacol 32:101–102

Boobis AR, Brodie MJ, Kahn GC, Fletcher DR, Saunders JH, Davies DS (1980) Monooxygenase activity of human liver in microsomal fractions of needle biopsy specimens. Br J Clin Pharmacol 9:11–19

Breimer DD, Schellens JHM, Soons PA (1988) Assessment of in vivo oxidative drug metabolizing enzyme activity in man by applying a cocktail approach. In: Proceedings of the 8th International Symposium on Microsomes and Drug Oxidation. Taylor and Francis, London, pp 232–240

Brøsen K, Gram LF (1988) First-pass metabolism of imipramine and desipramine: impact of the sparteine oxidation phenotype. Clin Pharmacol Ther 43:400–406

Brøsen K, Gram LF, Klysner R, Bech P (1986) Steady-state levels of imipramine and its metabolites: significance of dose-dependent kinetics. Eur J Clin Pharmacol 30:43–49

Dayer P, Balant L, Kupfer A, Striberni R, Leemann T (1985) Effect of oxidative polymorphism (debrisoquine/sparteine type) on hepatic first-pass metabolism of bufuralol. Eur J Clin Pharmacol 28:317–320

Eichelbaum M (1982) Defective oxidation of drugs: pharmacokinetic and therapeutic implications. Clin Pharmacokinet 7:1–22

Evans DAP, Mahgoub A, Sloan TP, Idle JR, Smith RL (1980) A family and population study of the genetic polymorphism of debrisoquine in a white British population. J Med Genet 17:102–105

Inaba T, Tyndale RE, Mahon WA (1986) Quinidine: potent inhibition of sparteine and debrisoquine oxidation in vivo. Br J Clin Pharmacol 22:199–200

Lennard MS, Tucker GT, Wood HF (1986) The polymorphic oxidation of beta-adrenoceptor antagonists. Clinical pharmacokinetic considerations. Clin Pharmacokinet 11:1–17

Meier PJ, Mueller HK, Dick B, Meyer UA (1983) Hepatic monooxygenase activities in subjects with a genetic defect in drug oxidation. Gastroenterology 85:682–692

Sheiner LB, Benet LZ (1985) Premarketing observational studies of population pharmacokinetics of new drugs. Clin Pharmacol Ther 38:481–487

Speirs CJ, Murray S, Boobis AR, Seddon CE, Davies DS (1986) Quinidine and the identification of drugs whose elimination is impaired in subjects classified as poor metabolizers of debrisoquine. Br J Clin Pharmacol 22:739–743

Temple R (1983) Discussion paper on the testing of drugs in the elderly. Memorandum of the Food and Drug Administration of DHHS, Washington

Von Bahr C, Groth CG, Jansson H, Lundgren G, Lind M, Glaumann H (1980) Drug metabolism in human livers in vitro: establishment of a human liver bank. Clin Pharmacol Ther 27:711–725

Clinical Significance of Pharmacokinetic Variability

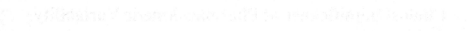

Clinical Implications of the Pharmacokinetics of Tricyclic Antidepressants

J. C. Nelson, C. Mazure, and P. I. Jatlow[1]

Knowledge gained during the past 20 years about the pharmacokinetics of tricyclic antidepressant drugs has helped to refine clinical practice. This discussion will focus on kinetic features of tricyclic antidepressants which appear to have important implications for clinical practice.

1 Relationship of Plasma Concentrations to Clinical Outcome

Plasma concentrations of tricyclic antidepressants vary 40-fold among patients receiving comparable dosage. This observation led to the hypothesis that the variability in plasma levels might account for the differences in response and side effects encountered during treatment. It is beyond the scope of this discussion to review all of the studies in this area; nevertheless, the issue warrants acknowledgement since the clinical relevance of tricyclic antidepressant kinetics is dependent on the assumption that drug levels affect outcome.

Studies of the relationship to tricyclic antidepressant drug concentrations and clinical response have been mixed and controversial. However, the American Psychiatric Association Task Force on Use of Laboratory Tests in Psychiatry (1985) concluded that relationships of drug concentrations and response appear to be established in severe endogenous inpatients for nortriptyline, imipramine, and desipramine. Although effective levels vary from drug to drug, considering the broad range of plasma concentrations observed, there is some consistency if the higher levels of hydroxynortriptyline are taken into account. These drugs are effective generally in the 100–300 ng/ml range. While this range is not precise, it does define drug levels which are clearly low and those which are clearly high.

The reduced effectiveness of nortriptyline at higher levels remains an interesting question. Why should a window occur with one tricyclic antidepressant and not with others? This issue is further complicated by the problem of distinguishing side effects from symptoms. Some somatic symptoms may reflect both adverse drug effect and severity of depression (Nelson et al. 1984). Determining that elevated drug levels are truly less effective is more difficult than it seems.

[1] Yale University School of Medicine, Department of Psychiatry, Yale-New Haven Hospital, 20 York Street, New Haven, CT 06504, USA

Clinical Pharmacology in Psychiatry
Editors: S. G. Dahl and L. F. Gram
(Psychopharmacology Series 7)
© Springer-Verlag Berlin Heidelberg 1989

Tricyclic antidepressant blood levels have frequently not been associated with response in outpatient studies of depression. Possible explanations include the following: that drug levels have no relationship to response in these patients, that drug levels may be related to response in individuals but have no common threshold for the group, and that the threshold for true antidepressant effect is similar, but factors other than the drug have a greater effect on outcome. The latter possibility seems likely, given the high placebo response rate observed in these patients and reports that benzodiazepines, neuroleptics, and psychotherapy are of value in this group.

The other important question is whether elevated drug levels are associated with toxicity. Correlations of side effect and blood levels have been reported (Asberg et al. 1970), but the side effects noted seldom required discontinuation of treatment. There have not been many studies of severe adverse reactions which interrupted treatment. Delirium has been reported in patients with high levels of amitriptyline (Preskorn and Simpson 1982; Livingston et al. 1983). Preskorn et al. (1988) have also suggested that such a relationship might hold for the other tricyclic antidepressants, but this is less well established. In several sizable studies of imipramine, delirium was not reported. During treatment with nortriptyline, levels above 450 ng/ml are less common. We reported an increased frequency of delirium in patients receiving desipramine with concomitant neuroleptic treatment, but delirium rarely occurred in patients on desipramine alone, regardless of blood levels (Nelson et al. 1982a). The increased frequency in patients on neuroleptics was not explained by higher plasma levels of desipramine but by the presence of neuroleptic. Severe tremors have been associated with elevated desipramine plasma levels (Nelson et al. 1984), but it is not clear whether this has a similar basis. It does suggest that toxicity may be associated with elevated drug concentrations.

2 Effects of Other Drugs on Concentrations of Tricyclic Antidepressants

The effect of neuroleptics on tricyclic antidepressant plasma levels was one of the first common drug interactions in psychiatry to be well described (Gram and Overo 1972). The mechanism was the inhibition of hydroxylation. We noted that the magnitude of this effect was substantial; desipramine levels commonly doubled following the addition of a neuroleptic (Nelson and Jatlow 1980). Many drugs have now been demonstrated to raise or lower tricyclic antidepressant blood levels. In our experience one of the most problematic interactions is the profound lowering of tricyclic antidepressant levels by barbiturates, which can make effective treatment with tricyclic antidepressants very difficult. Quinidine has a twofold effect. Not only does it have an apparent additive effect with tricyclic antidepressant to slow cardiac conduction, but it also inhibits the metabolism of the tricyclic antidepressants (Steiner et al. 1987). The effects of tricyclic antidepressants on the metabolism of other drugs has been less often reported, but inhibition of perphenazine metabolism by amitriptyline has been noted (Spiker et al. 1986).

3 Use of Timed Samples for Rapid Dose Adjustment

The possibility of adjusting dose on the basis of timed drug levels after a standard dose was suggested by several studies demonstrating a relationship between steady-state levels and single or multiple blood levels obtained after a single dose. While multiple sampling may be more precise, single samples are simpler to obtain and appear to be adequate for clinical purposes. The feasibility of this method was first reported for antitriptyline (Dawling et al. 1984; Madakasira and Khazanie 1985). Use of timed samples resulted in steady-state levels of amitriptyline and nortriptyline within the desired range and a high rate of response in the latter study.

We recently completed a study using 24-h plasma desipramine levels to calculate the dose necessary to obtain a target steady-state plasma level of 140 ng/ml. Dose adjustment employed the regression equation determined in a previous sample, linking single timed levels to steady-state levels (Nelson et al. 1987). When the dose was determined (50–500 mg/day), the full amount was administered the next day and then continued for 4 weeks. Unlike the experience with amitriptyline, rapid dose adjustment with desipramine was not accompanied by sedation. Forty-four of 48 patients achieved steady state levels within the range of 115–300 ng/ml. This differed significantly from a sample of 83 patients who received a fixed dose of 2.5 mg/kg, and in whom only 19 of 83 had levels in the 115–300 range (44/48 versus 19/83; $p < 0.01$).

Response rates for the rapid dose adjustment study were compared with a previous fixed dose efficacy study using a similar Hamilton cutoff score to define response (Nelson et al. 1982b). The patients in both studies were relatively similar, having unipolar nonpsychotic major depression which failed to respond to 1 week of hospitalization off antidepressants. In the current dose adjustment study 31 of 33 patients attained levels above 115 ng/ml, and at 3 weeks 17 of 33 responded (52%); at 4 weeks 21 of 32 (66%) responded. In the prior study employing a fixed dose of 2.5 mg/kg desipramine, 9 of 30 patients achieved levels above 115 ng/ml, and 11 of 30 (37%) responded at 3 weeks. The study terminated at this point, but most nonresponding patients continued on this dose for varying periods. No new responders were identified. Response rates in the two studies were not significantly different at 3 weeks, and this was not a parallel randomized comparison, but the results suggested a higher rate of response using the dose adjustment method.

The impact of rapid dose adjustment on the timing of response was also examined. Quitkin et al. (1984) previously suggested that 6 weeks of tricyclic antidepressant treatment is necessary to achieve the maximum response rate. In that study response rates rose slowly, reaching 20% by the 4th week and 55% by the 6th week. However, dosage was increased gradually, reaching the full dose by the 18th day. We examined our sample using a similar method of rating cumulative response on the Clinical Global Improvement scale. In the dose adjustment study the full dose was reached by the 3rd day of drug administration, and response rates began to ascend during week 2. At 2 weeks 18 of 35 responded (51%), at 3 weeks 22 of 33 responded (58%), and at 4 weeks 27 of 33 responded (82%), which was the maximal rate of response. Six nonresponding patients continued on desipramine but without further change. The maximal response rate in this sample was reached 2 weeks earlier than in the Quitkin study. It was our impression that the difference was explained by the rapid institution of the full dose in our study. It might be argued that rapid institution of 300 mg/day of desipramine might achieve similar results. However, in a study using a fixed dose of 300 mg/day of desipramine (Stewart et al. 1980), 7 of 20 patients had desipramine levels above 300 ng/ml. Use of a 24-h level provides the assurance that a full dose of 300–400 mg/day is necessary, and that slow metabolizers can be identified and given lower doses.

This technique does require that the clinical laboratory be prepared with appropriate internal standards to assay samples at low concentration and to provide rapid turnaround time for results. The potential savings in time of treatment justifies the effort.

4 Do Tricyclic Antidepressants Demonstrate Linear Kinetics?

Early reports indicated that the kinetics of tricyclic antidepressants were linear during dose adjustment. Recent reports, however, in small samples (Bjerre et al. 1981; Cooke et al. 1984) indicated nonlinear changes in desipramine. To assess the frequency and magnitude of nonlinear changes we examined 42 inpatients treated to steady state on a low and on a higher dose (Nelson and Jatlow 1987). We found that one-third of the sample had linear kinetics, another third demonstrated nonlinear changes, but the magnitude appeared to be of little importance. The final third had substantial nonlinear changes, that is, concentration rose 50% more than that predicted by the dose change. Marked nonlinear changes were most likely to occur in rapid metabolizers. The findings are very similar to those reported by Brøsen et al. (1986), who described steady-state concentration/dose ratios for desipramine and imipramine at two different imipramine doses in 17 patients. Nonlinear increases were noted particularly for desipramine. This findings differ for amitriptyline and nortriptyline, for which linear changes have been reported.

The findings would appear to raise questions about the value of rapid dose adjustment based on timed samples since these methods assume linear kinetics. However, since one is usually attempting to obtain a plasma level within a reasonably broad therapeutic range, the degree of nonlinear change encountered is usually not of sufficient magnitude to compromise the rapid dose method. Since marked nonlinear changes were most likely to occur in rapid metabolizers, these patients can be identified with the 24-h level and the dose reduced accordingly.

5 Activity of the Hydroxy Metabolites

Studies in vitro and in animals have suggested pharmacological activity for the hydroxy metabolites of tricyclic antidepressants, although antidepressant activity in human subjects has only recently been studied. Concentrations of hydroxyimipramine and hydroxyamitriptyline are low in human subjects relative to their parent compounds (Potter et al. 1982; Bock et al. 1982), but levels of hydroxydesipramine are commonly about half those of the parent drug (Bock et al. 1983), and levels of hydroxynortriptyline usually exceed those of the parent compound (Bertilsson et al. 1979).

Studies of hydroxynortriptyline during administration of amitriptyline suggested that these compounds might contribute to an upper limit of effectiveness (Breyer-Pfaff et al. 1982; Robinson et al. 1985). However, these analyses were complicated by the presence of three compounds – amitriptyline, nortriptyline and hydroxynortriptyline. Recently Nordin et al. (1987a) administered nortriptyline to 30 depressed inpatients and found that responders had nortriptyline levels within a window bounded by 358–728 nM (94–191 ng/ml) and hydroxynortriptyline levels between 428 nM and 688 nM (119–191 ng/ml), although these thresholds were based on retrospective inspection of the distribution.

Three studies have investigated the antidepressant activity of hydroxydesipramine during fixed dose trials, and all three were negative (Nelson et al. 1983; Amsterdam et al. 1985; Kutcher et al. 1986b). However, the effects of hydroxydesipramine may be obscured by the parent drug in a fixed dose study, since total drug levels are highly dependent on desipramine levels but not hydroxydesipramine (Bock et al. 1983). Patients with high ratios of hydroxydesipramine to desipramine (OH-DMI/DMI) rapidly metabolize the drug and thus have low desipramine and low total drug levels. In our sample (Bock et al. 1983) and that of Amsterdam et al. (1985) OH-DMI/DMI ratios inversely correlated with desipramine levels ($r = -0.63$ and $r = -0.75$, respectively).

We reexamined the relationship of hydroxydesipramine plasma levels and response in a prospective desipramine study in which 24-h plasma levels were used to achieve a relatively uniform desipramine plasma level (Nelson et al. 1988a). We hypothesized that the contribution of hydroxydesipramine to response might become apparent since desipramine levels were relatively constant. Twenty-seven nonpsychotic, unipolar inpatients with major depression completed a 4-week trial. On every measure of response, total drug levels (desipramine plus hydroxydesipramine) were more strongly correlated with outcome than were desipramine levels alone. Using multiple regression, both desipramine and hydroxydesipramine levels were independently and significantly associated with response on the Clinical Global Improvement scale and together accounted for 40% of the variance in response while desipramine levels alone explained 20% of the variance. These findings suggest that hydroxydesipramine has antidepressant activity. We noted that few patients in the current study had high OH-DMI/DMI ratios. In our fixed dose study

(Nelson et al. 1983), 7 of 45 patients had OH-DMI/DMI ratios greater than 0.7. In the dose adjustment study only 1 of 42 patients had a ratio above 0.7. We suspect that nonlinear changes in desipramine levels during dose adjustment resulted in lower OH-DMI/DMI ratios. This effect may diminish the clinical importance of hydroxydesipramine at therapeutic levels.

Research to date has explored the activity of the hydroxylated tricyclic antidepressants in the presence of the parent drug. The activity of the hydroxy metabolites could be more directly studied by administration of the hydroxy compounds themselves. This has only recently been attempted by Bertilsson et al. (this volume). Direct evidence of antidepressant activity would support the use of hydroxylated tricyclic antidepressants for the treatment of depression. Since hydroxydesipramine and hydroxynortriptyline are substantially less anticholinergic than their parent drugs (Nordin et al. 1987b), these metabolites might offer advantages over currently available tricyclic antidepressants.

6 Kinetic Changes in the Elderly

It is well known that the elderly are likely to show alterations in pharmacokinetics, but specific information about tricyclic antidepressants is only recently emerging. Early studies noted an association of age with drug levels (Nies et al. 1977), but recent large studies for desipramine (Nelson 1982a; Amsterdam et al. 1985) and for nortriptyline (Bertilsson et al. 1979) indicate little evidence of a relationship.

Elevation of the hydroxy metabolites of antidepressants in the elderly has been noted and is of particular concern since levels of such metabolites have been associated with ECG abnormalities (Young et al. 1985; Kutcher et al. 1986a). Increases in concentrations of hydroxynortriptyline in the elderly appears well established. In 16 elderly patients, on comparable doses, Young et al. (1984) found mean levels of hydroxynortriptyline to be almost twice as high as those in a younger sample, and in some cases, hydroxynortriptyline levels were four times higher than the level of nortriptyline.

Elevated hydroxydesipramine plasma levels were first reported by Kitanaka et al. in 1982. The mean OH-DMI/DMI ratio in the four elderly patients studies was 0.86 versus 0.38 in younger patients. However, the four older patients received lower doses (62 versus 183 mg/day) and achieved lower desipramine levels (44 versus 135 ng/ml) than the younger patients. Nonlinear kinetics of desipramine may have influenced these findings.

We examined two larger samples of depressed elderly patients who received doses comparable to younger patients, in order to determine the magnitude of the increase in hydroxydesipramine, if present (Nelson et al. 1988b). Sample 1, which received a fixed dose of desipramine, consisted of 68 patients, of whom 23 were over 60 years of age. Sample 2 received a dose adjusted to attain a target desipramine blood level; 20 of the 56 patients in this group were over 60. The mean age of the elderly patients was 69 and 72 in the two samples, respectively, and ranged up to 85. Hydroxydesipramine levels were higher in patients over 60 than in younger patients, but the differences were not significant in either sample individually. In the two samples combined, average hydroxydesipramine levels were 11 ng/ml higher in patients over 60 (55 versus 44 ng/ml) and the difference was significant ($p = 0.02$).

Unlike the Kitanaka study, OH-DMI/DMI ratios were not higher in the patients over 60, but our elderly patients received doses comparable to the younger patients. We suspect that if comparable dosage is administered, nonlinear increases in desipramine levels result in lower OH-DMI/DMI ratios (Nelson et al. 1987).

Our findings indicate that levels of hydroxy metabolites are elevated in the elderly, but the magnitude of the difference is not large in relation to total drug levels, averaging 220 ng/ml. However, other kinetic changes in this group may magnify this increase in hydroxy metabolites of tricyclic antidepressants.

Plasma protein binding of the tricyclic antidepressants has generally not been considered to be a major factor since protein binding is much less variable than total plasma concentration. However, Javaid et al. (1985) reported that plasma protein binding of tricyclic antidepressants may be reduced in the elderly. In addition, the hydroxy metabolites appear to be less protein bound in plasma than their parent compounds. For hydroxynortriptyline, free fractions of 35% have been reported (Breyer-Pfaff et al. 1982). Ratios of OH-DMI/DMI and of hydroxynortriptyline to nortriptyline are higher in CSF than in plasma (Potter et al. 1982; Nordin et al. 1985), probably as result of decreased protein binding of these compounds. If hydroxy metabolites of tricyclic antidepressants are less protein bound than their parent compounds, and protein binding is further decreased in the elderly, and, furthermore, concentrations of hydroxy metabolites are higher in the elderly, then free concentrations of hydroxy metabolites might be substantially elevated in older patients. Further study of kinetics in the elderly would not only be clinically useful but might further clarify the pharmacodynamic implications of these kinetic changes.

References

Amsterdam JD, Brunswick DJ, Potter L et al. (1985) Desipramine and 2-hydroxy-desipramine plasma levels in endogenous depressed patients: lack of correlation with therapeutic response. Arch Gen Psychiatry 42:361–364

APA Task Force on the Use of Laboratory Tests in Psychiatry (1985) Tricyclic antidepressants – blood level measurements and clinical outcome: an APA task force report. Am J Psychiatry 142:155–162

Asberg M, Chronholm B, Sjöqvist F et al. (1970) Correlation of subjective side effects with plasma concentration of nortriptyline. Br Med J 4:18–21

Bertilsson L, Mellstrom B, Sjöqvist F (1979) Pronounced inhibition of noradrenaline uptake by 10-hydroxy-metabolites of nortriptyline. Life Sci 25:1285–1292

Bjerre M, Gram LF, Kragh-Sorensen P et al. (1981) Dose-dependent kinetics of imipramine in elderly patients. Psychopharmacology (Berlin) 75:354–357

Bock JL, Giller E, Gray S et al. (1982) Steady-state plasma concentrations of cis and trans-10-OH amitriptyline metabolites. Clin Pharmacol Ther 31:609–616

Bock JL, Nelson JC, Gray S et al. (1983) Desipramine hydroxylation: variability and effect of antipsychotic drugs. Clin Pharmacol Ther 33:190–197

Breyer-Pfaff U, Gaertner HJ, Kreuter F et al. (1982) Antidepressive effect and pharmacokinetics of amitriptyline with consideration of unbound drug and 10-hydroxynortriptyline plasma levels. Psychopharmacology (Berlin) 76:240–244

Brøsen K, Gram LF, Klysner R, Bech P (1986) Steady-state levels of imipramine and its metabolites: significance of dose-dependent kinetics. Eur J Clin Pharmacol 30:43–49

Cooke RG, Warsh JJ, Stancer HC et al. (1984) The nonlinear kinetics of desipramine and 2-hydroxydesipramine in plasma. Clin Pharmacol Ther 36:343–349

Dawling S, Ford S, Rangedara DC, Lewis RR (1984) Amitriptyline dosage prediction in elderly patients from plasma concentration at 24 hours after a single 100 mg dose. Clin Pharmacokinet 9:261–266

Gram LF, Overo KF (1972) Drug interaction: inhibitory effect of neuroleptics on metabolism of tricyclic antidepressants in man. Br Med J 1:463–465

Javaid JI, Matuzas W, Davis JM, Fawcett J (1985) Plasma protein binding of tricyclic antidepressants in young and elderly. Presented at the American College of Neuropsychopharmacology, Annual Meeting, December 1985

Kitanaka I, Ross RJ, Cutler NR et al. (1982) Altered hydroxydesipramine concentrations in elderly depressed patients. Clin Pharmacol Ther 31:51–55

Kutcher SP, Reid K, Dubbin JD et al. (1986a) Electrocardiogram changes and therapeutic desipramine and 2-hydroxy-desipramine concentrations in elderly depressives. Br J Psychiatry 148:676–679

Kutcher SP, Shulman KI, Reed K (1986b) Desipramine plasma concentration and therapeutic response in elderly depressives: a naturalistic pilot study. Can J Psychiatry 31:752–754

Livingston RL, Zucker DK, Isenberg K, Wetzel RD (1983) Tricyclic antidepressants and delirium. J Clin Psychiatry 44:173–176

Madakasira S, Khazanie PG (1985) Reliability of amitriptyline dose prediction based on single-dose plasma levels. Clin Pharmacol Ther 37:145–149

Nelson JC, Jatlow P (1980) Neuroleptic effect on desipramine steady state plasma concentrations. Am J Psychiatry 137:1232–1234

Nelson JC, Jatlow PI (1987) Nonlinear desipramine kinetics: prevalence and importance. Clin Pharmacol Ther 41:666–670

Nelson JC, Jatlow PI, Bock J, Quinlan DM, Bowers MB (1982a) Major adverse reactions during desipramine treatment. Arch Gen Psychiatry 39:1055–1061

Nelson JC, Jatlow PI, Quinlan DM, Bowers MB (1982b) Desipramine plasma concentration and antidepressant response. Arch Gen Psychiatry 39:1419–1422

Nelson JC, Bock J, Jatlow P (1983) The clinical implications of 2-hydroxydesipramine in plasma. Clin Pharmacol Ther 33:183–189

Nelson JC, Jatlow P, Quinlan DM (1984) Subjective side effects during desipramine treatment. Arch Gen Psychiatry 41:55–59

Nelson JC, Jatlow PI, Mazure C (1987) Rapid desipramine dose adjustment using 24-hour levels. J Clin Psychopharmacol 7:72–77

Nelson JC, Mazure C, Jatlow PI (1988a) Antidepressant activity of 2-hydroxy-desipramine. Clin Pharmacol Ther 44:283–288

Nelson JC, Atillasoy E, Mazure C, Jatlow PI (1988b) Hydroxydesipramine in the elderly. J Clin Psychopharmacol 8:428–433

Nies A, Robinson DS, Friedman MJ et al. (1977) Relationship between age and tricyclic antidepressant plasma levels. Am J Psychiatry 134:790–793

Nordin C, Bertilsson L, Siwers B (1985) CSF and plasma levels of nortriptyline and its 10-hydroxy metabolite. Br J Clin Pharmacol 20:411–413

Nordin C, Bertilsson L, Siwers B (1987a) Clinical and biochemical effects during treatment of depression with nortriptyline – the role of 10-hydroxynortriptyline. Clin Pharmacol Ther 42:10–19

Nordin C, Bertilsson L, Otani K et al. (1987b) Little anticholinergic effect of E-10-hydroxynortriptyline compared with nortriptyline in healthy subjects. Clin Pharmacol Ther 41:97–102

Potter WZ, Calil HM, Sutfin TA et al. (1982) Active metabolites of imipramine and desipramine in man. Clin Pharmacol Ther 31:393–401

Preskorn SH, Simpson S (1982) Tricyclic antidepressant induced delirium and plasma drug concentration. Am J Psychiatry 139:822–823

Preskorn SH, Dorey RC, Jerkovich GS (1988) Therapeutic drug monitoring of tricyclic antidepressants. Clin Chem 34:822–828

Quitkin FM et al. (1984) Duration of antidepressant drug treatment. Arch Gen Psychiatry 41:238–245

Robinson DS, Cooper TB, Howard D et al. (1985) Amitriptyline and hydroxylated metabolite plasma levels in depressed outpatients. J Clin Psychopharmacol 5:83–88

Spiker DG, Perel JM, Hanin I et al. (1986) The pharmacological treatment of delusional depression: part II. J Clin Psychopharmacol 6:339–342

Steiner E, Dumont E, Spina E, Dahlqvist R (1987) Inhibition of desipramine 2-hydroxylation by quinidine and quinine. Clin Pharmacol Ther 43:577–581

Stewart JW, Quitkin F, Fyer A, Rifkin A, McGrath P, Liebowitz M, Rosnick L, Klein D (1980) Efficacy of desipramine in endogenously depressed patients. J Affect Dis 2:165–176

Young RC, Alexopoulos GS, Shamoian CA et al. (1984) Plasma 10-hydroxynortriptyline in elderly depressed patients. Clin Pharmacol Ther 35:540–544

Young RC, Alexopoulos GS, Shamoian CA et al. (1985) Plasma 10-hydroxynortriptyline and ECG changes in elderly depressed patients. Am J Psychiatry 142:866–868

Detection of Populations at Risk
Using Drug Monitoring Data

A. E. BALANT-GORGIA [1], M. GEX-FABRY [2], and L. P. BALANT [2]

1 Introduction

One of the aims of clinical pharmacokinetics is to detect patient subpopulations at risk of showing abnormally high or abnormally low blood concentrations when given normal doses of a drug. Numerous publications have reported that factors such as age (Nies et al. 1977), phenothiazine co-medication (Brøsen et al. 1986a; Balant-Gorgia et al. 1986), tobacco and alcohol (Sutfin et al. 1988; Vandel et al. 1982) as well as genetic factors (Brøsen et al. 1986b) are responsible for the large inter-individual variability affecting steady-state concentrations of tricyclic antidepressants. The clinical relevance of this information is clear since concentration-response curves of these drugs tend to be biphasic, with clinical deterioration and more frequent and severe side effects with increasing blood levels (Molnar and Gupta 1980).

The purpose of the present study was twofold. Its first aim was to show the feasibility of identifying subgroups of patients at risk, on the basis of drug monitoring data. The second goal was to determine the metabolic processes affected, using a model-based approach.

2 Patients and Methods

A total of 150 patients treated with clomipramine (Anafranil) for depressive illness at in- and out-patient units of the Geneva University Psychiatric Institution were included in the study. Their distribution according to sex, age, smoking, chronic alcohol intake and neuroleptic co-medication is given in Table 1. Patients suspected of non-compliance with their antidepressant medication were excluded. Doses of clomipramine were administered orally and ranged from 25 to 200 mg per day (median value, 100 mg per day). The corresponding range of concentrations was 32–621 ng/ml for the sum of clomipramine and desmethylclomipramine. Assuming a therapeutic range between 160 and 450 ng/ml (Faravelli et al. 1984; Preskorn and Irwin 1982), 63% of the patient population were within this range.

[1] Therapeutic Drug Monitoring Unit, Department of Psychiatry, University Medical Center, 1211 Geneva 4, Switzerland
[2] Clinical Research Unit, Department of Psychiatry, P.O. Box 79, 1211 Geneva 8, Switzerland

Clinical Pharmacology in Psychiatry
Editors: S. G. Dahl and L. F. Gram
(Psychopharmacology Series 7)
© Springer-Verlag Berlin Heidelberg 1989

Table 1. Deviations from the grand mean for hydroxylation and demethylation pseudo-clearances obtained by analysis of variance

	n	Hydroxylation (log clearance)		Demethylation clearance	
		Deviation from grand mean (1.19)	Statistical significance	Deviation from grand mean (22.3)	Statistical significance
Sex			$p < 0.05$		ns
Men	54	+0.04			
Women	93	−0.02			
Age (years)			$p < 0.005$		$p < 0.005$
<40	39	+0.09		+2.4	
40–64	71	+0.01		+2.1	
65–74	13	+0.03		−5.5	
≧75	24	−0.20		−6.9	
Smoking			ns		$p < 0.005$
No	97			−2.3	
Yes	50			+4.4	
Alcohol			ns		$p < 0.005$
No	134			+0.9	
Yes	13			−8.9	
Neuroleptics			$p < 0.05$		ns
No	136	+0.01			
Yes	11	−0.11			

Clomipramine and desmethylclomipramine blood monitoring was performed according to clinical routine, whenever the attending psychiatrist had clinical reasons to demand it (Sjöqvist et al. 1980). Blood samples were taken at steady-state, i.e. at least after 3 weeks at the same dosage regimen. Blood concentrations of clomipramine, desmethylclomipramine and their hydroxylated metabolites hydroxyclomipramine and hydroxydesmethylclomipramine were determined by HPLC and electrochemical detection (Balant-Gorgia et al. 1986).

The statistical analysis was performed by means of the ANOVA (analysis of variance) procedure of SPSS-X (Statistical Package for the Social Sciences).

3 Results

Visual inspection of concentration versus daily dose plots reveals that age may be an influential parameter in two ways: lower doses are generally administered to elderly patients, and fairly high blood concentrations are often reached despite the low doses. A pharmacokinetic model was developed in order to investigate the metabolic pathway involved in such an effect. Equal rates were assumed for demethylation of clomipramine to desmethyl-

clomipramine and of hydroxyclomipramine to hydroxydesmethylclomipramine. Similar rates were also postulated for hydroxylation of clomi-
pramine to hydroxyclomipramine and of desmethylclomipramine to hydroxydesmethylclomipramine. Identical rates of conjugation with glucuronic acid
and excretion were similarly postulated for the two hydroxy metabolites. In
addition, a hepatic first-pass effect was included for demethylation to desmethylclomipramine and hydroxylation to hydroxyclomipramine. Pseudo-
clearance values were then calculated on the basis of trough steady-state con-
centrations according to equations of the form: $C_{ss,trough} = F \times dose/\tau \times CL_{pseudo}$, where F is the systemic availability and τ the dosing interval. Clearance and first-pass effect were linked by the formulae:
$CL = Q_H \times \varepsilon$ and $F = 1 - \varepsilon$, where Q_H is the liver blood flow and ε is the hepatic
extraction ratio. This model was applicable since whole-blood concentrations
were available.

Model predictions indicate that reduced hydroxylation capacity results in
marked accumulation of desmethylclomipramine, accompanied by a smaller
increase of clomipramine levels. Demethylation does not affect the sum of
these two compounds. A plot relating the concentrations of clomipramine and
desmethylclomipramine measured during routine drug monitoring to the
clearances was constructed in order to identify patients exhibiting very slow
hydroxylation and/or demethylation rates (not shown). For a typical subject,
receiving 100 mg clomipramine per day, measured concentrations of 60 ng/ml
clomipramine and 150 ng/ml desmethylclomipramine lead to pseudo-
clearance values of 16 l per hour for hydroxylation and 23 l per hour for
demethylation.

Analysis of the pseudo-clearances for the 150 patients entering the study
reveals that hydroxylation clearance exhibits a strongly skewed distribution
(range, 5.5–42.5; median value, 15.7 l per hour), whereas demethylation
clearance is close to normal (range, 1.9–50.4; median value, 22.0 l per hour).
These values were further analysed for differences according to sex, age group,
smoking, chronic alcohol drinking and phenothiazine co-medication (Table
1). Hydroxylation as well as demethylation capacities decrease significantly
with age: the effect becomes apparent at about 75 years for the former process
and at about 65 years for the latter. Tobacco and alcohol seem to affect only
demethylation: smoking leads to an average 20% increase of demethylation
capacity, and strong inhibition follows chronic alcohol intake. Phenothiazine
co-medication is found to decrease hydroxylation clearance. Finally, women
show slightly reduced hydroxylation capacity compared to men.

4 Discussion

The present study indicates that very simple statistical techniques applied to
routine drug monitoring data may be of great help in identifying groups of
patients at risk of excessively low or high concentrations of clomipramine.
Results are in keeping with previous studies reporting increased tricyclic
antidepressant concentrations among the elderly (Nies et al. 1977), inhibition

of hydroxylation by levomepromazine (Brøsen et al. 1986a; Balant-Gorgia et al. 1986) and induction of liver enzymes by tobacco smoke (Sutfin et al. 1988). Reduced demethylation capacity following chronic alcohol intake is also expected as a likely result of liver damage. A possible effect of sex remains to be further investigated.

By considering pseudo-clearances, our model-based approach allows identification of the metabolic pathway affected by a given factor. The repercussions of this effect on drug concentrations are then easily predicted. By contrast, analysing either blood concentrations directly or metabolic ratios, which are under the combined influence of various processes, often leads to interpretation difficulties.

The prediction of extremely important accumulation of desmethyl-clomipramine as a result of poor hydroxylation capacity may be interpreted with respect to genetic polymorphism. Similarly, very high levels of desipramine have been reported in subjects phenotyped as poor metabolizers of debrisoquine or sparteine (Brøsen et al. 1986b). A recent series of case reports from our group further emphasizes the clinical relevance of such an observation: among eight patients characterized by excessively high antidepressant concentrations, three were later identified as poor metabolizers of debrisoquine, while three had neuroleptic co-medication not suspected before.

References

Balant-Gorgia AE, Balant LP, Genet C, Dayer P, Aeschlimann JM, Garrone G (1986) Importance of oxidative polymorphism and levomepromazine treatment on the steady-state blood concentrations of clomipramine and its major metabolites. Eur J Clin Pharmacol 31:449–455

Brøsen K, Gram LF, Klysner R, Bech P (1986a) Steady-state levels of imipramine and its metabolites: significance of dose-dependent kinetics. Eur J Clin Pharmacol 30:43–49

Brøsen K, Klysner R, Gram LF, Otton SV, Bech P, Bertilsson L (1986b) Steady-state concentrations of imipramine and its metabolites in relation to the sparteine/debrisoquine polymorphism. Eur J Clin Pharmacol 30:679–684

Faravelli C, Ballerini A, Ambonetti A, Broadhurst A, Das M (1984) Plasma levels and clinical response during treatment with clomipramine. J Affect Dis 6:95–107

Molnar G, Gupta RN (1980) Plasma levels and tricyclic antidepressant therapy. II. Pharmacokinetic, clinical and toxicologic aspects. Biopharm Drug Dispos 1:283–305

Nies A, Robinson DS, Friedman MJ, Green R, Cooper TB, Ravaris CL, Ives JO (1977) Relationship between age and tricyclic antidepressant plasma levels. Am J Psychiatry 134:790–793

Preskorn SH, Irwin H (1982) Toxicity of tricyclic antidepressants – kinetics, mechanism, intervention: a review. J Clin Psychiatry 43:151–156

Sjöqvist F, Bertilsson L, Äsberg M (1980) Monitoring tricyclic antidepressants. Ther Drug Monit 2:85–93

Sutfin TA, Perini GI, Molnar G, Jusko WJ (1988) Multiple-dose pharmacokinetics of imipramine and its major active and conjugated metabolites in depressed patients. J Clin Psychopharmacol 8:48–53

Vandel B, Vandel S, Jounet JM, Allers G, Volmat R (1982) Relationship between plasma concentration of clomipramine and desmethylclomipramine in depressive patients and the clinical response. Eur J Clin Pharmacol 22:15–20

Hydroxy Metabolites of Tricyclic Antidepressants: Evaluation of Relative Cardiotoxicity *

B. G. Pollock and J. M. Perel [1]

1 Clinical Studies

Patients treated with nortriptyline and imipramine also have considerable plasma levels of pharmacologically active hydroxy metabolites. Hydroxylation controls the clearance of tricyclic antidepressants; 2-hydroxyimipramine and 2-hydroxydesipramine each comprise about 30% of their respective parent drug levels, whereas unconjugated E-10-hydroxynortriptyline (E-10-OH-NT) constitutes 150%–300% of nortriptyline levels, and its geometrical isomer Z-10-hydroxynortriptyline (Z-10-OH-NT) constitutes only 5%–22% of the total hydroxynortriptyline formed (DeVane and Jusko 1981; Mellstrom et al. 1981). Since the renal clearance of these metabolites determines their steady-state concentrations, it is not surprising that disproportionate increases in hydroxy metabolite levels, relative to their parent compounds, have been demonstrated in patients suffering from chronic renal failure (Lieberman et al. 1985). Moreover a decrease in renal clearance in old age could also account for the disproportionately high concentration of 10-hydroxynortriptyline (Young et al. 1985) and 2-hydroxydesipramine (Kitanaka et al. 1982) observed in elderly patients. This may be of particular concern because in the aged the cardiovascular system may already be compromised.

Attempts have been made to draw conclusions about the cardiovascular effects of hydroxy metabolites from plasma level monitoring for these metabolites in patients treated with nortriptyline. In 1984, Young et al. reported on a patient who developed congestive heart failure, and who had a therapeutic plasma level of nortriptyline (112 ng/ml) but a high plasma concentration of E-10-OH-NT (426 ng/ml). In contrast, Bertilsson et al. (1985) reported on a patient who was a fast hydroxylator of debrisoquine, with extremely high E-10-OH-NT levels (980 ng/ml), and who exhibited remarkably few side effects. Cardiographic changes (significant prolongation of the PR interval) which occurred in 8 of 18 elderly patients treated with nortriptyline were, however, correlated with E-10-OH-NT concentrations (Young et al. 1985). In this study, no relationship could be found using plasma nortriptyline, age, drug dose, or baseline cardiovascular status. In a similar investiga-

* This work was supported in part by a Merck Fellowship from the American Federation for Aging Research and NIMH grant 30915.
[1] Department of Psychiatry, Clinical Pharmacology Program, University of Pittsburgh School of Medicine, Western Psychiatric Institute and Clinic, Pittsburgh, PA 15213, USA

tion of 21 elderly depressed patients, Schneider (1986) found a significant association between QRS prolongation and combined E-10-OH-NT and nortriptyline levels greater than 300 ng/ml. This relationship could not be discerned when only nortriptyline plasma levels were considered. There have been no comparable investigations with imipramine, but Kutcher et al. (1986) found significant prolongation of PR and QRS intervals correlated only with 2-hydroxydesipramine plasma levels in ten elderly patients.

2 Previous Animal Cardiovascular Studies

The lack of sufficient quantities of these metabolites in a pure form has limited research on their direct pharmacological effects. There has been only one study previously reported in the world literature which compared the direct hemodynamic effects of the hydroxylated metabolite of imipramine to that of its parent compound (Jandhyala et al. 1977). This study used mongrel dogs anesthetized with sodium pentobarbital; left ventricular pressure catheters and flow probes were placed by highly invasive procedures; thoracotomy and pericardial resection were performed. It should be noted that electrocardiograms and plasma levels were not determined in this pioneering work. It was found that 2-hydroxyimipramine (1.25 mg/kg) reduced left ventricular function markedly within 10 min of intravenous administration and caused reductions in cardiac output. In contrast, imipramine at 2.5 mg/kg did not cause significant myocardial depression until 90 min after administration, suggesting either animal fatigue or a possible contribution of a metabolite. Subsequently, Wilkerson (1978), showed that 2-hydroxyimipramine was twice as potent as imipramine in counteracting ouabain-induced arrhythmias in dogs.

3 Current Experiments

The hemodynamic, cardiographic, and pharmacokinetic characteristics of the de novo hydroxy metabolites of imipramine and nortriptyline, relative to their parent compounds, were studied in an unanesthetized swine preparation (Pollock et al. 1987a, b). Increasingly, the pig has been recognized as a highly appropriate cardiovascular model. Cardiac output, arterial and left ventricular end-diastolic pressures, left ventricular peak dP/dT, and the continuous electrocardiogram were assessed after the intravenous administration of the drug or metabolite. Plasma, sampled over 120 min, and CSF, sampled at 60 min, were analyzed by reverse-phase HPLC with spectrofluorometric detection for imipramine and 2-hydroxyimipramine, and ultraviolet detection for nortriptyline and its hydroxy metabolites. Equilibrium dialysis was performed on plasma sampled at 60 min. Pharmacokinetic calculations were assisted by computer modeling.

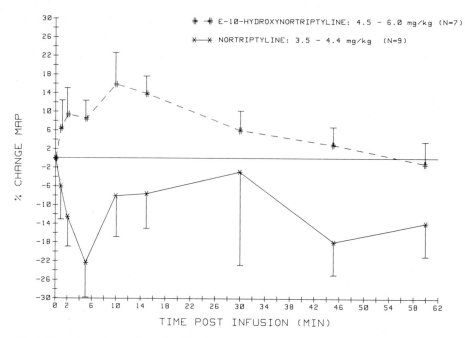

Fig. 1. Percentage change from baseline in mean arterial pressure (*MAP*) in unanesthetized swine

Administration of 5–6 mg/kg 2-hydroxyimipramine in animals, as contrasted to that of 8.5 mg/kg imipramine, produced a significantly greater incidence of life-threatening arrhythmias and caused profound and significant decreases in contractility, blood pressure, and cardiac output. Nortriptyline caused significantly more severe arrhythmias than did *E*-10-OH-NT at all dosage intervals (4–8 mg/kg) but was not significantly different from *Z*-10-OH-NT in this effect. Nortriptyline also caused profound and significant hypotension when compared with higher doses of *E*-10-OH-NT (Fig. 1). *Z*-10-OH-NT, in contrast to its geometrical isomer at the same dose, caused marked bradycardia and decrements in contractility, blood pressure, and cardiac output. All compounds studied, except *E*-10-OH-NT, produced dose-related declines in cardiac output. The hydroxy metabolites, compared with their parent compounds, had smaller volumes of distribution and shorter half-lives. CNS penetration, as estimated by CSF/plasma ratios, was significantly greater for 2-hydroxyimipramine (0.19 ± 0.05) and *E*-10-OH-NT (0.36 ± 0.06) but not for *Z*-10-OH-NT (0.13 ± 0.03), when compared with the respective parent compounds imipramine (0.07 ± 0.03) and nortriptyline (0.14 ± 0.06). This phenomenon was partially accounted for by significantly less plasma protein binding for the hydroxy metabolites, as determined by equilibrium dialysis.

4 Conclusions

Although *E*-10-OH-NT and 2-hydroxyimipramine possess comparable pharmacokinetic properties relative to their parent compounds, these two hydroxy metabolites have now been demonstrated to show vastly differing relative cardioactivities. Moreover, the *Z*-10-OH-NT metabolites has been shown to be more cardiotoxic than its geometrical isomer, while at the same time being less "free" than it. These findings argue against a simple pharmacokinetic explanation for the differing cardiotoxicities of the metabolites.

There are clear implications for vigilance, with regard to the potential toxic effects of 2-hydroxyimipramine. Especially in the context of co-administration with drugs that induce hepatic microsomal enzymes and in the aged or patients with compromised renal functioning. Recognizing the cardiotoxicity of 2-hydroxyimipramine may lead to innovative approaches in managing overdoses of imipramine, through tactics targeted at either minimizing 2-hydroxyimipramine formation or enhancing its extraction.

In contrast, recognizing the relatively benign cardiovascular profile of *E*-10-OH-NT, while not detracting from the need for plasma monitoring in older nortriptyline-treated patients, lends support to Bertilsson et al.'s (1986) contention that this metabolite may be a potentially useful antidepressant in its own right. Theoretically, this agent might be particularly advantageous for an elderly population.

Acknowledgements. We are very grateful to Drs. A. A. Manian, A. Jorgensen, L. Bertilsson, and B. Resul for providing samples of the hydroxy metabolites.

References

Bertilsson L, Aberg-Wistedt A, Gustafsson LL, Nordin C (1985) Extremely rapid hydroxylation of debrisoquine: a case report with implication for treatment with nortriptyline and other tricyclic antidepressants. Ther Drug Monit 7:478–480

Bertilsson L, Nordin C, Otani K, Resul B, Scheinin M, Siwers B, Sjöqvist F (1986) Disposition of single oral doses of E-10-hydroxynortriptyline in healthy subjects, with some observations on pharmacodynamic effects. Clin Pharmacol Ther 40:261–267

DeVane CL, Jusko W (1981) Plasma concentration monitoring of hydroxylated metabolites of imipramine and desipramine. Drug Intell Clin Pharm 15:263–266

Jandhyala B, Steenberg M, Perel JM, Manian AA, Buckley J (1977) Effects of several tricyclic antidepressants on the hemodynamics and myocardial contractility of anesthetized dogs. Eur J Pharmacol 42:403–410

Kitanaka I, Ross RJ, Cutler N, Zavadil AP, Potter WZ (1982) Altered hydroxydesipramine concentrations in elderly depressed patients. Clin Pharmacol Ther 31:51–55

Kutcher SP, Reid K, Dubbin JD, Shulman KI (1986) Electrocardiogram changes and therapeutic desipramine and 2-hydroxy-desipramine concentrations in elderly depressives. Br J Psychiatry 148:676–679

Lieberman JA, Cooper TB, Suckow RF, Steinberg H, Borenstein M, Brenner R, Kane JM (1985) Tricyclic antidepressant and metabolite levels in chronic renal failure. Clin Pharmacol Ther 37:301–307

Mellstrom B, Bertilsson L, Sawe J, Schulz H, Sjöqvist F (1981) E- and Z-10-hydroxylation of nortriptyline: relationship to polymorphic debrisoquine hydroxylation. Clin Pharmacol Ther 30:189–193

Pollock BG, Perel JM, Stiller RL, Birder RL, Manian A (1987a) Comparative cardiotoxicity and pharmacokinetics of imipramine and 2-hydroxyimipramine in unanesthetized swine. Clin Res 35:380

Pollock BG, Perel JM, Stiller RL, Foglia JP (1987b) Comparative cardiotoxicity and pharmacokinetics of nortriptyline and its isomeric hydroxymetabolites in unanesthetized swine. Fed Proc 46:305

Schneider LS (1986) Monitoring hydroxymetabolites of nortriptyline (Letter). N Engl J Med 314:989

Wilkerson RD (1978) Antiarrhythmic effects of tricyclic antidepressant drugs in ouabain-induced arrhythmias in the dog. J Pharmacol Exp Ther 206:666–674

Young RC, Alexopoulos G, Shamoian CA, Dhar A, Kutt H (1984) Heart failure associated with high plasma 10-hydroxynortriptyline levels. Am J Psychiatry 141:432–433

Young RC, Alexopoulos G, Shamoian CA, Kent E, Dhar A, Kutt H (1985) Plasma 10-hydroxynortriptyline and ECG changes in elderly depressed patients. Am J Psychiatry 142:866–868

Therapeutic Drug Monitoring of Tricyclic Antidepressants: A Means of Avoiding Toxicity *

S. H. Preskorn [1]

1 Introduction

Therapeutic drug monitoring of tricyclic antidepressants has become a standard-of-care issue. The value of such monitoring has been a topic of discussion for almost 20 years, since the substantial interindividual differences in tricyclic antidepressant metabolism were first described (Hammer et al. 1967). Unfortunately, widespread acceptance of this tool in practice was delayed by an almost exclusive focus on the relationship between tricyclic antidepressant concentration in plasma and antidepressant efficacy. Debates abounded about whether such relationships were linear or curvilinear, to the exclusion of other important issues, particularly the relationship between tricyclic antidepressant concentration in plasma and toxicity.

These debates were not only pedantic, but they also obscured these more substantive concerns. When using a drug, the physician and the patient are interested in safety as well as efficacy. They are also interested in the rapidity and predictability of response.

In comparison to simple dosage titration based on clinical response, adjustment based on therapeutic drug monitiring has many advantages: (a) it hastens response by reducing the time needed to optimize the dose; (b) it improves overall efficacy by ensuring that all patients achieve optimum drug concentration; (c) it increases the confidence that a patient needs alternative therapy when he fails to respond to a trial of a tricyclic antidepressant; (d) it provides a means of assessing whether nonresponse is due to poor compliance; and (e) it reduces the risk that patients will develop iatrogenic toxicity due to a chronic accumulation resulting in toxic concentrations on conventional doses, due to slow tricyclic antidepressant metabolism. The chapter by Nelson (this volume) addresses the first four of these issues. This chapter focuses on the last one.

Tricyclic antidepressants have a narrow therapeutic index, particularly tertiary amine tricyclic antidepressants (e.g., amitriptyline, doxepin, and imipramine). Generally, optimum response requires a tricyclic antidepressant

* This research was supported in part by Psychiatric Research Institute at St. Francis Regional Medical Center, Veterans Administration Merit Review Program, and NINCDS Grant NS23645-02.
[1] Psychiatric Research Institute, University of Kansas School of Medicine, and Veterans Administration Medical Center, Wichita, KS 67214, USA

Table 1. Evolution of CNS toxicity

Affective symptoms	Motor symptoms	Psychotic symptoms	Organic symptoms
Mood	Tremor	Thought disorder	Disorientation
↓Concentration	Ataxia	Hallucination	↓Memory
Lethargy	Seizures[a]	Delusions	Agitation
Social W/D			Confusion

W/D, withdrawal.
[a] Seizures typically occur late but can occur earlier in the evolution.

concentration in plasma on the order of 100–300 ng/ml (APA Task Force Report 1985). Above 450 ng/ml there is a high incidence of tricyclic antidepressant induced delirium which can lead to grand mal seizures (Preskorn et al. 1988a). Above 1000 ng/ml, virtually all patients show electrocardiographic evidence of tricyclic antidepressant induced slowing of intracardiac conduction, which can lead to sudden death (Spiker et al. 1975).

Central nervous system (CNS) toxicity is of particular interest for two reasons (Preskorn et al. 1988a). First, it occurs at concentrations only 50% higher than the upper limit of the optimum range for tertiary amine tricyclic antidepressants. Second, it has an insidious prodrome (Table 1) which may be misinterpreted by the clinician as a worsening of the underlying psychiatric disorder. Hence, the clinician may make decisions which will increase the seriousness of the toxicity, such as (a) increasing the dose of tricyclic antidepressant or (b) adding a neuroleptic which can inhibit the metabolism of tricyclic antidepressants (Gram and Brøsen, this volume). The symptoms and signs of tricyclic antidepressant induced CNS toxicity are listed in Table 1, with the earliest ones on the left and the later ones on the right.

2 CNS Toxicity and Plasma Levels

Amitriptyline is the tricyclic antidepressant with the most substantial data base demonstrating a relationship between drug concentrations in plasma and CNS toxicity. Preskorn and Biggs (1978) first described the relationship in a patient receiving amitriptyline. The first large-scale population study was conducted by Preskorn and Simpson (1982), with 100 patients being treated with amitriptyline. They found that there was an 86% chance of developing amitriptyline-induced delirium when the amitriptyline concentration in plasma exceeded 450 ng/ml. Livingston et al. (1983) examined 135 patients treated predominantly with amitriptyline and found that 35% of patients with levels above 300 ng/ml developed delirium versus 5% in patients with levels below 300 ng/ml. Preskorn et al. (1984) found that 88% of amitriptyline-treated patients with levels above 250 ng/ml had drug-induced EEG abnormalities, and that 14% developed delirium whereas neither EEG abnormalities nor delirium occurred below 250 ng/ml.

The next best studied tricyclic antidepressant is imipramine. Meador-Woodruff et al. (1988) found that 56% of 15 patients with tricyclic antidepressant concentration in plasma above 450 ng/ml developed delirium, versus 0% in 16 patients below 450 ng/ml. In this study, 94% of the patients were on imipramine. Preskorn et al. (1988 b) reported the first prospective study of this phenomenon in children with prepubertal major depressive disorder treated with imipramine. Of children with levels above 450 ng/ml ($n=4$), 75% developed delirium, versus 0% below 450 ng/ml ($n=61$) and 0% in patients treated with placebo ($n=15$). In the latter study, the treatment team was blind to the tricyclic antidepressant concentration in plasma. In two of the three cases, they misidentified the prodrome of the delirium as a worsening of the underlying depressive disorder. In both cases, the team decided to alter therapy based on this misidentification in such a way that the toxicity would have been increased. The monitoring laboratory, which was not blind to the results of therapeutic drug monitoring, aborted these decisions and prevented two potential tragedies.

Thus, a body of studies have accumulated over a 10-year period documenting a relationship between tricyclic antidepressant concentration in plasma and tricyclic antidepressant induced delirium. To put these figures in perspective, Preskorn et al. (1988 a) reviewed the published population studies of tricyclic antidepressant induced CNS toxicity and performed a meta-analysis of the above reports on the relationship between concentration and CNS toxicity. There have been seven large studies of adverse CNS effects of tertiary tricyclic antidepressants in depressed patients treated with conventional daily doses (100–300 mg/day; Table 2). These studies represented 959 patients, of whom 57 (or 6%) developed tricyclic antidepressant induced delirium. Based on the meta-analysis of the concentration: response studies,

Table 2. Incidence of CNS toxicity in patients treated with tricyclic antidepressants

Authors	Total	n	Percent
Davies et al. (1971)	150	20	13.3
Boston Collaborative Study (1972)	260	12	4.6
Schulderbrandt et al. (1974)	201	3	1.5
Preskorn and Simpson (1982)	100	6	6.0
Livingston et al. (1983)	125	10	8.0
Meyers and Mei-tal (1983)	43	3	7.0
Preskorn et al. (1978 c)	80	3	4.0
	959	57	6.0
Range for all studies:			1.5%–13.3%
Range omitting highest and lowest:			4.0%– 8.0%
Overall frequency			6.0%

this risk was three to six times higher than in patients whose tricyclic antidepressant concentration in plasma was below 450 ng/ml. This same meta-analysis showed that the risk increased to 33% and 67% if the tricyclic antidepressant plasma concentration exceeded 300 and 450 ng/ml, respectively. Thus, a direct relationship exists between tricyclic antidepressant concentration in plasma and the risk of tricyclic antidepressant induced delirium, at least for tertiary amine tricyclic antidepressants.

There is now sufficient data to conclude that the overall risk of 6% for tricyclic antidepressant induced delirium from the population studies is due to the development of toxic concentrations in slow metabolizers receiving conventional daily doses. Preskorn and Kent (1984) reported that 7% of patients treated with conventional daily doses of amitriptyline developed tricyclic antidepressant concentrations in plasma in excess of 450 ng/ml. Studies reviewed elsewhere in this volume show that 4%–7% of Caucasians are slow metabolizers of tricyclic antidepressants and will develop drug concentration in plasma associated with a high risk of toxicity, despite being treated with conventional doses. Thus, the clinician who employs tricyclic antidepressants without using therapeutic drug monitoring runs a predictable risk of encountering toxicity in his patients.

3 CNS Toxicity: Course and Risk Factors

In addition to population studies, a number of case reports of tricyclic antidepressant induced CNS toxicity have been published in the past 10 years. Preskorn and Jerkovich (1988) reviewed 36 such cases to determine course and risk factors. Of these 36 cases, 15 patients were treated with amitriptyline, 12 with imipramine, and 9 with desipramine. The course of tricyclic antidepressant induced delirium was found to evolve over a 14-day period following initiation of the dose on which the toxicity would occur. The evolution over that period started with a protean prodrome (Table 1). In almost 50% of cases, the clinician interpreted this prodrome as a worsening of the underlying depressive disorder and, hence, often made decisions (increasing the tricyclic antidepressant dose or adding a neuroleptic) which only worsened the situation. The most reliable signs to emerge were tremor, especially of the upper extremities, and ataxia. Physicians should monitor for such signs in their patients, especially if they do not use therapeutic drug monitoring to optimize dosage of tricyclic antidepressants.

The review for risk factors supported the conclusion that high tricyclic antidepressant concentration in plasma was the major predictor of tricyclic antidepressant induced CNS toxicity. The concentration for each drug was as follows: 462 ± 362 for amitriptyline, 624 ± 170 for imitriptyline, and 430 ± 272 for desipramine. Tertiary amine tricyclic antidepressants (amitriptyline and imipramine) had more florid toxicity than did desmethylimipramine. Other risk factors included age (the older the patient the lower the threshold for tricyclic antidepressant induced CNS toxicity), sex (women at higher risk than men), and concomitantly administered medications. The latter effect was due to both pharmacokinetic (e.g., neuroleptics which inhibit tricyclic antidepressant metabolism) and pharmacodynamic interactions (e.g. from anticholinergic agents which have additive effects).

4 Catastrophic Outcomes

Given the above knowledge, the failure to employ therapeutic drug monitoring during tricyclic antidepressant pharmacotherapy is becoming a standard-of-care issue in the United States. Coroners, at least in larger cities, are quantitating tricyclic antidepressant concentration in plasma when performing postmortems in cases of unexpected deaths during tricyclic antidepressant pharmacotherapy. Through consultation with physicians, this author has collected five cases in which a catastrophic outcome resulted from the chronic accumulation of toxic tricyclic antidepressant concentrations in plasma (Table 3). In four of the five cases, a malpractice suit was filed alleging negligence and failure in diagnosis. In all cases, the failure to employ therapeutic drug monitoring when using pharmacotherapy with tricyclic antidepressants was an issue.

All five patients were on conventional daily doses of tertiary amine tricyclic antidepressants (i.e., amitriptyline and imipramine). In only one case was there any identifiable risk factors for the development of tricyclic antidepressant toxicity. This patient was a 62-year-old man with a history of past myocardial infarction with resultant decreased left ventricular function

Table 3. Summary of catastrophic outcomes due to failure to monitor plasma levels of tricylic antidepressants

Age (years)	Sex	Drug	Dose	Levels[f]	Outcome
5	Male	Imipramine IMI[a]	50	10.0	Sudden death
30	Female	Imipramine IMI[b]	100	1.2	Sudden death
34	Male	Amitriptyline AMI[c]	375	5.5	Sudden death
52	Female	Amitriptyline AMI[d]	350	Unknown	Paralytic ileus with bowel infarction and resection
62	Male	Amitriptyline AMI[e]	100	0.95	Ventricular arrythmia

[a] No other drugs given or detected.
[b] Also taking propranolol 60 mg/day, diazepam 20 mg/day, flurazepam 30 mg/day p.r.n.
[c] Phenelzine 60 mg/day added due to worsening of depression, disulfiram 250 mg/day.
[d] Thioridazine 600 mg/day and benztropine 2 mg/day were added due to psychotic component and development of neurological symptoms, respectively.
[e] Haloperidol 10 mg/day added 7 days earlier due to suspected psychotic decompensation.
[f] Levels of parent compound plus desmethyl metabolite (mg/l).

and liver disease. In retrospect, all five were slow metabolizers, which could only be detected through the use of therapeutic drug monitoring. In four of the cases, the clinician detected early symptoms and signs of tricyclic antidepressant induced CNS toxicity but concluded that these phenomena were due to worsening of the depressive disorder. In response to this interpretation, tricyclic antidepressant doses were increased and/or neuroleptics added. The correct diagnosis was not made until after the catastrophe had occurred.

5 Comment

The rationale behind therapeutic drug monitoring is to improve the safety and efficacy of pharmacotherapy when feasible. In psychiatry, therapeutic drug monitoring is an accepted requirement for the proper use of lithium pharmacotherapy. Therapeutic drug monitoring in the case of lithium is done in order to improve safety, perhaps more so than to improve efficacy. However, the use of therapeutic drug monitoring for pharmacotherapy with tricyclic antidepressants is still being debated. Unfortunately, this controversy is in part due to an almost exclusive focus on efficacy in such debates. Data accumulated on the relationship between tricyclic antidepressant concentration in plasma and toxicity are generally not well known. Such data, nevertheless do exist and provide a compelling argument for employing therapeutic drug monitoring as a standard aspect of tricyclic antidepressant pharmacotherapy. This chapter has focused on CNS toxicity, but data also exist relating cardiotoxicity to tricyclic antidepressant concentrations in plasma.

Acknowledgements. The author gratefully acknowledges Ms. Pam Widener and Ms. Dee Alligood for manuscript preparation. A modified version of this chapter appeared in an article in *Psychopharmacology Bulletin.*

References

APA Task Force on Use of Laboratory Tests in Psychiatry (1985) Tricyclic antidepressants – blood level measurements and clinical outcome. An APA Task Force Report. Am J Psychiatry 142:155–162

Boston Collaborative Drug Surveillance Program (1972) Adverse reactions to the tricyclic antidepressant drugs. Lancet 1:529

Davies RK, Tucker GJ, Harrow M, Detre TP (1971) Confusional episodes and antidepressant medication. Am J Psychiatry 128:127–131

Hammer W, Idestrom C-M, Sjöqvist F (1967) Chemical control of antidepressant drug therapy. Excerpta Med Int Congr Ser 122:301–310

Livingston RL, Zucker DK, Isenberg K, Wetzel RD (1983) Tricyclic antidepressants and delirium. J Clin Psychiatry 44:173–176

Meador-Woodruff JH, Abil M, Wisner-Carlson, Grunhaus L (1988) Behavioral and cognitive toxicity related to elevated plasma tricyclic antidepresssant levels. J Clin Psychopharmacol 8:28–32

Meyers BS, Mei-Tal V (1983) Psychiatric reactions during tricyclic treatment of elderly reconsidered. J Clin Psychopharmacol 3:2–6

Preskorn SH, Biggs JT (1978) Use of tricyclic antidepressant blood levels. N Engl J Med 298:166

Preskorn SH, Kent TA (1984) Mechanisms and interventions in tricyclic antidepressants overdoses. In: Stancer HC et al. (eds) Guidelines for the use of psychotropic drugs. Spectrum, New York, pp 63–75

Preskorn SH, Jerkovich GS (1988) The role of plasma monitoring in avoiding central nervous system toxicity of tricyclic antidepressants. J Clin Psychopharmacol (in press)

Preskorn SH, Simpson S (1982) Tricyclic-antidepressant-induced delirium and plasma drug concentration. Am J Psychiatry 139:6

Preskorn SH, Othmer SC, Lai C, Othmer E (1984) Tricyclic-induced electroencephalogram abnormalities and plasma drug concentrations. J Clin Psychopharmacol 4:262–264

Preskorn SH, Dorey RC, Jerkovich GS (1988a) Therapeutic drug monitoring of tricyclic antidepressants. Clin Chem 34:822–828

Preskorn SH, Weller EB, Jerkovich G, Hughes CW, Weller RA (1988b) Depression in children: concentration dependent CNS toxicity of tricyclic antidepressants. Psychopharmacol Bull 24:140–142

Preskorn SH, Weller EB, Jerkovich G, Hughes CW, Weller RA (1988c) Depression in children: concentration dependent CNS toxicity of tricyclic antidepressants. Psychopharmacol Bull 24:140–142

Schulterbrandt JC, Raskin A, Reatig N (1974) True and apparent side effects in a controlled trial of chlorpromazine and imipramine in depression. Psychopharmacologia 38:236–239

Spiker DG, Weiss AN, Chang SS, Ruwitch JF, Biggs JT (1975) Tricyclic antidepressant overdose: clinical presentation and plasma levels. Clin Pharmacol Ther 18:539–546

Neuroleptic Drug Levels in Erythrocytes and in Plasma: Implications for Therapeutic Drug Monitoring

D. L. GARVER [1]

1 Introduction

Brodie (1967) first suggested that drug levels of antipsychotic drugs might be related to therapeutic response. Since then, a host of investigators have developed and refined techniques of measuring neuroleptic drugs in various body fluids and of relating such levels of drug to antipsychotic response during systematic pharmacologic trials in psychotic disorders.

The development of clinical methodology equal to the task of demonstrating relationships between drug levels and therapeutic response is beyond the scope of the present chapter, but we may observe that state-of-the-art clinical methodology for such trials needs to address the following:

- Selection of psychotic subjects known to respond to psychotropic medication.
- Use of predetermined fixed dose(s) of drug so as to achieve drug levels below, within, and above the expected therapeutic range.
- A stable, drug-free period at baseline with which to compare quantitative changes in psychotic symptoms associated with drug treatment.
- Systematic quantitative assessment of psychotic symptoms and behavior affected by drug treatment.
- Attention to heterogeneity within psychotic populations, which may be associated with different drug level-response relationships among psychotic patient groups.

Techniques for monitoring neuroleptic drugs have focused upon assessment of drug concentrations in one of four compartments: in cerebrospinal fluid (CSF), in total plasma, free (in plasma water), and within blood cells (Fig. 1).

2 CSF Drug Levels and Antipsychotic Response

Whatever the relevant mechanism of action of the neuroleptic drugs is – dopamine D_2 receptor blockade (Seeman et al. 1976) or presynaptic depolarization inactivation (Chiodo and Bunney 1983) – such action is

[1] University of Alabama at Birmingham, School of Medicine, UAB Station Birmingham, AL 35294, USA

Clinical Pharmacology in Psychiatry
Editors: S. G. Dahl and L. F. Gram
(Psychopharmacology Series 7)
© Springer-Verlag Berlin Heidelberg 1989

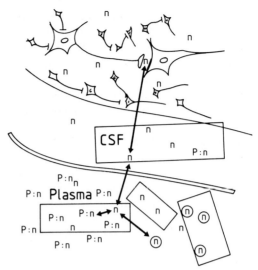

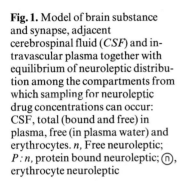

Fig. 1. Model of brain substance and synapse, adjacent cerebrospinal fluid (*CSF*) and intravascular plasma together with equilibrium of neuroleptic distribution among the compartments from which sampling for neuroleptic drug concentrations can occur: CSF, total (bound and free) in plasma, free (in plasma water) and erythrocytes. *n*, Free neuroleptic; *P:n*, protein bound neuroleptic; ⓝ, erythrocyte neuroleptic

presumably related to the concentration of free (unbound) drug and active metabolites in the vicinity of critical neuronal systems. Ideally, one would want to measure the free (unbound) drug at critical receptors and relate such concentrations to clinical response parameters. Practically, the CSF and the concentrations of the drug in it is the closest access point to such receptors. In contrast to plasma, the CSF contains only a small amount of protein, and CSF neuroleptic concentrations are primarily the concentrations of free (unbound) drug. CSF drug levels may have another advantage in contrast to monitoring drug concentrations in the periphery for assessing such drug level-response relationships: CSF drug levels reflect the consequence to the central nervous system (CNS) of the partition of drugs by the blood-brain barrier. Such partition is a result of continuous phospholipid (cellular) membranes associated with most capillaries and differential lipid solubility of drugs and their metabolites. Relatively more polar drugs and their metabolites, even though present in the periphery and active in in vitro models of neuroleptic action, may be differentially denied access to the CNS. CSF measurements of psychotropic drug concentrations in most cases need to reflect both parent drug and active metabolites which get into the CNS.

Unfortunately, only one systematic study has been reported which relates CSF neuroleptic levels to antipsychotic response. Performance of such studies is complicated by CSF drug levels which are frequently below the limit of the sensitivity of assays. Wode-Helgodt et al. (1978) found that antipsychotic effects of chlorpromazine at 2 weeks of treatment were positively and significantly ($p < 0.001$) related to the concentrations of chlorpromazine measured by gas chromatograph/mass spectroscopy in the CSF, but only a trend was found with plasma. (At 4 weeks of such treatment, even the significant relationship between CSF chlorpromazine levels and morbidity score dissolved). Wode-Helgodt et al. (1978) found CSF concentrations of chlorpromazine were about 3% of that found in plasma. Patients with CSF chlorpromazine concentrations above 1 ng/ml did significantly better at 2 weeks than those with lower levels; a similar trend was found for patients with plasma concentrations over 40 ng/ml as opposed to those whose levels were lower. While 27% of the variance in antipsychotic response could be accounted for by CSF chlorpromazine levels, only 15% could be accounted for with plasma chlorpromazine concentrations.

Rimon et al. (1981) attempted a similar study with megadoses (60 mg per day) of haloperidol in treatment-resistant schizophrenics. He reported that CSF concentrations of haloperidol (measured by radioimmunoassay) were 5.3% of that found in plasma. Rimon et al. (1981) found no relationship between CSF haloperidol concentrations and therapeutic effects of the drug. Here the use of treatment-resistant subjects and the use of doses of haloperidol which produce serum levels of 50–200 ng/ml (all above the linear portion of the dose response curve) mitigate against finding a relationship between drug level and response. Forsman and Öhman (1977), using gas chromatography, had previously reported that CSF concentrations of haloperidol were 8.8% that of plasma in patients whose plasma levels were 4.3–60 ng/ml, but they did not attempt to relate such concentrations to treatment effects. However, using equilibrium dialysis and ultrafiltration, they reported that the free fraction of haloperidol in plasma was virtually identical to the concentration of haloperidol found in the CSF of the same patients (7.9% versus 8.8% of total plasma concentrations, respectively).

3 Free Drug (in Plasma Water) and Antipsychotic Response

There has been one study examining the relationship between drug (and active metabolites) free in plasma water (unbound) and therapeutic response. Tang et al. (1984), using equilibrium dialysis, found preliminary evidence that free chlorpromazine and active metabolites (assayed by the radioreceptor assay of Creese and Snyder 1977) correlated with response at the end of 25 days of treatment ($r=0.83$; $n=6$). Total plasma neuroleptic activity of chlorpromazine and active metabolites also correlated with response but at a somewhat lower level ($r=0.70$). As against the 69% of variance in antipsychotic response that could be accounted for by free chlorpromazine levels, only 49% could be accounted for with plasma chlorpromazine concentrations. In the Tang et al. (1984) study an attempt to study free and total haloperidol and its relationship to therapeutic response was confounded by megadose (60 mg haloperidol per day), which, as in the Rimon et al. (1981) study, does not distribute drug levels of patients on the linear portion of the drug response curve; no significant relationships were found with haloperidol. In the Tang et al. (1984) data, free chlorpromazine and metabolites represented 2.1% of total plasma-binding activity; free haloperidol and metabolites were 4.6% of total binding activity. There was considerable between-patient (but little within-patient) variance in the proportion of free drug, which varied from 1.4% to 9.4% for chlorpromazine, and from 1.1% to 3.1% for haloperidol. The Tang et al. (1984) study used a radioreceptor assay for neuroleptic drug which measures total dopamine D_2 receptor blocking activity (parent drug as well as active metabolite; Creese and Snyder 1977).

4 Erythrocyte Drug Levels and Antipsychotic Response

In studies on the relationship of drug levels to therapeutic response, a third strategy to approximate the relative quantity of free drug is to utilize the concentration of drug in a standard volume of tissue which itself equilibrates with the free drug. If the tissue to be assayed is identical between patients with respect to composition and volume, one could anticipate a linear relationship between the free drug and that found assayed in the tissue, providing, of course, that the availability of free drug remains constant (and is not significantly decreased by its transfer to the tissue).

Human erythrocytes generally meet the requirement for such a tissue – virtually identical in composition between patients, in equilibrium with the free drug in plasma water, and easily compacted to achieve identical volumes for assay. In vivo animal experiments carried out by Dekirmenjian and coworkers (Garver et al. 1978) indicated that concentrations of the phenothiazine butaperazine in packed erythrocytes is correlated more strongly ($r = 0.90$) than the total plasma butaperazine ($r = 0.69$) with brain butaperazine concentrations. In vitro studies showed a linear relationship between free drug and that found in packed erythrocytes suspended with the butaperazine (24% to 63%) as varying dilutions of plasma (1 : 1 to 1 : 5) were added to butaperazine and erythrocytes.

4.1 Butaperazine

The first studies attempting to relate neuroleptic concentrations of erythrocytes and clinical effects utilized butaperazine, since this was found to be without significant confounding metabolites and to have a simple fluorometric assay. Garver et al. (1977), with replication by Casper et al. (1980), found clear relationships between erythrocyte (as contrasted to plasma) concentrations of butaperazine and therapeutic response in a 2-week study with a fixed, steady dose design (Fig. 2). In these studies, a clear "therapeutic window" was found for erythrocyte butaperazine and its antipsychotic effect. However, no clear relationship could be found between plasma butaperazine concentrations and therapeutic effects. Whereas 52% of the variance in antipsychotic response could be accounted for by erythrocyte butaperazine levels, only 1% of the variance could be accounted for by plasma butaperazine levels.

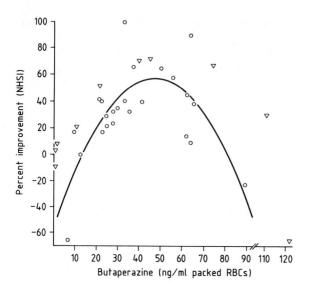

Fig. 2. Therapeutic response as rated by New Haven Schizophrenic Index (*NHSI*) as function of mean steady-state erythrocyte levels of butaperazine (ng/ml). *Inverted triangles* denote results from pilot study by Garver et al. (1977). (From Casper et al. 1980)

4.2 Haloperidol

Attempts to relate neuroleptic levels to therapeutic response using other neuroleptic drugs have, in general, met with limited success. Smith et al. (1982) reported that maximal therapeutic effects of haloperidol at the end of 24 days of predetermined fixed-dose treatment occurred in patients who had an inter-

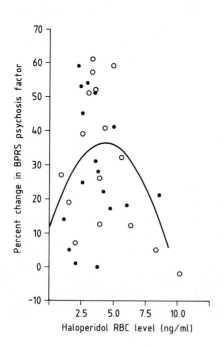

Fig. 3. Therapeutic response as rated by Brief Psychiatric Rating Scale (*BPRS*) psychosis factor as a function of mean steady-state erythrocyte levels of haloperidol (ng/ml). $R^2 = 0.32; p < 0.005$. (From Smith et al. 1985)

mediate range of 2.4–5.4 ng haloperidol per milliliter packed erythrocytes (as opposed to above or below the range). In a subsequent study, Garver et al. (1984) found that erythrocyte haloperidol levels of 1.0–2.2 ng/ml (rather than higher) were associated with greater therapeutic response at day 7 of fixed-dose haloperidol treatment, but by day 14 of treatment, a meaningful erythrocyte drug level-response relationship virtually disappeared. In an expanded study, Smith et al. (1984a, 1985) confirmed their initial (1982) finding, and reported that a curvilinear fit of erythrocyte haloperidol levels (with maximal response at 2.2–6.8 ng haloperidol per milliliter packed erythrocytes) correlated slightly better with therapeutic response at the end of 24 days of treatment than did plasma haloperidol levels (Fig. 3). Erythrocyte haloperidol levels accounted for 32% of the variance in antipsychotic response, and plasma haloperidol levels accounted for 27%. All of the erythrocyte studies of haloperidol used gas chromatographic assays.

4.3 Thioridazine

Using a radioreceptor assay (Creese and Snyder 1977) for erythrocyte thioridazine, Cohen et al. (1980b) found that erythrocyte neuroleptic activity correlated linearly ($r=0.88$; $p<0.01$) with therapeutic response in patients treated with a fixed dose of 200 or 400 mg of thioridazine. Plasma neuroleptic activity correlated even slightly better ($r=0.91$; $p<0.01$) with response parameters. In a predetermined, fixed dose study using 150–750 mg thioridazine per day for 24 days, Smith et al. (1984b) found little relationship between therapeutic response and erythrocyte thioridazine ($r=0.13$), its metabolite mesoridazine ($r=0.16$), or the sum of the two ($r=0.17$) using gas chromatographic assays. In each case, however, the linear correlation of response with erythrocyte drug measurement (above) was slightly better than for plasma measurements ($r=0.11$, $r=0.09$, and $r=0.11$, respectively). Using a spectrofluorometric assay for "thioridazine and metabolites," Smith et al. (1984b) also described a significant linear relationship between response and erythrocyte thioridazine ($r=0.41$; $p<0.05$) and only a trend toward response and plasma thioridazine ($r=0.35$; $p<0.10$). Although erythrocyte neuroleptic activity was not assessed with the radioreceptor assay by Smith et al. (1985), plasma neuroleptic activity with thioridazine correlated with response more strongly ($r=0.47$; $p<0.05$) than did gas chromatographic or spectrofluorometric assays. In the thioridazine studies of Smith et al. (1984b, 1985) on the same patients, it is striking that each chemically less specific assay produced higher correlations of drug levels with antipsychotic effects: for plasma, gas chromatographic $r=0.16$, fluorometric $r=0.35$, radioreceptor $r=47$; for erythrocyte, gas chromatographic $r=0.16$ and fluorometric $r=0.41$. Using gas chromatographic methods only 3% of the variance in antipsychotic response could be accounted for by erythrocyte or plasma thioridazine levels. Using spectrofluorometric assays the variance in response which could be accounted for was 17% for erythrocyte drug levels and 12% for plasma drug levels (Smith et al. 1985). Using the radioreceptor assay, Cohen et al. (1980 b) accounted for 77% of the response variance with erythrocyte neuroleptic activity of thioridazine and metabolites; total plasma neuroleptic activity accounted for even more (83%) of the variance in antipsychotic response.

4.4 Fluphenazine

A single study attempting to relate fluphenazine erythrocyte concentrations measured by gas chromatography to therapeutic effects showed little apparent relationship at 2 weeks of treatment following fixed doses of 2.5–10 mg fluphenazine per day (Mavroidis et al. 1984c). In this same group of patients, plasma fluphenazine levels were also poorly related to antipsychotic concentrations when drug levels were measured by gas chromatography (Mavroidis et al. 1984a). However, the use of a radioreceptor assay on the same patient plasmas, showed more typical drug level-response curves (Hitzemann et al. 1986). In the Mavroidis et al. (1984c) data, 30% of the variance of response parameters could be accounted for by erythrocyte fluphenazine concentrations, while but 22% of this variance could be accounted for by plasma fluphenazine levels.

In summary, the early hope that simple, clear relationships would emerge between erythrocyte neuroleptic levels and therapeutic response has born little fruit except with the infrequently used phenothiazine butaperazine, for which 52% of the variance in the drug level-response relationship can be attributed to factors associated with the erythrocyte butaperazine level (Table 1). Erythrocyte haloperidol levels, which appear to account for about 32% of the

Table 1. Variance in antipsychotic response accounted for by neuroleptic drug concentrations in cerebrospinal fluid, free in plasma water or in erythrocytes, and in total plasma

Drug	Investigator	Assay	Cerebro-spinal fluid	Free in plasma water	Red blood cells	Total plasma
Chlorpromazine	Wode-Helgodt et al. (1978)	GC/MS	27%	–	–	15%
	Tang et al. (1984)	RR	–	69%	–	49%
Thioridazine	Smith et al. (1984b, 1985)	GC	–	–	3%	2%
	Smith et al. (1985)	SF	–	–	17%	12%
	Smith et al. (1985)	RR	–	–	–	22%
	Cohen et al. (1980b)	RR	–	–	77%	83%
Fluphenazine	Mavroidis et al. (1984c)	GC	–	–	30%	22%
Haloperidol	Smith et al. (1985)	GC	–	–	32%	27%
Butaperazine	Casper et al. (1980)	SF	–	–	52%	1%

GC, Gas chromatography; GC/MS, gaschromatography/mass spectrometry; SF, spectrofluoroscopy; RR, radioreceptor assay.

variance in the haloperidol-response relationship, are only slightly more superior to plasma haloperidol levels (27% of variance) when measured by gas chromatography. Erythrocyte thioridazine concentration is only slightly better than plasma thioridazine concentration for such drug-response relationships, but neither appears to account for more than 3% of the variance when thioridazine and mesoridazine are measured by gas chromatograhic methods. When assayed in the same study with fluorometric methods, which presumably monitor greater numbers of thioridazine metabolites, erythrocyte thioridazine concentration accounted for 17% of the variance in response. When erythrocytes were analyzed with the radioreceptor assay in a different study by Cohen et al. (1980b), 77% of the variance in response could be accounted for by erythrocyte neuroleptic activity; however, 83% could be accounted for by plasma neuroleptic activity. The chlorpromazine and thioridazine data, which permit contrasts between the use of specific (gas chromatography/mass spectrometry or gas chromatography) and that of functional assays (radioreceptor), suggest that metabolites of at least some of the parent neuroleptic do play a major role in the functional antipsychotic effects of some neuroleptics. The data suggest the possibility that the type of assay itself may be a critical element in relating both peripheral and central measures of drug concentrations/activity to antipsychotic response. In seven of eight studies (Table 1), measurements of free drug directly (free in plasma water or in CSF) or indirectly (in the erythrocytes) improved the fit (as compared with total plasma levels) between drug level measurements and therapeutic effects. Clearly, additional studies are needed, examining the relationships of erythrocyte concentration of drugs, concentrations of the free drug (in plasma water), and CSF drug levels in the same patients – all in relationship to one another and to therapeutic response. The additional assessment of plasma or serum levels should also be undertaken in the same patients to determine under what circumstances between-patient variance in response parameters can be reduced by utilizing compartments other than the total (bound and free) drug in plasma or serum for drug level determinations. Neuroleptic drugs without active metabolites should be utilized in such initial studies until an assay that meaningfully integrates the activity of all active components of drug can be perfected. Despite its theoretical advantages, there clearly are difficulties with the present-day radioreceptor assay, which appears to require standardization for each neuroleptic drug separately (Cohen et al. 1980a) and may behave erratically in the presence of unpredictable plasma constituents (Mailman et al. 1984).

5 Plasma Drug Levels and Antipsychotic Response

Most of the studies relating neuroleptic levels to therapeutic response have utilized serum or plasma as the compartment for drug concentration measurement. As noted previously, free drug in plasma water is in equilibrium not only with erythrocytes, but also with plasma proteins. Both between-subject and, sometimes, within-subject variance in the ratio of total bound to free concentrations of drug can be introduced by quantitative and qualitative differences in the binding of drugs by plasma protein. Variations in quantity of plasma albumins effect the ratio of free versus bound neuroleptic (Bevilacqua et al. 1979). Wide swings in α_1 glycoproteins may similarly alter the free/total ratio of many psychotropic drugs despite the comparatively low affinity of some neuroleptics for α_1 glycoproteins (Schley and Muller-Oerlinghausen 1983).

5.1 Chlorpromazine

As noted previously, the Wode-Healgodt et al. (1978) study of chlorpromazine and therapeutic response suggested that patients with blood levels above 40 ng chlorpromazine per milliliter by gas chromatography/mass spectroscopy did significantly better than subjects with lower chlorpromazine levels after 2 but not after 4 weeks of treatment.

5.2 Haloperidol

Eight predetermined fixed-dose drug level-response studies have been reported for plasma haloperidol. Wistedt et al. (1984) related plasma haloperidol levels (assayed by high pressure liquid chromatography) and response at the end of 4 weeks of treatment. They found a positive linear correlation of symptom amelioration and haloperidol plasma levels ranging from 2 to 12 ng/ml. Mavroidis et al. (1983), Smith et al. (1984a) and Potkin et al. (1985) each gave up to approximately 25 mg haloperidol per day to schizophrenic patients. At 2, 3, or 6 weeks of drug treatment, respectively, each of these three studies found diminished response at lower haloperidol plasma concentrations, generally below 7–8 ng/ml either by gas chromatography or by radioimmunoassay specific for haloperidol. Each of these studies also delineated an intermediate drug concentration at which maximal response tended to occur: at approximately 7–13 ng/ml (Mavroidis et al. 1983; Smith et al. 1984a) or at 10–22 ng/ml (Potkin et al. 1985). Each of these three studies also documented diminished response associated with higher haloperidol levels: at approximately 14–18 ng/ml (Mavroidis et al. 1983), at 14–22 ng/ml (Smith et al. 1984a), and at 23–75 ng/ml (Potkin et al. 1985). Diminished response associated with higher haloperidol levels monitored by radioreceptor assay were also reported by Contreras et al. (1987). After 2 weeks of treatment with 20 mg haloperidol per day, 12 of 14 patients with neuroleptic activity the equivalent of 22 ng haloperidol/ml or lower were responders, whereas 5 of 13 patients with levels higher than 22 ng/ml were responders.

In contrast to the four above described studies which suggested diminished response at high haloperidol plasma levels, two other fixed-dose studies have found sustained antipsychotic response at high plasma haloperidol levels. In the study by Linkowski et al. (1984) patients received 30 mg per day and in one by Bigelow et al. (1985) up to 28 mg per day. Plasma haloperidol levels were assayed by radioimmunoassay (Linkowski et al. 1984) or high-pressure liquid chromatography (Bigelow et al. 1985). Both investigators found sustained antipsychotic responses associated with plasma haloperidol levels of 8–25 ng/ml (Linkowski et al. 1984) and 10–28 ng/ml (Bigelow et al. 1985) at the end of 6 weeks of treatment.

Finally, in a preliminary study van Putten et al. (1985), administering 5–20 mg haloperidol per day and assaying plasma haloperidol by radioimmunoassay, failed to find any systematic relationship between drug level and response (over plasma haloperidol levels ranging from 0.2 to 18 ng/ml) after the 1st week of treatment.

5.3 Thiothixene

Only one predetermined, fixed dose study of plasma thiothixene and response has been reported which used chemical assays. In this study by Mavroidis et al. (1984b), doses of thiothixene ranged from 16 to 60 mg per day. At the end of 2 weeks of drug treatment, greater improvement was associated with plasma thiothixene levels (by gas chromatography) above 2 ng/ml; a plateau of continued antipsychotic response was found in patients whose plasma thiothixene levels were between 2 and 10.5 ng/ml.

Van Putten et al. (1983) also reported a predetermined, fixed dose (0.44 mg/kg) study of thiothixene treatment and response during 4 weeks of treatment. Van Putten et al. (1983) measured each patient's total dopamine D_2 receptor blocking activity using the radioreceptor assay (Creese and Snyder 1977). Although Van Putten et al. (1983) found improvement occurring over the entire range of plasma levels, the chances of substantial improvement appear greater at higher total neuroleptic levels (above 40 neuroleptic units) than at lower levels.

5.4 Fluphenazine

Two predetermined fixed-dose studies with fluphenazine and gas chromatography assays found strikingly similar results: diminished antipsychotic response at high plasma fluphenazine levels. Dysken et al. (1981) gave 5–20 mg fluphenazine orally for 2 weeks to recently admitted schizophrenics. Maximum improvement (48.8%) occurred in the patients whose plasma fluphenazine levels were between 0.2 and 2.7 ng/ml as determined by gas chromatography. Three of the patients with plasma fluphenazine levels above and three patients below this range showed 7.3% and 10.0% deterioration from baseline, respectively. Mavroidis et al. (1984a) using both a similar design and assay found that nine schizophrenic patients at 0.1–0.7 ng fluphenazine per milliliter plasma had a mean 59% response at 2 weeks of treatment, while ten patients with higher fluphenazine levels (0.8–2.3 ng/ml) had significantly less improvement (34.0%). Both studies found diminished response at high fluphenazine levels. Hitzemann et al. (1986), reporting on the same group of patients as in the Mavroidis et al. (1984a) study, found strikingly different patterns of drug levels and response when radioreceptor assays were used on the same samples of plasma previously assayed by gas chromatography. Using the radioreceptor assay (Creese and Snyder 1977), nonresponders who had high levels of fluphenazine (by gas chromatography) had virtually no active metabolites in the radioreceptor assay. Most good fluphenazine responders had total plasma neuroleptic activity of 3–6 ng fluphenazine equivalents per milliliter plasma. The shape of the drug level-response curve was transformed by the radioreceptor assay to a more typical sigmoidal curve.

5.5 Thioridazine

As noted previously, Cohen et al. (1980b) used a radioreceptor assay to assess the relationship between plasma thioridazine and response at 2 weeks in a predetermined, fixed dose study. The study used low doses (200–400 mg/day) of thioridazine. They found response to be linearly correlated ($r = 0.95$) with plasma neuroleptic activity. As also previously noted, Smith et al. (1984b), utilizing a gas chromatography assay for detection of plasma thioridazine and mesoridazine and using fixed, predetermined doses of thioridazine ranging from 150 to 750 mg daily for 24 days, showed little relationship between thioridazine drug levels and therapeutic response.

In summary, the data from these 15 predetermined, fixed dose studies of chlorpromazine, thioridazine, fluphenazine, haloperidol, and thiothixene generally paint a rather consistent pattern with respect to the lower portion of the relationship between plasma drug level and antipsychotic response: increasing drug levels appear, within limits, to be associated with increased antipsychotic responses. This is particularly convincing in the data for haloperidol with gas chromatographic assays and for thioridazine when measured by receptor binding assay. In contrast, a relatively inconsistent picture is painted with respect to response at higher levels of the neuroleptic drugs. Both studies of patients receiving fluphenazine showed diminished antipsychotic response at high fluphenazine levels, and four of seven relevant studies of haloperidol similarly show diminished response at high drug levels. The study which used chemical assays with thiothixene had insufficient data points at high drug concentrations to describe the upper portion of the thiothixene level-response curve. However, with the radioreceptor assay, it appears as though there may be continued response at high levels of thiothixene and of fluphenazine and their active metabolites. The studies with chlorpromazine and thioridazine may not have used sufficiently high doses of the drug with which to evaluate the upper arm of the drug level-response pattern.

6 Conclusion

The attempt to use antipsychotic drug concentrations for routine drug monitoring and dosage adjustment is premature at this time. Major difficulties remain with the choice of relevant assays, with the choice of compartment from which to measure drug levels, and in interpreting presently available studies. In particular, it is unclear whether advantages of utilizing free levels of drug (or derivatives thereof, as in CSF or erythrocytes) outweigh the added time and expense required to gather the sample and perform the assay. It is also unclear which drugs need to be studied with assays that monitor a host of metabolites, as well as the parent drug, in order to find meaningful relationships between drug levels and response, which can be used to guide treatment. Such issues remain to be solved before widespread therapeutic drug monitoring programs can be established for the antipsychotic drugs.

References

Bevilacqua R, Benassi CA, Largajolli R, Veronese FM (1979) Psychoactive butyrophenones: binding to human and bovine serum albumin. Pharmacol Res Commun 11:447–454

Bigelow LB, Hirsch DG, Braun T, Korpi ER, Wagner RL, Zaleman S, Wyatt RJ (1985) Absence of a relationship of serum haloperidol concentration and clinical response in chronic schizophrenia: a fixed dose study. Psychopharmacol Bull 21:66–68

Brodie BB (1967) Psychochemical and biochemical basis of pharmacology. JAMA 202:600–609

Casper R, Garver DL, Dekirmenjian H, Chang S, Davis JM (1980) Phenothiazine levels in plasma and red blood cells. Arch Gen Psychiatry 37:301–305

Chiodo LA, Bunney BS (1983) Typical and atypical neuroleptics: different effects of chronic administration on the activity of A_9 and A_{10} midbrain dopaminergic neurons. J Neurosci 3:1607–1619

Cohen BM, Lapinski JF, Harris PQ, Pope HG, Friedman M (1980a) Clinical use of the radioreceptor assay for neuroleptics. Psychiatry Res 1:173–178

Cohen BM, Lapinski JF, Pope HG, Harris PQ, Allesman RI (1980b) Neuroleptic blood levels and therapeutic effect. Psychopharmacology (Berlin) 70:191–193

Contreras S, Alexander H, Faber R, Bowden C (1987) Neuroleptic radioreceptor activity and clinical outcome in schizophrenia. J Clin Psychopharmacol 7:95–98

Creese I, Snyder SH (1977) A simple and sensitive radioreceptor assay for antischizophrenic drugs in blood. Nature 270:180–182

Dysken NW, Javaid JI, Chang SS, Shaffer C, Shahid A, Davis JM (1981) Fluphenazine pharmacokinetics and therapeutic response. Psychopharmacology (Berlin) 73:205–210

Forsman A, Öhman R (1977) Studies on serum protein binding of haloperidol. Curr Ther Res 21:245–255

Garver DL, Dekirmenjian H, Davis JM, Casper R, Ericsen S (1977) Neuroleptic drug levels and therapeutic response: preliminary observations with red blood cell bound butaperazine. Am J Psychiatry 134:304–307

Garver DL, Dekirmenjian H, Davis JM (1978) Phenothiazine red blood cell levels and clinical response. Psychopharmacol Bull 14:27–29

Garver DL, Hirschowitz J, Glickstein GA, Canter DR, Mavroidis ML (1984) Haloperidol plasma and RBC levels and clinical antipsychotic response. J Clin Psychopharmacol 4:133–137

Hitzemann RJ, Garver DL, Mavroidis M, Hirschowitz J, Zemlan FP (1986) Fluphenazine activity and antipsychotic response. Psychopharmacology (Berlin) 90:270–273

Linkowski P, Hubain P, von Frenckell R, Mendlewicz J (1984) Haloperidol plasma levels and clinical response in paranoid schizophrenics. Eur Arch Psychiatry Neurol Sci 234:231–236

Mailman RB, Dehaven DL, Halpern EA, Lewis MH (1984) Serum effects confound the neuroleptic radioreceptor assay. Life Sci 34:1057–1064

Mavroidis ML, Kanter DR, Hirschowitz J, Garver DL (1983) Clinical response and plasma haloperidol levels in schizophrenia. Psychopharmacology (Berlin) 81:354–356

Mavroidis ML, Garver DL, Kanter DR, Hirschowitz J (1984a) Fluphenazine plasma levels and clinical response. J Clin Psychiatry 45:370–373

Mavroidis ML, Kanter DR, Hirschowitz J, Garver DL (1984b) Clinical relevance of thiothixene plasma levels. J Clin Psychopharmacol 4:155–157

Mavroidis ML, Kanter DR, Hirschowitz J, Garver DL (1984c) Therapeutic blood levels of fluphenazine: plasma or RBC determinations. Psychopharmacol Bull 20:168–170

Potkin SG, Shen Y, Zhou D, Pardes H, Shu L, Phelps B, Poland B (1985) Does a therapeutic window for plasma haloperidol exist? Preliminary Chinese data. Psychopharmacol Bull 24:59–61

Rimon R, Averbuch I, Rozick P, Fijman-Danilovich L, Kara T, Dasperg H, Epstein RP, Belmaker RH (1981) Serum and CSF levels of haloperidol by radioimmunoassay and radioreceptor assay during high-dose therapy of resistant schizophrenic patients. Psychopharmacology (Berlin) 73:197–199

Schley J, Muller-Oerlinghausen B (1983) The binding of chemically different psychotropic drugs to acid glycoprotein. Pharmacopsychiatry 16:82–85

Seeman P, Lee T, Chau-Wong M, Wong K (1976) Antipsychotic drug doses and neuroleptic/dopamine receptors. Nature 261:717–719

Smith RC, Broules G, Shvartsburd A, Allen R, Lewis N, Schoolar JC, Chojnecki M, Johnson R (1982) RBC and plasma levels of haloperidol and clinical response in schizophrenia. Am J Psychiatry 139:154–156

Smith RC, Baumgartner R, Misra CH, Mauldin M, Shvartsburd A, Ho BT, DeJohn C (1984a) Haloperidol plasma levels and prolactin response as predictors of clinical improvement in schizophrenia: chemical versus radioreceptor plasma level assays. Arch Gen Psychiatry 41:1044–1049

Smith RC, Baumgartner R, Ravajondron GK, Shvartsburd A, Schoolar JC, Allen R, Johnson R (1984b) Plasma and red cell levels of thioridazine and clinical response in schizophrenia. Psychiatry Res 12:287–296

Smith RC, Baumgartner R, Burd A, Ravichandran GK, Mauldin M (1985) Haloperidol and thioridazine drug levels and clinical response in schizophrenia: comparison of gas-liquid chromatography and radioreceptor drug level assays. Psychopharmacol Bull 21:52–59

Tang SW, Glaister J, Davidson L, Toth R, Jeffries JJ, Seeman P (1984) Total and free plasma neuroleptic levels in schizophrenic patients. Psychiatry Res 13:285–293

Van Putten T, May PRA, Marder SR, Wilkens JN, Rosenberg BJ (1983) Plasma levels of thiothixene by radioreceptor assay: clinical usefulness. Psychopharmacology (Berlin) 79:40–44

Van Putten T, Marder SR, May PRA, Poland RE, O'Brien RP (1985) Plasma levels of haloperidol and clinical response. Psychopharmacol Bull 21:69–72

Wistedt B, Johanivesz G, Omerhodzic M, Arthur H, Bertilsson L, Petters I (1984) Plasma haloperidol levels and clinical response in acute schizophrenia. Nord Psykiat Tidsskr 9:13

Wode-Helgodt B, Borg S, Fyro B, Sedvall G (1978) Clinical effects and drug concentrations in plasma and cerebrospinal fluid in psychiatric patients treated with fixed doses of chlorpromazine. Acta Psychiatr Scand 58:149–173

Active Metabolites of Neuroleptics in Plasma and CSF: Implications for Therapeutic Drug Monitoring

E. Mårtensson and G. Nyberg [1]

Neuroleptic drugs, particularly those of the phenothiazine type, give rise to metabolites that are pharmacologically active and may contribute to the clinical effects of the drugs. In a drug-monitoring situation one must therefore consider not only the concentration of the parent drug but also that of one or several metabolites, depending on their contribution to the total clinical effect. Chlorpromazine and thioridazine are the two neuroleptic drugs that have been most thoroughly studied in this respect. Since we have been involved in studies of thioridazine, the present discussion is limited to this drug. A similar discussion would also be relevant to other neuroleptic drugs.

A large number of unconjugated thioridazine metabolites have been identified in blood and urine from patients treated with thioridazine (Mårtensson et al. 1975). Unconjugated and glucoronic acid conjugated hydroxy metabolites have been found in urine and faeces, but their presence in blood has not been reported (Papadopoulos et al. 1985). The structural formula of thioridazine and its main metabolites is shown in Fig. 1. Thioridazine and two of its main metabolites, the side-chain sulphoxide and the side-chain sulphone, have affinities to dopamine D_2 receptors. The two metabolites also have a clinically demonstrated antipsychotic effect. Consequently, these three substances are of interest to assay in a drug-monitoring situation. One question is, however, how much each of these contributes to the antipsychotic effect.

Figure 2 shows the average relative concentration patterns of thioridazine and the antipsychotically active metabolites in the serum and CSF of patients. The concentrations of thioridazine and those of its side-chain sulphoxide are about equal, while the concentrations of the side-chain sulphone are much lower. Thioridazine and its main metabolites are highly protein bound in plasma (Nyberg et al. 1978). The mean free fractions are 0.18% for thioridazine, 1.6% for side-chain sulphoxide, and 0.94% for side-chain sulphone, with more than ten-fold inter-individual variations. The fact that the unbound plasma concentrations are of the same magnitude as the CSF concentrations, and that it is generally assumed that they are in equilibrium with each other, has led some researchers to advocate the use of unbound plasma concentrations as ideal for drug monitoring of psychoactive drugs.

---

[1] Department of Psychiatry, University of Gothenburg, Lillhagen Hospital, 422 03 Hisings Backa, Sweden

Clinical Pharmacology in Psychiatry
Editors: S. G. Dahl and L. F. Gram
(Psychopharmacology Series 7)
© Springer-Verlag Berlin Heidelberg 1989

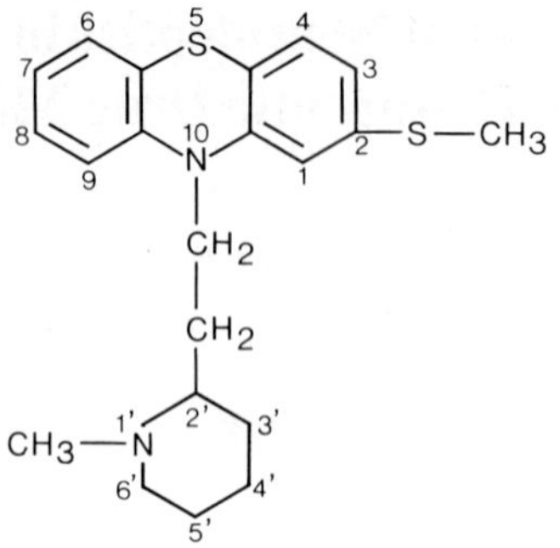

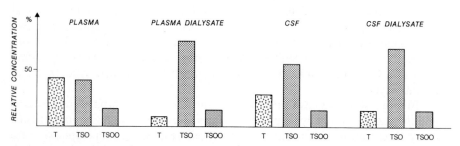

Position in thioridazine formula

	2	5	7	1'
Thioridazine side-chain sulphoxide	$\overset{\displaystyle O}{\overset{\displaystyle \|}{-S}}-CH_3$		—H	—CH₃
Thioridazine side-chain sulphone	$\overset{\displaystyle O}{\underset{\displaystyle O}{\overset{\displaystyle \|}{\underset{\displaystyle \|}{-S}}}}-CH_3$		—H	—CH₃
Thioridazine ring sulphoxide	—S—CH₃	=O	—H	—CH₃
7-hydroxy-thioridazine	—S—CH₃		—OH	—CH₃
Nor-thioridazine	—S—CH₃		—H	—H

Fig. 1. Structural formula of thioridazine and some of its metabolites in man

Fig. 2. Average relative concentrations of thioridazine, (*T*) thioridazine side-chain sulphoxide (*TSO*) and thioridazine side-chain sulphone (*TSOO*) in plasma, plasma dialysate, CSF, and CSF dialysate of thioridazine-treated patients

The unbound concentration profile of the three substances is strikingly different from the total plasma concentration profile, in which the side-chain sulphoxide is very dominant (Fig. 2). The CSF concentration profile is some-what different, mainly due to the fact that particularly thioridazine is to some extent protein bound in the CSF. If we look at the unbound CSF concentra-tions, we have essentially the same pattern as for unbound plasma concentra-tions. From these data one may suspect that the side-chain sulphoxide con-

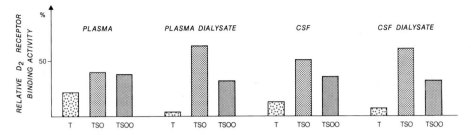

Fig. 3. Average relative dopamine D_2 receptor binding activities of thioridazine (*T*), thioridazine side-chain sulphoxide (*TSO*) and thioridazine side-chain sulphone (*TSOO*) in plasma, plasma dialysate, CSF and CSF dialysate in patients treated with thioridazine. The values were obtained by multiplying the relative concentrations with corresponding relative dopamine D_2 receptor affinities

tributes most to the antipsychotic effect and should therefore be monitored in the first place.

In in vitro experiments the two side-chain oxidized metabolites have higher affinities to dopamine D_2 receptors than the parent drug. Results obtained with receptor preparations from rat, hamster, sheep and calf brain, indicate that the side-chain sulphoxide and the side-chain sulphone are, respectively, on average about two and five times more potent than thioridazine (Bylund 1981; Kilts et al. 1984). If we assume that the same relative potencies are valid for human brain, we may construct dopamine D_2 receptor blocking profiles for plasma and CSF by multiplying the relative concentration values with the corresponding relative dopamine D_2 receptor affinity (Fig. 3). The relative contribution from thioridazine then appears to be very small, particularly in the dialysates from plasma and CSF, while the side-chain sulphoxide still appears to be the most important substance. The contribution from the side-chain sulphone may, however, also be considerable.

We do not know whether the drug concentrations available to the receptors in the brain are the same as in the CSF; although many believe that there is probably a fairly close relationship. For several neuroleptic drugs, the concentrations in the brain tissue are higher than in the plasma, and thus enormously much higher than in the CSF. Data concerning drug concentrations in human brain are scarce, but post-mortem analysis of brains from thioridazine-treated patients showed that the concentration of thioridazine was much higher than the concentrations of the side-chain sulphoxide and side-chain sulphone (Divono et al. 1978). We have found a similar human brain concentration pattern (thioridazine 89%, side-chain sulphoxide 10%, side-chain sulphone 1%; unpublished data).

Figure 4 shows the concentration profile and the corresponding dopamine D_2 receptor blocking activity profiles constructed from these data. These profiles are quite different from the CSF profiles, with thioridazine as the dominant substance. If we assume that the concentration profile of the whole brain gives a good reflection of the concentrations available at the receptors,

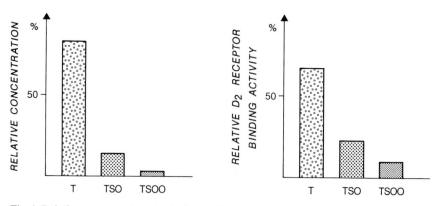

Fig. 4. Relative concentrations in the human brain and relative dopamine D_2 receptor binding activities calculated as described in the legends to Figs. 2 and 3, from the concentrations reported by Dinovo et al. (1978). *T*, Thioridazine; *TSO*, thioridazine side-chain sulphoxide; *TSOO*, thioridazine side-chain sulphone

the concentration of thioridazine itself would be the most important to consider by therapeutic drug monitoring. The differences between the contributions from the side-chain oxides to the total dopamine D_2 receptor blocking activities in the plasma, CSF and brain are illustrated in Table 1.

How do these theoretical considerations accord with data available from clinical studies? Axelsson (1977) compared the relative antipsychotic effect of the side-chain sulphoxide and the side-chain sulphone with that of thioridazine by treating ten patients with each of the three compounds in equipotent doses and determined plasma concentrations at steady state. It was estimated that the two side-chain metabolites together accounted for only 37% (with a wide range, from 17% to 97%) of the total antipsychotic effect of thioridazine treatment. This figure agrees with the relative dopamine D_2 receptor blocking activity of the two metabolites that could be calculated for brain tissue (Table 1).

Table 1. Calculated relative dopamine D_2 receptor blocking activity of side-chain sulphoxide and sulphone

	Percent of total
Plasma total	75
Plasma dialysate	95
CSF	87
CSF dialysate	93
Brain	32

A study of the relationship between serum concentrations of thioridazine and its metabolites and the clinical response indicated that therapeutically optimal serum concentration intervals are age dependent both for thioridazine and for the side-chain sulphoxide. It was also quite clear that there was no relationship between the ring sulphoxide concentrations and the clinical effect (Axelsson and Mårtensson 1983).

Determining the metabolite concentrations in plasma may be of value for assessment of the risk of side effects. Particularly the ring sulphoxide, which appears to have no antipsychotic effect but often attains plasma concentrations several times higher than that of thioridazine (Mårtensson et al. 1975), is of interest in this respect. In an experiment with dogs given either thioridazine or one of the metabolites (Heath et al. 1985), profound changes in cardiac output and blood pressure were seen in those receiving thioridazine ring sulphoxide but not in those receiving thioridazine or the side-chain sulphoxide or sulphone. Although all four compounds increased the QRS and the Q-t$_c$ interval, ventricular arrythmias were seen only in dogs receiving the ring sulphoxide. In a study on thioridazine-treated patients, the decrease in blood pressure induced by the treatment was correlated to the serum concentration of the ring sulphoxide but not to the concentrations of thioridazine, the side-chain sulphoxide or the side-chain sulphone. These findings indicate that the ring sulphoxide may play an important role in the development of serious cardiac side effects by thioridazine treatment (Axelsson and Mårtensson 1983).

In summary, we may conclude that the concentration patterns of thioridazine and its two antipsychotically active metabolites are different in the plasma, CSF and brain. If we look at the dopamine D$_2$ receptor binding activities, thioridazine itself represents only a minor fraction in the CSF compared to those of the two side-chain oxidized metabolites, while the opposite is true for brain tissue. We do not know, however, the concentration ratios between the substances that are directly available to the various receptors in the brain. The few clinical data so far available indicate a concentration-effect relationship, at least for thioridazine and for the side-chain sulphoxide. We can not say whether the concentration of one or the other of these two substances is more related to the antipsychotic effect. Determination of the plasma levels of the metabolites, particularly the ring sulphoxide, may however be of value in assessing the risk for serious side effects.

References

Axelsson R (1977) On the serum concentration and antipsychotic effects of thioridazine, thioridazine side-chain sulfoxide and thioridazine side-chain sulfone in chronic psychotic patient. Curr Ther Res 21:587–605

Axelsson R, Mårtensson E (1983) Clinical effects related to the serum concentration of thioridazine and its metabolites. In: Gram LF, Usdin E, Dahl SG, Kragh-Sörensen P, Sjöqvist I, Morselli PL (eds) Clinical pharmacology in psychiatry. Macmillan, London

Bylund DB (1981) Interaction of neuroleptic metabolites with dopaminergic, α-adrenergic muscarinic and cholinergic receptors. J Pharmacol Exp Ther 217:81–86

Dinovo EC, Rost RO, Sunshine I, Gottschalk LA (1978) Distribution of thioridazine and its metabolites in human tissues and fluids obtained post mortem. Clin Chem 24:1828–1830

Heath A, Svensson C, Mårtensson E (1985) Thioridazine toxicity – an experimental cardiovascular study of thioridazine and its major metabolites in overdose. Vet Hum Toxicol 27:101–105

Kilts CD, Knight DL, Mailman RB, Widerlöv E, Breese GR (1984) Effects of thioridazine and its metabolites on dopaminergic function. Drug metabolism as a determinant of the antidopaminergic actions of thioridazine. J Pharmacol Exp Ther 231:334–342

Mårtensson E, Nyberg G, Axelsson R, Serck-Hansen K (1975) Quantitative determination of thioridazine and non-conjugated thioridazine metabolites in serum and urine of psychiatric patients. Curr Ther Res 18:667–700

Nyberg G, Axelsson R, Mårtensson E (1978) Binding of thioridazine and thioridazine metabolites to serum proteins in psychiatric patients. Eur J Clin Pharmacol 14:341–350

Papadopoulus AS, Carammer L, Cowan DA (1985) Phenolic metabolites of thioridazine in man. Xenobiotica 15(4):309–316

Hydroxyhaloperidol and Clinical Outcome in Schizophrenia

A. C. Altamura[1], M. Mauri[1], R. Cavallaro[1],
M. G. Regazzetti[1], and S. R. Bareggi[2]

1 Introduction

Poor results in the pharmacotherapy of schizophrenic disorders may be attributed both to pharmacometabolic and to pharmacokinetic patterns. Studies on the relationship of plasma level to clinical response have contributed to the rationalization of treatment, although the evidence of a clear-cut plasma level-response relationship is controversial for most neuroleptics (Dahl 1986).

In many such studies the measurement of neuroleptic drug metabolites has been hampered by poor sensitivity and specificity of the methods used. For this reason, an important variable affecting clinical response, the metabolic patterns, often has been omitted or misinterpreted. More recently, progress in analytical assays has partly solved these problems and made it possible to perform more sensitive and specific determinations of neuroleptics and their metabolites.

For haloperidol, one of the most widely prescribed neuroleptics, a correlation between plasma levels and clinical outcome has not been clearly demonstrated. A relationship between plasma levels and clinical response to haloperidol treatment or a therapeutic plasma level range has been reported by some authors (Mavroidis et al. 1983; Smith et al. 1985) but not by others (Bigelow et al. 1985; Dahl 1986 for review). This lack of homogeneity may stem from various sources, such as differences in patient populations, different times of evaluation of clinical and pharmacokinetic parameters, and non-detection of the main metabolite of haloperidol.

Haloperidol metabolism seems to follow two different pathways, the first of which results in the formation of small inactive fragments of the molecule, while the other produces a reduced compound, hydroxyhaloperidol, which seems to be less active (25%) and to have less affinity (1/400) to dopamine D_2 receptors than the parent drug, both in vitro and in vivo (Browning et al. 1982; Korpi and Wyatt 1984).

The small number of studies on hydroxyhaloperidol which have been performed so far have found variable concentrations of this compound in the plasma of patients treated with haloperidol (Larson et al. 1983; Ereshefsky et

[1] Institute of Clinical Psychiatry, University of Milan, Via F. Sforza 35, 20122 Milan, Italy
[2] Department of Pharmacology, University of Milan, Via L. Vanvitelli 32, 20100 Milan, Italy

Clinical Pharmacology in Psychiatry
Editors: S. G. Dahl and L. F. Gram
(Psychopharmacology Series 7)
© Springer-Verlag Berlin Heidelberg 1989

al. 1984; Shostack et al. 1988) and in post-mortem brain tissue of schizophrenic patients (Korpi et al. 1984). In a preliminary study, Ereshefsky et al. (1984) showed that a higher ratio between plasma levels of hydroxyhaloperidol and those of haloperidol (RHL/HL ratio) was associated with poor clinical response. Our first data showed a similar relationship between the clinical outcome and the plasma levels ratio (Altamura et al. 1987; 1988). The aim of this further study was to evaluate relationships between hydroxyhaloperidol plasma levels, the RHL/HL ratio, and the clinical outcome and side effects in a larger sample of schizophrenic patients.

2 Methods

A total of 30 patients (24 men and 6 women), aged 17–52 years (mean, 30 ± 1.8 SE) and diagnosed as schizophrenics according to DSM-III criteria (12 disorganized, 5 paranoid, 13 undifferentiated), were treated with conventional haloperidol doses ranging from 8 to 18 mg per day (mean, 10.6 mg ± 0.6 SE), for 6 weeks. The daily dosage was unchanged for each patient after the 1st week of treatment. The clinical outcome and the extrapyramidal side effects were assessed, respectively, by means of the Brief Psychiatric Rating Scale (BPRS; Overall and Gorham 1962) and the Extrapyramidal Side Effects Rating Scale (EPSE; Simpson and Angus 1970). Evaluations were made at admission (time 0), after 3 weeks (time 1) and after 6 weeks of treatment (time 2). EEG, ECG and routine haematochemical investigations were performed at time 0 and time 2. Plasma haloperidol and hydroxyhaloperidol levels were determined by high-performance liquid chromatography (HPLC) with electrochemical detection (Korpi et al. 1983) and a gas-chromatography/mass-spectrometry assay, to confirm HPLC data, after the 3rd week of treatment. Statistical analysis of the data was performed by regression analysis.

3 Results

The plasma levels ranged from 1.3 to 16.8 ng/ml (mean, 4.8 ± 0.6 SE) for haloperidol and from 0 to 16.8 ng/ml (mean, 4.7 ± 0.8 SE) for the metabolite (Fig. 1). The RHL/HL ratios ranged from 0 to 4.3 (mean, 1.1 ± 0.2 SE). The haloperidol and haloperidol plus hydrxoyhaloperidol plasma levels were significantly correlated with the daily dose of haloperidol ($r = 0.4$, $p < 0.05$; $r = 0.38$, $p < 0.05$). A linear positive correlation was found between haloperidol and hydroxyhaloperidol plasma levels ($r = 0.39$; $p < 0.05$). There was no correlation between haloperidol plasma levels and clinical response, evaluated as percentage improvement in BPRS ratings after 3 and 6 weeks of treatment. No significant correlation was found between hydroxyhaloperidol plasma levels or RHL/HL ratios and the clinical outcome after 3 weeks of treatment. However, a significant negative correlation was found between

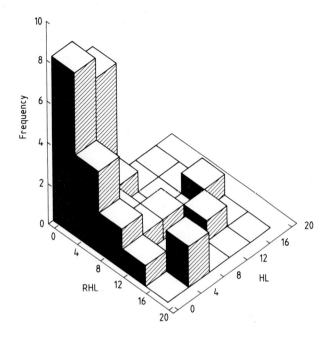

Fig. 1. Distribution of haloperidol (*HL*) and hydroxyhaloperidol (*RHL*) plasma levels (ng/ml) among 30 patients

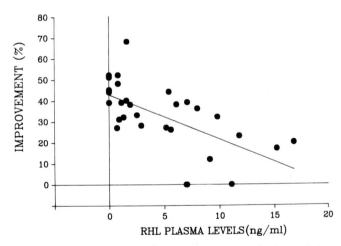

Fig. 2. Relationship between hydroxyhaloperidol (*RHL*) plasma levels and therapeutic improvement, assessed by the Brief Psychiatric Rating Scale (*BPRS*), after 6 weeks of treatment (% of basal values). $r = -0.62$; $p < 0.01$

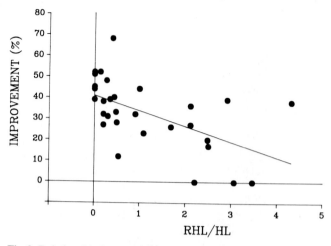

Fig. 3. Relationship between RHL/HL ratios and therapeutic improvement, assessed by the Brief Psychiatric Rating Scale (*BPRS*), after 6 weeks of treatment (% of basal values). $r = -0.55; p < 0.01$

hydroxyhaloperidol plasma levels ($r = -0.62$, $p < 0.01$; Fig. 2), RHL/HL ratios ($r = -0.55$, $p < 0.01$; Fig. 3) and clinical outcome after 6 weeks of treatment. No correlation between haloperidol, hydroxyhaloperidol, or haloperidol plus hydroxyhaloperidol plasma levels and EPSE scores was observed.

4 Discussion

The results of this study are consistent with the hypothesis that hydroxyhaloperidol, the main metabolite of haloperidol, significantly influences the clinical response to haloperidol treatment. Our data do not show any relationship between haloperidol plasma levels and clinical response, in agreement with other studies (see Dahl 1986 for review). However, a significant negative correlation was found between hydroxyhaloperidol plasma levels, RHL/HL ratios and clinical outcome at the end of the study. In other words, higher hydroxyhaloperidol plasma levels were associated with an absent or poor clinical improvement, in accordance with previously published data (Ereshefsky et al. 1984) and our own findings (Altamura et al. 1987, 1988).

The reason for this relationship might be that hydroxyhaloperidol exerts a lower antipsychotic activity than haloperidol. The antipsychotic potency of hydroxyhaloperidol was estimated to be 25% of that of haloperidol, based on behavioural effects in animals (Browning et al. 1982). Moreover, in in vitro dopamine D_2 receptor binding, hydroxyhaloperidol was reported to have a relative activity of 25% compared to that of haloperidol and one of 40% in the platelet enzyme inhibition test (Rubin and Poland 1981). Korpi and Wyatt

(1984) found the in vitro dopamine D_2 receptor binding affinity of hydroxyhaloperidol to be 0.25% of that of haloperidol. On the other hand, our data showed a correlation between hydroxyhaloperidol plasma levels, RHL/HL ratio and improvement after 6 weeks of treatment, but not after 3 weeks. Side effects were not shown to be related to the plasma levels of the two compounds.

These observations suggest that studies on the relationship between plasma level and clinical response should be extended to more than 3 weeks in order to assess true antipsychotic effect (Cotes et al. 1978), and, furthermore, that hydroxyhaloperidol plasma levels and/or RHL/HL ratios could be used as an early indicator of response to treatment with haloperidol. Further research is being undertaken to study the possible, more specific relationship between psychopathological aspects (i.e. single or clustered schizophrenic symptoms) and the metabolic patterns in patients treated with HL in order to closer evaluate the influence of variability in HL metabolism in determining clinical response in schizophrenia. Moreover, the role of the HL metabolism in the development of neuroleptic-induced, short- and long-term reactions (parkinsonism, tardive dyskinesia) must be considered. Preliminary results seem to indicate that patients with high RHL/HL ratio tend to develop few, acute or chronic, extrapyramidal symptoms.

References

Altamura AC, Mauri MC, Cavallaro R, Gorni A (1987) Haloperidol metabolism and anti-psychotic effect in schizophrenia. Lancet 1:814

Altamura AC, Mauri MC, Cavallaro R, Colacurcio F, Gorni A, Bareggi S (1988) Reduced haloperidol/haloperidol ratio and clinical outcome in schizophrenia: preliminary evidences. Prog Neuropsychopharmacol Biol Psychiatry 12(5):689–694

Bigelow LB, Kirch DG, Braun T, Korpi ER, Wagner RL, Zalkman S, Wyatt RJ (1985) Absence of relationship of serum haloperidol concentration and clinical response in chronic schizophrenia: a fixed dose study. Psychopharmacol Bull 21(1):66–68

Browning JL, Silverman PB, Harrington CA, Davis LM (1982) Preliminary behavioural and pharmacological studies on the haloperidol metabolite reduced haloperidol. Abstr Soc Neurosci 8:470

Cotes PM, Crow TJ, Johnstone EC, Bartlett W, Bourne RC (1978) Neuroendocrine changes in acute schizophrenia as a function of clinical state and neuroleptic medication. Psychol Med 8:657–665

Dahl SG (1986) Plasma level monitoring of antipsychotic drugs. Clin Pharmacokinet 11:36–61

Ereshefsky L, Davis CM, Harrington CA, Jann MW, Browning JL, Saklad SR, Burch NR (1984) Haloperidol and reduced haloperidol plasma levels in selected schizophrenic patients. J Clin Pharmacol 4:138–142

Korpi ER, Wyatt RJ (1984) Reduced haloperidol: effects on striatal dopamine metabolism and conversion to haloperidol in the rat. Psychopharmacology (Berlin) 83:34–37

Korpi ER, Phelps BH, Granger H, Chang W, Linnoila M, Meek JL, Wyatt RJ (1983) Simultaneous determination of haloperidol and its reduced metabolite in serum and plasma by isocratic liquid chromatography with electrochemical detection. Clin Chem 29:624–628

Korpi ER, Kleinman JE, Costakos DT, Linnoila M, Wyatt RJ (1984) Reduced haloperidol in the post mortem brains of haloperidol treated patients. Psychiatry Res 11:259–269

Lavsson M, Forsman A, Ohman RA (1983) A high performance liquid chromatographic method for the determination of haloperidol and reduced haloperidol in serum. Curr Ther Res 34(6):999–1008

Mavroidis ML, Hirschowitz J, Kanter DR, Garver DL (1983) Clinical response and plasma haloperidol levels in schizophrenia. Psychopharmacology (Berlin) 81:354–356

Overall J, Gorham D (1962) Brief psychiatric rating scale. Psychol Rep 10:799–812

Rubin RT, Poland RE (1981) Serum haloperidol determination and their contribution to the treatment of schizophrenia. In: Dahl S, Usdin E (eds) Clinical pharmacology in psychiatry. Macmillan, London, pp 217–225

Shostak M, Perel JM, Stiller RL, Wyman W, Curran S (1987) Plasma haloperidol and clinical response: a role for reduced haloperidol in antipsychotic activity? J Clin Psychopharmacol 7(6):394–400

Simpson RM, Angus JSW (1970) A rating scale for extrapyramidal side effects. Acta Psychiatr Scand [Suppl] 212:11–19

Smith RG, Baumgartner R, Burd A, Ravichandran GK, Maudlin M (1985) Haloperidol and thioridazine drug levels and clinical response in schizophrenia: comparison of gas-liquid chromatography and radioreceptor drug level assay. Psychopharmacol Bull 21(1):52–58

Plasma Level Monitoring
for Maintenance Neuroleptic Therapy *

S. R. MARDER, T. VAN PUTTEN, and M. ARAVAGIRI [1]

1 Introduction

Schizophrenic patients differ markedly in the dose of neuroleptic that is necessary to treat their acute exacerbations of illness and to maintain their remis-
sions once they have been adequately treated. Decisions about drug dosage
during the maintenance phase are particularly problematic because the
clinician is unable to assess a clinical response in individuals who are clinically
stable. During this phase, the monitoring of plasma levels of neuroleptic drugs
could provide an objective method of assessing a patient's pharmacotherapy.
Unfortunately, there have been very few studies of plasma level measurement
in maintenance therapy. However, the available studies (Brown et al. 1982;
Wistedt et al. 1982) suggest that patients with lower plasma levels are more
vulnerable to relapse.

   This report focuses on some of the problems that plague researchers who
study relationships between clinical outcome and plasma levels in patients
receiving long-term maintenance therapy. Particular emphasis is placed on
studies that utilize long-acting depot drugs since these may be the preferred
compounds (Freeman 1980) for this stage of treatment. We demonstrate that
some of the thorniest problems associated with finding relationships between
clinical response and plasma levels are exaggerated in studies of maintenance
therapy and depot drugs.

2 Defining Outcome for Maintenance Treatment

The maintenance phase of treatment in schizophrenia begins after a patient
has recovered from an acute psychotic episode. At that time point, one of the
important clinical goals is to prevent the recurrence of another episode.
Numerous clinical studies have firmly established that when stabilized
schizophrenic patients are continued on neuroleptic medications, their rates of

* Supported by the Veterans Administration Medical Research Service and the UCLA Mental Health Clinical Research Center for the Study of Schizophrenia (NIMH).
[1] West Los Angeles Veterans Administration Medical Center, Brentwood Division, and
Department of Psychiatry and Biobehavioral Sciences, 11301 Wilshire Boulevard, UCLA,
Los Angeles, CA 90073, USA

Clinical Pharmacology in Psychiatry
Editors: S. G. Dahl and L. F. Gram
(Psychopharmacology Series 7)
© Springer-Verlag Berlin Heidelberg 1989

relapse are considerably lower than those of patients who are changed to a placebo. There is much less evidence about the appropriate dose of maintenance neuroleptic or the optimal plasma level for this stage of treatment. Clinical experience suggests that the best dosage and plasma level for maintenance therapy is considerably lower than that for the treatment of acute schizophrenia, but methodological problems make the comparison difficult. These methodological problems may have resulted in the relative lack of well designed studies of plasma levels in maintenance therapy and in the tendency of clinicians often to prescribe doses of neuroleptic for well stabilized patients that are probably more appropriate for the treatment of acute psychosis.

Among the problems in maintenance studies is the measurement of outcome. In acute studies, clinicians can compare the amount of improvement or the lack of it that occurs at different plasma levels. In maintenance therapy, patients begin the study in a stable condition, and the clinician is forced to measure a negative outcome – psychotic relapse or exacerbation. Another problem is the length of time which the observer must wait between the time when a dose is measured and the time when the outcome is evaluated. Whereas the clinical response in acute treatment occurs relatively rapidly, in days or weeks, the response in maintenance treatment requires a much longer period of time. When well stabilized patients have their medications discontinued, the majority of relapses occur 4–6 months later. Therefore, most maintenance studies require at least 1 year, and perhaps 2 or 3, for measuring outcome.

The importance of the manner in which outcome is defined is demonstrated by the following study from our laboratory (Marder et al. 1987). We evaluated clinical outcome in a study in which schizophrenic patients were randomly assigned to receive either 5 mg or 25 mg fluphenazine decanoate. Patients were followed for 2 years, and outcome was measured at frequent intervals using measures of clinical psychopathology and side effects. We struggled to find the best definition of relapse, since the most common definition, rehospitalization, appeared to us to be unsatisfactory. This is because the decision to hospitalize is often influenced by social factors that are only peripherally related to psychopathology. We resolved the issue by using two separate definitions of negative outcome. The first we called psychotic exacerbation, defined as a worsening of 3 or more points on the Brief Psychiatric Rating Scale (BPRS) factor scores for thought disturbance or paranoia. This is a rather sensitive measure and defines minor features of clinical worsening that are rather common for schizophrenic patients. The more serious negative outcome was called psychotic relapse, defined as a psychotic exacerbation that could not be controlled within a few days when the dose of fluphenazine decanoate was increased to as high as 10 mg in the low-dose group or 50 mg in the high-dose group.

Defining these two levels of outcome was important because the clinical results were very different. Figure 1 demonstrates a survival analysis in which the vertical axis represents the percentage of patients who remain in the study

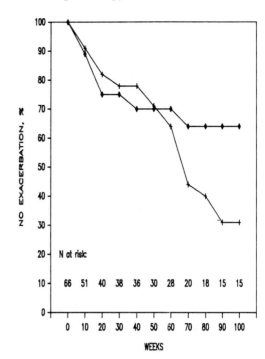

Fig. 1. Two-year survival analysis of patients without exacerbation. Patients received fixed doses of fluphenazine, either 5 mg (*crosses*) or 25 mg (*diamonds*). (From Marder et al. 1986)

without exacerbations at any given time on the original fixed dose. During the 2nd year, the two doses demonstrated very different survival rates. Although the patients receiving 5 mg continued to relapse at approximately the same rat as they did during the 1st year, patients receiving the conventional dose had a negligible exacerbation rate. The actual 2-year survival rates were 31% on 5 mg and 64% on 25 mg. The end-point survival rates were significantly different ($p < 0.05$). The analysis shown in Fig. 2, on the other hand, uses psychotic relapse as the indicator of negative outcome. In this case, the two doses appear approximately equal. The slight difference between the two dosage groups is not statistically significant.

Our findings also indicate other problems associated with outcome measurement. Even though the low-dose patients were more vulnerable to psychotic exacerbations, we found that these patients felt better, as indicated by lower scores on items from the SCL-90R (Hopkins Symptom Checklist-90, Revised), a self-report measure for subjective distress. These scores were highly correlated with scores for akathisia and retardation, suggesting that patients on the higher doses experienced more extrapyramidal side effects, as manifested in increased anxiety and depression. Thus, in evaluating outcome in maintenance therapy the clinician may be performing a complex cost-benefit analysis in which the amount of protection that a patient receives is weighed against the discomfort resulting from the treatment itself.

There are other problems associated with the long intervals during which maintenance patients need to be evaluated. During this period of time, usually

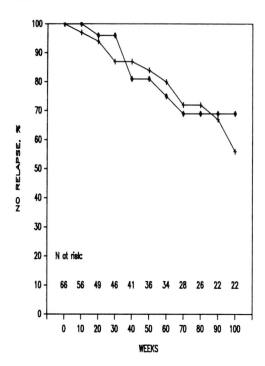

Fig. 2. Two-year survival analysis of patients without relapse. Patients received dose ranges of fluphenazine, either 5–10 mg (*crosses*) or 25–50 mg (*diamonds*). (From Marder et al. 1986)

1–2 years, patients are likely to be exposed to numerous environmental factors that can have an important effect on outcome. These are different than the relatively controlled conditions that exist in a psychiatric hospital. Studies from a number of cultures reveal that environmental stress, particularly criticism expressed within the patient's family, can have powerful effects on relapse rates. This results in an important source of variance in outcome that is uncontrolled by the research team.

3 Plasma Level Measurement in Maintenance Therapy

As mentioned previously, patients are usually treated with much lower drug doses during maintenance therapy. This creates an obvious problem for measuring plasma levels of certain neuroleptics, which may have been low for patients treated with conventional levels. The most obvious example is fluphenazine. A number of studies indicate that acutely ill patients commonly have a clinical response with plasma levels below the nanogram range (Dysken et al. 1981; Mavroidis et al. 1984; Tune et al. 1980; Dudley et al. 1983). Plasma levels may be considerably lower for patients treated with fluphenazine decanoate. For this reason, studies of fluphenazine plasma levels have often required the sensitivity of a radioimmunoassay.

4 Problems for Studies of Depot Neuroleptics

Long-acting injectable neuroleptics, or depot neuroleptics, have certain characteristics that make studying these drugs considerably more difficult when compared with oral drugs. Among these is the length of time it takes these drugs to reach a steady state. Figure 3 is from the aforementioned study (Marder et al. 1986) in which chronic schizophrenic patients were randomized to either 5 or 25 mg fluphenazine decanoate administered every 2 weeks. Fluphenazine levels were measured at regular intervals using a radioimmunoassay developed by Midha and his colleagues at the University of Saskatchewan. The most important data comes from the group randomized to the higher dose. On the 25-mg dose, patients required as long as 3–6 months to reach a steady state. Others (McCreadie et al. 1986; Gelders 1986) have reported similar results for haloperidol decanoate, although Deberdt et al. (1980) reported that haloperidol reached a steady state after only two monthly injections.

The length of time that it takes for depot neuroleptics to reach a steady state can be a significant problem for researchers and clinicians. The researcher should be cautious about interpreting a plasma level during the first several weeks of treatment since the patient may not be at steady state, resulting in the conclusion that the dosage is too low. It is important, there-

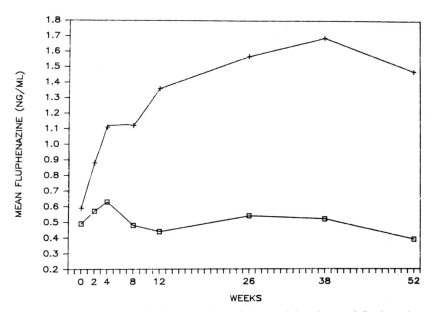

Fig. 3. Mean plasma levels of fluphenazine in patients receiving doses of fluphenazine decanoate every 14 days, either 5 mg (*squares; n = 12–26*) or 25 mg (*crosses; n = 9–19*). Differences between the two dosage groups are statistically significant at 8 weeks and thereafter. (From Marder et al. 1986)

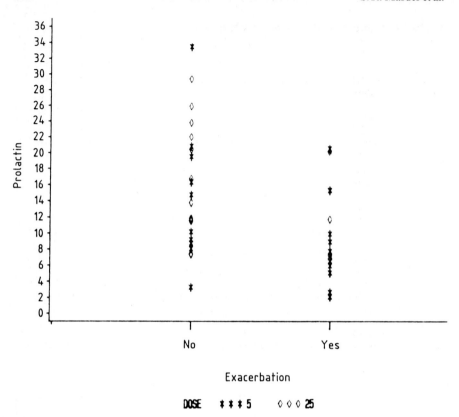

Fig. 4. Six-month prolactin levels in patients who exacerbated (*n* = 22) and those who did not (*n* = 15). Fluphenazine dose was either 5 mg (*asterisks; n* = 23) or 25 mg (*diamonds; n* = 14). (From Wilkins et al. 1987)

fore, that clinicians design studies with a duration that is long enough that all subjects will have a sufficient number of observations following steady state. For the clinician, the problems are somewhat different. If the clinician is cautious and starts a patient's treatment at a relatively low dose, there is likely to be a significant period of time – perhaps 1–3 months – during which the patient may be significantly undertreated. This would result in the patient being more vulnerable to relapse. If too high a dose is selected, the patient may gradually become exposed to a dose which is higher than necessary and perhaps even toxic. There are three possible solutions to this dilemma: (a) supplement the patient with oral medication during the vulnerable months when the depot drug is reaching a stable steady state; (b) start the patient at a high or loading dose of depot drug during the first injections and decrease the dose during subsequent injections; and (c) use a shorter inter-injection interval during the first several months. Currently, there is inadequate information available to guide clinicians during the early days of depot treatment.

In our studies, we confronted this problem by analyzing data on blood levels after patients reached steady state (Wilkins et al. 1987). This is illustrated by our method for evaluating the relationship between prolactin levels and clinical outcome, using the same study previously mentioned in which doses of 5 and 25 mg fluphenazine decanoate were compared. In order to analyze the relationship between these levels and subsequent exacerbations, we chose the 6-month level as the index since this appeared to be the point at which patients had reached a reliable steady state. We then compared this level with exacerbation rates during the next 18 months. Figure 4 displays the 6-month prolactin levels for patients who exacerbated and those who did not during the subsequent 18 months. The values for patients who exacerbated were significantly lower ($p = 0.017$). It is also notable that there is a wide range of prolactin levels among the patients receiving 5 mg. This suggests that even with depot drugs there is considerable variability in plasma levels for patients receiving the same dose. Figure 5 demonstrates the respective rates of exacerbation-free survival among patients who had 6-month prolactin levels above and below the mean of 11.5 ng/ml. Survival was significantly higher among those with the higher prolactin levels.

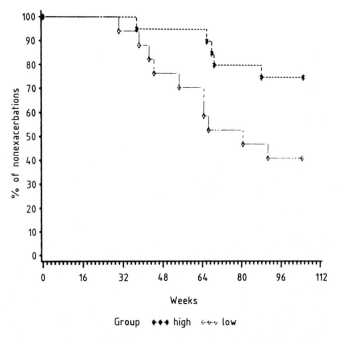

Fig. 5. Survival analysis for psychotic exacerbations in patients treated with fluphenazine, with 6-month prolactin levels either above (*asterisks*) or below (*diamonds*) the mean of 11.5 mg/nl. Differences are statistically significant ($p = 0.03$, Wilcoxon x^2; $p = 0.05$, log-rank x^2). (From Wilkins et al. 1987)

We also studied the relationship between 6-month fluphenazine levels and exacerbation. Although the mean fluphenazine level at 6 months was lower for patients who exacerbated during the subsequent 18 months (0.57 ng/ml for exacerbators versus 1.01 ng/ml for patients who remained stable), this difference was not statistically significant. It may be that with a larger sample size a significant difference would have been found.

5 Drug Metabolism for Depot Neuroleptics

Some of the antipsychotic effect of neuroleptics may be related to psychoactive metabolites. For example, important major metabolic pathways of phenothiazine neuroleptics include sulfoxidation, N oxidation, oxidative N dealkylation, ring hydroxylation, and glucuronidation. It is likely that a considerable amount of the variance among patients in plasma levels, dosage, and clinical response is related to differences in metabolism. Drug metabolism probably differs substantially when patients are changed from the oral to the depot form of the same drug, since the depot form avoids first-pass hepatic metabolism.

Perhaps the best studied metabolic pathway for the phenothiazines involves the oxygenation of the ring sulfur atom to form sulfoxide derivatives. Early reports (Dahl 1976; Dahl and Strandjord 1977) suggested that sulfoxide metabolites could be found in plasma after the oral administration of phenothiazines but not after their parenteral administration. However, Hartmann et al. (1983) have reported that sulfoxidation of chlorpromazine can occur in the small intestine, suggesting that this metabolic pathway may be a factor for patients treated parenterally. Evidence that sulfoxidation actually takes place in patients treated with fluphenazine decanoate is provided in a recent report by Midha et al. (1987). Using a radioimmunoassay method which had been confirmed by gas chromatography/mass spectrometry, they found fluphenazine sulfoxide in 97% of samples taken from 30 schizophrenic patients who had been maintained on chronic fluphenazine decanoate without any administration of oral fluphenazine. Interestingly, the levels of fluphenazine sulfoxide were nearly as high as those of the parent drug. Since there was a considerable amount of variation in sulfoxide levels among patients, it is conceivable that differences among patients in metabolism may be clinically important. We are currently involved in ongoing studies to determine the utility of measuring other metabolites in addition to the parent drug and its sulfoxide metabolite. Our collaborators have already developed radioimmunoassay methods for measuring 7-hydroxyfluphenazine and fluphenazine N-oxide. We have found these metabolites in the plasma of patients on both oral and depot fluphenazine in quantities that are similar to that of the parent drug. Determining the clinical importance of these substances will be a difficult statistical challenge.

The impact on plasma levels due to changing a patient from oral to depot fluphenazine was demonstrated in a recent study from our laboratory. We

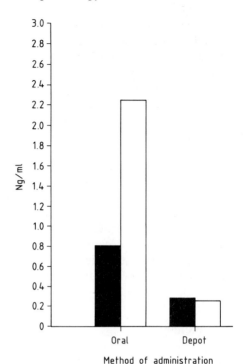

Fig. 6. Mean fluphenazine and fluphenazine sulfoxide levels in eight patients treated with oral and depot fluphenazine. Ratio of fluphenazine to fluphenazine sulfoxide: oral, 2.99; depot, 1.01. Differences are statistically significant ($p = 0.0002$, t test)

were interested in differences in drug metabolism between the oral and depot forms and whether there was a relationship between how an individual patient metabolized a drug and its route of its administration. Eight newly admitted psychotic patients were first stabilized on oral fluphenazine for at least 4 weeks. Following stabilization, the oral drug was discontinued, and fluphenazine decanoate was administered in doses between 5 and 25 mg every 2 weeks. Plasma levels of fluphenazine and fluphenazine sulfoxide were measured at regular intervals, but only after patients had been on the same dose of the oral drug for 1 week and the depot drug for 3 months. As noted in Fig. 6, the levels of both substances were higher for the oral route. This is not very interesting since the intention of the clinician was to use the lowest effective dose for maintenance therapy. More interesting is the difference in the ratios of the parent drug to its sulfoxide metabolite. In the orally treated patients, the concentration of the sulfoxide metabolite was approximately three times the concentration of the parent drug, whereas the patients on depot drugs had levels of parent drug and metabolite that were similar ($p = 0.0002$). This supports the view that sulfoxidation of the parent compound is likely to be a much more important factor for patients treated with an oral as opposed to a depot phenothiazine.

The presence of these metabolites may explain why studies which have investigated the relationship between plasma level and dose of fluphenazine have generally not found a strong relationship. An exception is a study by

Cohen et al. (1985) which found a correlation of 0.75 ($p < 0.0001$) between blood level and dose for patients treated with decanoate and enanthate esters. This later study differed from others in that a radioreceptor assay method was used. Since this method measures the activity of both the parent compound (i.e., fluphenazine) as well as its active metabolites, it may be that the strong relationship which Cohen et al. (1985) found was present because a major source of variation between patients – the efficiency of drug metabolism – was decreased.

Haloperidol appears to have a simpler and less variable metabolism, and as a result relationships between plasma level and clinical outcome may be easier to identify. For haloperidol decanoate, there appears to be a relatively high correlation between dose and plasma level (De Buck et al. 1981; Reyntjens et al. 1982; De Cuyper et al. 1986). McCreadie et al. (1986) have reported less variation in neuroleptic plasma levels with haloperidol decanoate than with fluphenazine decanoate. This parallels studies with oral haloperidol which also demonstrate less variation in plasma levels when compared with oral fluphenazine (Van Putten et al. 1985).

6 Conclusions

Despite all of the problems associated with finding relationships between plasma level and clinical outcome in maintenance therapy, there are important reasons for researchers to continue studies in this area. The most important reason may be the cost of an error in dosing during maintenance therapy. If the clinician sets the dose at too high a level, patients may be at a greater risk for tardive dyskinesia. In addition, manifestations of extrapyramidal side effects such as akathisia and akinesia can be tormenting and may interfere with a schizophrenic patient's rehabilitation. If the dose is set at too low a level, the patient may be more vulnerable to psychotic relapses, which can be costly in terms of lost jobs, unfulfilled family responsibilities, and diminished self-esteem. These clinical realities may help to sustain researchers who are frustrated by all of the problems associated with studying this phase of treatment.

References

Brown WA, Laughren T, Chisholm E, Williams BW (1982) Low serum neuroleptic levels predict relapse in schizophrenic patients. Arch Gen Psychiatry 39:998–1000
Cohen BM, Waternaux C, Chouinard G, Sommer BR, Jones B (1985) Plasma levels of neuroleptic in patients receiving depot fluphenazine. J Clin Psychopharmacol 5:328–332
Dahl SG (1976) Pharmacokinetics of methotrimeprazine after single and multiple doses. Clin Pharmacol Ther 19:435–442
Dahl SG, Strandjord RE (1977) Pharmacokinetics of chlorpromazine after single and chronic dosage. Clin Pharmacol Ther 21:409–414

Deberdt R, Elens W, Berghmans J, Heykants R, Woesterborghs R, Driesens F, Reyntjens A, van Wijngaarden I (1980) Intramuscular haloperidol decanoate for neuroleptic maintenance therapy: efficacy, dosage schedule, and plasma levels. Acta Psychiatr Scand 62:356–363

De Buck RP, Zelaschi N, Gilles C, Durdu J, Brauman H (1981) Theoretical and practical importance of plasma levels of haloperidol. Correlations with clinical and computerized EEG data. Prog Neuro Psychopharmacol 5:499–502

De Cuyper H, Bollen J, van Praag HM, Verstraeten D (1986) Pharmacokinetics and therapeutic efficacy of haloperidol decanoate after loading dose administration. Br J Psychiatry 148:560–566

Dudley J, Rauw G, Hawes EM, et al. (1983) Correlation of fluphenazine plasma levels versus clinical response in patients: a pilot study. Prog Neuro Psychopharmacol Biol Psychiatry 7:791–795

Dysken MW, Javaid JI, Chang SS, Schaffer C, Shahid A, Davis JM (1981) Fluphenazine pharmacokinetics and therapeutic response. Psychopharmacology (Berlin) 73:205–210

Freeman H (1980) Twelve years' experience with the total use of depot neuroleptics in a defined population. In: Cattabeni F et al. (eds) Long-term effects of neuroleptics. Raven, New York, pp 559–564

Gelders YG (1986) Pharmacology, pharmacokinetics and clinical development of haloperidol decanoate. Int Clin Psychopharmacol 1(s):1–11

Hartmann F, Gruenke LD, Craig JC, Bissell DM (1983) Chlorpromazine metabolism in extracts of liver and small intestine from guinea pig and from man. Drug Metab Dispos 11:244–248

Marder SR, Hawes EM, van Putten T, Hubbard JW, McKay G, Mintz J, May PRA, Midha KK (1986) Fluphenazine plasma levels in patients receiving low and conventional doses of fluphenazine decanoate. Psychopharmacology (Berlin) 88:480–483

Marder SR, van Putten T, Mintz J, Lebell M, McKenzie J, May PRA (1987) Low and conventional dose maintenance therapy with fluphenazine decanoate: two year outcome. Arch Gen Psychiatry 44:518–521

Mavroidis ML, Kanter DR, Hirschowitz J, Garver DL (1984) Fluphenazine plasma levels and clinical response. J Clin Psychiatry 45:370–373

McCreadie RG, McKane JP, Robinson ADT, Wiles DH, Stirling GS (1986) Depot neuroleptics as maintenance therapy in chronic schizophrenic in-patients. Int Clin Psychopharmacol 1(s):13–14

Midha KK, Hubbard JW, Marder SR, Hawes EM, van Putten T, McKay G, May PRA (1987) The sulfoxidation of fluphenazine in schizophrenic patients maintained on fluphenazine decanoate. Psychopharmacology (Berlin) 93:369–373

Reyntjens AJM, Heykants JJP, Woestenborghs RJH, Gelders YG, Aerts TUL (1982) Pharmacokinetics of haloperidol decanoate: a 2-year followup. Int Pharmacopsychiatry 17:238–246

Tune LE, Creese I, Depaulo JR, Slavney PR, Coyle JT, Snyder SH (1980) Clinical state and serum neuroleptic levels measured by radioreceptor assay in schizophrenia. Am J Psychiatry 137:187–190

Van Putten T, Marder SR, May PRA, Poland RE, O'Brien RP (1985) Plasma levels of haloperidol and clinical response. Psychopharmacol Bull 21:69–72

Wilkins JN, Marder SR, van Putten T, Midha KK, Mintz J, Setoda D, May PRA (1987) Circulating prolactin predicts risk of exacerbation in patients on depot fluphenazine. Psychopharmacol Bull 23:522–525

Wistedt B, Jorgensen A, Wiles D (1982) A depot neuroleptic withdrawal study: plasma concentration of fluphenazine and flupenthixol and relapse frequency. Psychopharmacology (Berlin) 78:301–304

Perphenazine Serum Levels in Patients on Standard Doses

F. HAFFNER [1]

1 Introduction

Concentration measurements of antipsychotic drugs may be useful in monitoring patient compliance and in evaluating adverse drug effects (Dahl 1986). Poor compliance seems to be underestimated as a source of drug failure (Hulka et al. 1976). The problem is of daily concern in psychiatric hospitals as well as at outpatient centres and in private practice. As a consequence, many physicians and psychiatrists are misled in their efforts to establish the right dose. Variable compliance, resulting in wide daily fluctuations of drug concentrations, may increase the risk of developing toxic symptoms and tardive dyskinesia (Kane et al. 1985), a hazard which seems to increase with dose and the length of treatment (Casey 1985). Poor compliance may also lead to abandoning a potentially good medicine on false premises.

Pronounced inter-individual variation in pharmacokinetics has been shown for several neuroleptics (Dahl and Strandjord 1977; Dahl 1982; Dahl and Hals 1986). A similar variability has been shown to be of clinical importance in treatment with antidepressants (Gram 1977; Sjøqvist et al. 1980; Gram et al. 1982; Brøsen and Gram 1988). There is no reason why these principles should not apply to neuroleptic drugs as well. High and very high doses of neuroleptics are still popular in many institutions. As recently pointed out, however, in a retrospective analysis of published results on drug therapeutic concentrations for different neuroleptics (Baldessarini et al. 1988), there is no solid evidence for the postulated good effect of high neuroleptic doses.

Much is known about the metabolism of antipsychotic drugs (Jørgensen 1986), but there is still disagreement concerning recommended serum concentrations of the drugs. Despite numerous studies on the use of antipsychotic drug concentrations in monitoring patient treatment, the value of such monitoring is still open to discussion. One reason for the lack of conclusive data is that the process of establishing therapeutic ranges is a tiresome and time-consuming task which requires drug concentration measurements in well designed studies with good analytical and biological precision and preferably with fixed doses at different levels.

The somewhat inconclusive and conflicting reports may partly be due to incongruent patient material, lack of correlating factors, or both. A re-

---

[1] Laboratory of Neurochemistry and Pharmacology, Department of Psychiatry, Buskerud County Hospital, Lier, Norway

Clinical Pharmacology in Psychiatry
Editors: S. G. Dahl and L. F. Gram
(Psychopharmacology Series 7)
© Springer-Verlag Berlin Heidelberg 1989

analysis of results from controlled studies of acute psychosis treated with fluphenazine (Kane et al. 1983; Kane 1985; Marder et al. 1984; Hogarty et al. 1976, 1979; Rifkin et al. 1977) leads to the conclusion that monitoring of serum concentrations of haloperidol and fluphenazine is of definite value. Similar results have been reported with perphenazine (Bolvig Hansen et al. 1982; Bolvig Hansen and Larsen 1985).

2 Serum Perphenazine Concentrations

The main objective of the present study was to evaluate the importance of determining serum concentration of perphenazine in the treatment of psychoses. Between June 1987 and February 1988, 431 sera from 292 patients were analysed. The samples (5–6 ml) were submitted by 53 different institutions, ranging from university psychiatric hospitals to private practices. Of these, 209 were single samples, and the remainder were two or more samples from 83 patients. The samples received from university hospital represented only a small fraction, about 10% of the total. The serum samples were received mostly by mail after 1–3 days and were analysed immediately upon arrival or stored at $-20\,°C$ until analysed. The mean time between sampling and reply to the clinicians for the first 100 samples was 12 days (range 3–19 days).

Along with the samples, a completed questionnaire was requested, giving information on previous neuroleptic treatment, duration of perphenazine treatment, dose, dosage form, concomitant drug use, clinical evaluation, antipsychotic and adverse drug effects, as well as results from earlier perphenazine assays. Serum perphenazine concentrations were determined using high-pressure liquid chromatography (HPLC), as described by Larsen et al. (1985). The clinicians were informed about the serum concentrations with a written comment for each patient, giving advice on dosage, also taking other drugs into consideration. The various institutions were encouraged to contact the laboratory to discuss unexpected results or difficult patients.

The concentrations in the first sample from each patient are presented in Fig. 1. Thirteen of the values in the column " > 30 nmol/l" represent sera with massive doses of other interfering substances, which made it impossible to obtain a concentration value. While 151 of the patients (52%) had serum values above the recommended range (2–6 nmol/l), 108 patients (36%) were within the recommended range, and 34 (12%) were below. In six of these cases noncompliance was suspected. In 41 patients dose changes were implemented following the information on perphenazine levels provided by the laboratory. This resulted in significantly more patients having levels below the upper limit of the therapeutic range. Twelve patients were reported to improve, in terms of fewer side effects ($n=4$) or better antipsychotic effect ($n=8$).

The observation that neuroleptics may be less effective at high doses is not commonly accepted, although this has been suggested for haloperidol

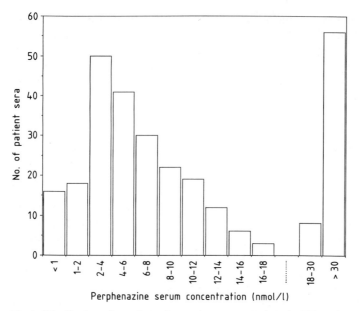

Fig. 1. Distribution of perphenazine serum concentrations in 292 patients examined during the 1st year of the study. The wide variation illustrates large differences in treatment strategies between different institutions and for different patients

(Neborsky et al. 1981), fluphenazine (Kane 1985; Marder et al. 1984) and perphenazine (Bolvig Hansen et al. 1982). There are also those who still ultrahigh doses, but, as pointed out by Baldessarini et al. (1988), there is a definite lack of evidence for the beneficial effect of this procedure.

The present study shows that a significant number of patients on conventional perphenazine doses have serum levels above the recommended range. Furthermore, the majority of patients showed no deterioration after dose reduction.

References

Baldessarini RJ, Cohen BM, Teicher MH (1988) Significance of neuroleptic dose and plasma level in the pharmacological treatment of psychoses. Arch Gen Psychiatry 45:79–91

Bolvig Hansen L, Larsen NE (1985) Therapeutic advantages of monitoring plasma concentrations of perphenazine in clinical practice. Psychopharmacology (Berlin) 87:16–19

Bolvig Hansen L, Larsen NE, Gulmann N (1982) Dose-response relationships of perphenazine in the treatment of acute psychoses. Psychopharmacology (Berlin) 78:112–115

Brøsen K, Gram LF (1988) First-pass metabolism of imipramine and desipramine: impact of the sparteine oxidation phenotype. Clin Pharmacol Ther 40:543–549

Casey DE (1985) Tardine dyskinesia: reversible and irreversible. In: Casey DE, Chase TN, Christensen AV, Gerlach J (eds) Dyskinesia research and treatment. Springer, Berlin Heidelberg New York, pp 88–97

Dahl SG (1982) Active metabolites of neuroleptic drugs: possible contribution to therapeutic and toxic effect. Ther Drug Monit 4:33–40

Dahl SG (1986) Plasma level monitoring of antipsychotic drugs. Clinical utility. Clin Pharmacokinet 11:36–61

Dahl SG, Hals PA (1986) Pharmacokinetic and pharmacodynamic factors causing variability in response to neuroleptic drugs. In: Dahl SG, Gram LF, Paul SM, Potter WZ (eds) Clinical pharmacology in psychiatry. Springer, Berlin Heidelberg New York, pp 266–274

Dahl SG, Strandjord RE (1977) Pharmacokinetics of chlorpromazine after single and chronic dosage. Clin Pharmacol Ther 21:437–448

Gram LF (1977) Plasma level monitoring of tricyclic antidepressant therapy. Clin Pharmacokinet 2:237–251

Gram LF, Pedersen OL, Kristensen CB, Bjerre M, Krag-Sørensen P (1982) Drug level monitoring in psychopharmacology: usefulness and clinical problems, with special reference to tricyclic antidepressants. Ther Drug Monit 4:17–25

Hogarty GE, Ulrich RF, Mussare F, Aristigueta N (1976) Drug discontinuation among long-term successfully maintained schizophrenic outpatients. Dis Nerv Syst 37:494–500

Hogarty GE, Schooler NR, Ulrich RF, Mussare F, Ferro P, Herron E (1979) Fluphenazine and social therapy in the aftercare of schizophrenic patients. Arch Gen Psychiatry 36:1283–1294

Hulka BS, Cassel JC, Kupper LL (1976) Disparities between medications prescribed and consumed among chronic disease patients. In: Lasagna L (ed) Patient compliance. Futura Mount Kisco, New York, pp 123–152

Jørgensen A (1986) Metabolism and pharmacokinetics of antipsychotic drugs. In: Bridges JW, Chassaud LF (eds) Progress in drug metabolism, vol 9. Taylor and Francis, London, pp 111–174

Kane JM (1985) Antipsychotic drug side effects: their relationship to dose. J Clin Psychiatry 46:16–21

Kane JM, Rifkin A, Woerner M, Reardon G, Sarantoakis S, Schibel D, Ramos-Lorenzi J (1983) Low dose neuroleptic treatment of outpatient schizophrenic patients. Arch Gen Psychiatry 40:893–896

Kane JM, Woerner M, Lieberman J (1985) Tardive dyskinesia: prevalence, incidence, and risk factors. In: Casey DE, Chase TN, Christensen AV, Gerlach J (eds) Dyskinesia research and treatment. Springer, Berlin Heidelberg New York, pp 72–78

Larsen NE, Bolving Hansen L, Knudsen P (1985) Quantitative determination of perphenazine and its dealkylated metabolite using high-performance liquid chromatography. J Chromatogr 341:244–250

Marder SR, van Putten T, Mintz J, McKenzie J, Lobell M, Faltico G, May PRA (1984) Costs and benefits of two doses of fluphenazine. Arch Gen Psychiatry 41:1025–1029

Neborsky RJ, Jankowski DS, Perel JM, Munson E, Depry DO (1984) Plasma/RBC haloperidol ratios and improvement in acute psychotic symptoms. J Clin Psychiatry 45:10–13

Rifkin A, Quitkin F, Robiner DJ, Klein DJ (1977) Fluphenazine decanoate, fluphenazine hydrochloride given orally, and placebo in remittent schizophrenics. I. Relapse after one year. Arch Gen Psychiatry 34:43–47

Sjøqvist F, Bertilsson L, Åsberg M (1980) Monitoring tricyclic antidepressants. Ther Drug Monit 25:85–93

Dose-Finding Problems with Psychotropic Drugs

From Animal Experiments to Clinical Dosing: Some Aspects of Preclinical Development of Antidepressants

A. Delini-Stula [1]

1 Introduction

In the preclinical evaluation of new drugs several questions must be answered before a drug can be released for administration to humans. Obviously, the first question is always: Does the drug possess the desired pharmacological activity at all? If such activity is identified, there are other important questions which may be answered only in more elaborate studies. During the various phases of preclinical evaluation of a new drug (Table 1) the potency and dose

Table 1. Experimental phases and decision steps in the preclinical evaluation of drugs

Preclinical phase	Decision criteria [a]
Phase I: First screening	Interesting (desired) activity Relative potency Approximate toxicity
Phase II: Elaborate screening	Confirmation of activity Dose dependency Side effect profile Bioavailability after oral treatment Acute/subacute toxicity
Phase III: Broader characterization	General pharmacology Metabolism, distribution, excretion Chronic toxicity Mutagenicity

[a] The decision criteria listed here may be modified, as they are largely dependent on the specific objective and the selected screening strategy (mechanistic, behavioural) for drug development. The criterion for deciding on further development at the end of phase I is usually that of sufficiently potent activity. The number of criteria relevant for decision increases with each stage.

dependency of effects, general and specific toxicity, its relationship to the desired activity, and additional pharmacological effects and their relation to the main effect must be established. The findings generated in each phase of

---

[1] Research and Development, Ciba-Geigy Ltd. Basel, Switzerland

Clinical Pharmacology in Psychiatry
Editors: S. G. Dahl and L. F. Gram
(Psychopharmacology Series 7)
© Springer-Verlag Berlin Heidelberg 1989

preclinical studies determined the decision as to further development of the drug for a particular indication. In other words, the pharmacological objectives of drug research in animals consist of the evaluation of the profile and mechanism of action and thus the prediction of the therapeutic properties, efficacy and side effect profile of a drug.

For every therapeutic indication extrapolations from animal experiments to man present various difficulties. Even if animal models that faithfully replicate the disease are available, and the pharmacodynamic principle of action is clearly defined and objectively quantified, there are still many other unknown or unpredictable factors which may invalidate such extrapolations. Often, for instance, the metabolism and disposition of the drug in the body of individual species and man are different. It is impossible to forecast such difference in advance. Obviously, these factors may interfere with the therapeutic efficacy of the drug even if the pharmacodynamic principle of action has been validated in animals and in man.

Research on psychotropic drugs encounters particular difficulties. For many psychiatric conditions, the adequacy of animal models has not been established beyond doubt. For some mental disorders there are not even any rationally designed models. The exact mechanism of action of psychotropic drugs is not always certain, and even if a pharmacodynamic principle is identified or presumed, objective criteria for identifying the corresponding functional responses in man may not be available, thus making direct correlations and validations of animal findings and findings in man impossible. In this respect, research on antidepressants presents a particularly illustrative example of the possibilities and the limitations which animal experiments offer in terms of the prediction of therapeutic potential and efficacy of drugs.

2 Preclinical Strategies in the Development of Antidepressants

In general, organization of the screening and selection of the battery of tests which should permit the assessment of drug activity in animals is dependent largely on the type of drug or the activity that one is looking for. In other words, the test battery is conceived to match the rationale for, or hypothesis about, the pharmacodynamic principle underlying therapeutic action in man. In this respect, in the preclinical evaluation of drugs serendipity is today largely replaced by a rational approach in which the search for desired activity is based on the a priori formulation of a biological hypothesis. Either of two major approaches may be selected for designing a screening battery aimed at detecting the desired type of pharmacological activity of a drug, the mechanistic and the behavioural. The mechanistic approach is based on the assumption that specific effect on a specific and defined brain structure or system (neuron, receptor, enzyme) constitutes a therapeutic principle of a drug action. The behavioural approach assumes that there are correlations between the behavioural responses in animals and in humans and that changes may be induced in animal behaviour which simulate psychopathological con-

Table 2. Examples of mechanistic strategies in the search of antidepressants

Desired specific action	Target structure system	Prototype drug
Selective inhibition of reuptake	Noradrenaline neuron	Maprotiline
	Serotonin neuron	Fluoxetine
	Dopamine neuron	Bupropion
Selective inhibition of MAO	MAO-A enzyme	Brofaromine
	MAO-B enzyme	MD 780 236
Release of noradrenaline	α_2-Receptor	Idazoxan
Increase of "second" messenger concentration	Adenylate cyclase	Rolipram

ditions in man; the particular effect of a drug on selected and defined categories of behavioural responses in animals should therefore be predictive of therapeutic activity in man.

These two approaches have been applied in the evaluation of antidepressant drug potential in animals. Under the assumption that the monoamine hypothesis of depression is true, a new drug would be sought that corrects the assumed monoamine deficit. Table 2 presents examples of concepts which may be applied in a mechanistic screening approach to new antidepressants. Classical behavioural models for the screening of antidepressants do not fol-

Table 3. Examples of the most common functional screening models (tests) used for the evaluation of antidepressants

Test system	Species	Validity
Reserpine-induced hypothermia	Mouse	Sensitive to noradrenaline-uptake inhibitors and directly acting sympathicomimetics, less sensitive to MAO inhibitors, insensitive to serotonin-uptake inhibitors and "atypical" antidepressants (trazodone)
Tetrabenazine-induced catalepsy	Rat	Sensitive to noradrenaline inibitors, MAO-inhibitors and dopamine-stimulant drugs, insensitive to serotonin-uptake inhibitors and "atypical" antidepressants
Amorphine-induced hypothermia	Mouse	Sensitive to noradrenaline-uptake inhibitors and mixed uptake inhibitors, β-agonists and serotonin agonists-inhibitors irregular response to MAO
Clonidine-induced hypothermia	Mouse	Sensitive to α_2-receptor blockers and β-agonists, insensitive to uptake blockers and MAO-inhibitors
Behavioural "despair"	Mouse	Sensitive to dopamine agonists, less sensitive to noradrenaline-uptake inhibitors, insensitive to serotonin-uptake inhibitors, MAO-inhibitors and β-agonists
Behavioural "despair"	Rat	Seems sensitive to all antidepressants after chronic administration

low a behaviouristic strategy but reflect the assumption essentially that impaired functions or behavioural responses induced by catecholamine depletion simulate a state of depression. The ability of a drug to correct for such deficit is then euqated with antidepressant potential. Table 3 presents examples of functional or behavioural models which are commonly used in the evaluation of antidepressant drug activity and an overview over their validity. It is evident that, with the possible exception of the behavioural despair test in the rat, biochemical and behavioural models are interdependent in that biochemical properties of drugs largely determine in which functional test a drug will exert its activity.

3 Limits of Extrapolations from Animals to Man

In the case of antidepressant drugs, the major problem in extrapolating findings from animals to man, however, is that their exact mechanism of action is still unknown. The hypothesis that the inhibition of the neuronal uptake process of monoamines is the essential prerequisite of antidepressant action was seriously challenged already when it was found that drugs such as iprindole, mianserin and trazodone, which do not appreciably influence uptake mechanisms, have therapeutic activity. However, since there are no convincing examples of drugs which exert monoamine uptake-inhibiting effects in animals and man and are not antidepressants, it seems reasonable to assume that such inhibition may play a role in determining the therapeutic efficacy of these drugs. However, as illustrated in Table 4 the potency of amine uptake inhibition, determined in various in vitro or in vivo systems (Maitre et a. 1980, 1982) does not seem to bear any relationship to the clinical potency of a large series of antidepressants with established therapeutic efficacy. It is striking that clinical dosing of all these drugs is about the same, although they are so different in terms of biochemical profiles and potency of action. Also, in clinical investigations the attempts to demonstrate correlations between the uptake inhibiting potency, measured either directly or indirectly (for instance, serotonin in platelets or 3-methoxy-4-hydroxyphenylglycol (MHPG) concentrations in blood or urine) and therapeutic outcome, have mostly failed (Lingjaerde 1980; Charney et al. 1981; Beckmann and Goodwin 1975). Some recent results suggest, however, that effectiveness of noradrenaline uptake blockade may be relatively more important for the recovery in bipolar than in unipolar patients (Bowden et al. 1987). It is also interesting that during treatment with clomipramine a correlation was recently reported between clinical improvement and reduced platelet serotonin content (indirect measure of serotonin uptake inhibition) in adolescent patients with obsessive-compulsive disorders (Flament et al. 1987).

Assuming that the global antidepressant effect is the sum of particular effects on various systems and on psychopathological signs, the combination of which is characteristic of depression, the failure to predict such therapeutic ef-

Table 4. Relative potencies of antidepressants in inhibiting noradrenaline and serotonin-uptake in relation to clinical therapeutic doses. (Modified from Delini-Stula 1986)

Drug	Inhibition of uptake in the rat brain (ED_{50} mg/kg p. o.)		Mean oral daily dose (mg)
	Noradrenaline	Serotonin	
Tricyclics			
Imipramine	17	50	150
Desipramine	11	180	100–150
Clomipramine	80	15	75–150
Amitriptyline	100	120	50–150
Nortriptyline	150	200	75–150
Doxepin	300	85	150
Trimipramine	$\gg 300$	$\gg 300$	100–400
Non-Tricyclics			
Mianserin	$> 100\,(32\%)$	$\gg 100$	60–150
Maprotiline	140	$\gg 300$	75–150
Oxaprotiline	10	$\gg 300$	150
Viloxazine	40	150	150–300
Nomifensine	14	60	150
Zimelidine	$\gg 100$	6	200
Citalopram	$\gg 100$	2	25– 60
Fluoxetine	$\gg 100$	8	20– 60
Fluvoxamine	$\gg 30$	5	100–300
Cinopramine	13	0.6	5– 11
Ifoxetine (CGP 15 210)	$\gg 100$	5	100–150[a]
Levoprotiline	$\gg 300$	$\gg 300$	75–150[a]

$\gg$ At given dose no inhibition.
[a] According to the first clinical results.

ficacy on the basis of only a few biochemical variables is understandable. According to this view, it might be expected that the effectiveness of antidepressants in functional or behavioural models would be better explained regarding therapeutic potency and profile of action. However, also the functional models of depression, commonly used for the evaluation of antidepressant properties, have their limitations. As noted above, these limitations relate to the fact that the biochemical and behavioural/functional tests commonly used for determining antidepressant activity of drugs are largely interdependent. The effects of antidepressants assessed in these models mostly reflect, therefore, their biochemical properties, which implies that certain tests detect only certain categories of antidepressants. For instance, selective inhibitors of noradrenaline uptake are effective in monoamine-depleted animals (antagonism of reserpine- or tetrabenazine-induced signs of depression), but inactive in tests based on interaction with clonidine or L-5-HTP. By contrast, selective inhibitors of serotonin are practically inactive in all models except those based on interaction with the serotonergic system. The behavioural despair model in mice (Porsolt 1981), which is of interest because it is conceptually independent of the catecholamine theory of depression, is rather insensitive to antidepressants if they are given in single doses. However, behavioural despair in rats appears to offer a paradigm which sensitively detects antidepressant type of activity if drugs are administered subchronically (Delini-Stula et al. 1988).

The limitations of the models discussed above must also be viewed in terms of the fact that they do not even fulfil all the necessary criteria for validity as proposed by McKinney and Bunney (1969). Four of the postulated criteria are: (a) similarity of inducing conditions, i.e. aetiology, (b) similarity of behavioural symptoms, (c) common underlying neurobiological mechanisms, and (d) reversal of abnormal behaviour by the same clinically effective techniques. Criteria (a) and (c) are certainly not fulfilled, and criteria (b) and (d) are fulfilled only in part.

Figure 1 illustrates the relative potency of several antidepressants assessed in various functional tests in comparison to imipramine. Again, great differences can be noted both with respect to their overall profiles of action and

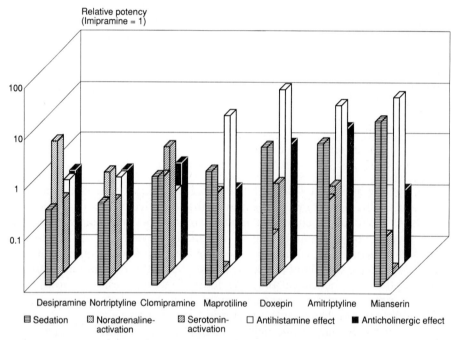

Fig. 1. Relative potencies of sedative, noradrenergic and serotonergic activation and antihistaminic and anticholinergic properties of antidepressants, in relation to that of imipramine. The potency of imipramine was arbitrarily normalized to 1. The ratios were calculated on the basis of in vivo ED_{50} (mg/kg p.o.) for inhibition of exploratory activity (rat), antagonism of reserpine ptosis and sedation (rat), potentiation of L-5-HTP excitation (rat), prevention of histamine toxicity (guinea-pigs) and antagonism of physostigmine toxicity (rat). (Modified from Delini-Stula 1983)

Table 5. Characteristics of the profiles of action of antidepressants and of levoprotiline

Drug	Uptake inhibition			Reversal of		Potentiation of responses to exogenous		
	Nor-adrena-line	Sero-tonin	Dopa-mine	Reser-pine hypo-thermia	Apo-mor-phine hypo-thermia	Nor-adrena-line	Sero-tonin	Dopa-mine
Imipramine	+	+	−	+	+	+	+	+
Desipramine	+	±	−	+	+	+	±	+
Clomipramine	+	+	−	+	+	+	+	+
Maprotiline	+	−	−	+	+	+	−	−
Oxaprotiline	+	−	−	+	+	+	−	+
Fluvoxamine	−	+	−	−	−	−	+	−
Levoprotiline	−	−	−	−	−	−	−	?

in terms of the potencies of individual actions in animals. Clinically these drugs differ, at best, with respect to their side effect profiles; there is at present no substantial evidence that, in terms of their overall therapeutic efficacy or specific effects on particular psychopathological signs in depression, these drugs can be clearly distinguished from each other. Nevertheless, it could be argued that all these drugs, at least in respect to one of the identified pharmacological or biochemical actions, fit one or the other current theoretical concept about the mechanism of action of antidepressants. In this sense, the effects assessed in biochemical or behavioural models have predicted, apart from the side effect profile, at least their global "antidepressant" potential.

The problems of prediction of antidepressant qualities of drugs and extrapolations from animal experiments to man are, however, strikingly illustrated by examples of drugs which have failed to show any action that fits an existing concept, but nevertheless have been clinically tested and discovered due to erroneous assumptions. One current example is that of levoprotiline, biochemically and in common screening tests a "silent" (−) or R enantiomer of oxaprotiline (Waldmeier et al. 1982; Delini-Stula et al. 1982; Mishra et al. 1982). Initial animal studies with this drug did not reveal any activity which would indicate its antidepressant potential (Table 5). However, in clinical studies levoprotiline was found to be therapeutically effective (Delini-Stula et al. 1983; Wendt, in press). Most interestingly also, according to findings to date, no distinction in clinical antidepressant efficacy of levoprotiline and established antidepressants could be demonstrated at equivalent daily doses (75–150 mg) of the drugs.

4 Conclusions

In the field of antidepressant research there are numerous problems and gaps in our knowledge which impede a rational prediction, on the basis of animal experiments, as to the therapeutic potential of a drug and thus the determination of dosing schedules. For the first clinical administration to humans, apart from toxicity studies, there is no clue which could serve as a guide for determining the dose levels which should be explored for therapeutic efficacy. Moreover, no specific objective criteria for "antidepressant" properties of drugs are currently established, either in healthy subjects or in patients, which would provide a reliable link between animal experiments and clinical findings. Predictions of antidepressant effectiveness of drugs from human pharmacological studies today are based mostly on comparisons with empirically established pharmaco-EEG profiles of antidepressants in healthy subjects. However, with the wider use of techniques such as positron-emission tomography and nuclear magnetic resonance, which may permit the identification of specific characteristics and sites of actions of antidepressants in the brain, new approaches could perhaps be expected within this field of research.

References

Beckmann H, Goodwin FK (1975) Antidepressant response to tricyclics and urinary MHPG in unipolar patients. Clinical response to imipramine or amitriptyline. Arch Gen Psychiatry 32(1):17–21

Bowden CL, Davis J, Garver DL, Hanin I, Koslow S, Maas JW (1987) Changes in urinary catecholamines and their metabolites in depressed patients treated with amitriptyline or imipramine. J Psychiatry Res 21(2):111–128

Charney DS, Heniger GR, Steinberg DE, Roth RH (1981) Plasma MHPG in depression: effects of acute and chronic desipramine treatment. Psychiatry 5(2):217–229

Delini-Stula A (1983) Pharmakologie der Antidepressiva. In: Langer G, Heimann H (eds) Psychopharmaka – Grundlagen und Therapie. Springer, Vienna New York, pp 81–95

Delini-Stula A (1986) New pharmacological findings in depression. Psychopathology 19 [Suppl 2]:94–102

Delini-Stula A, Hauser K, Baumann P, Olpe HR, Waldmeier PC, Storni A (1982) Stereospecificity of behavioural and biochemical response to oxaprotiline – a new antidepressant. Adv Biochem Psychopharmacol 31:265–275

Delini-Stula A, Vassout A, Hauser K, Bittiger H, Büch O, Olpe HR (1983) Oxaprotiline and its enantiomers: do they open new avenues in the research of the mode of action of antidepressants? In: Usdin E, Goldstein M, Friedhoff A, Georgotas A (eds) Frontiers in neuropsychiatric research. Mcmillan, London, pp 121–134

Flament MF, Rapoport IL, Murphy DL, Berg CJ, Lake CR (1987) Biochemical changes during clomipramine treatment of childhood, obsessive-compulsive disorder. Arch Gen Psychiatry 44(3):219–225

Lingjaerde D (1980) Antidepressants and serotonin uptake in platelets. Acta Psychiatr Scand [Suppl 280] 61:111–119

Maitre L, Moser P, Baumann PA, Waldmeier PC (1980) Amine uptake inhibitors: criteria of selectivity. Acta Psychiatr Scand [Suppl 280] 61:97–110

Maitre L, Baumann P, Jaekel J, Waldmeier PC (1982) 5-HT uptake inhibitors: psycho-pharmacological and neurobiological criteria of selectivity. Adv Biochem Psychopharmacol 34:229–246

McKinney WT, Bunney WE (1969) Animal models of depression. Arch Gen Psychiatry 21:240–248

Mishra R, Gillespie DD, Lovell R, Robson RD, Sulser F (1982) Oxaprotiline: induction of central noradrenergic subsensitivity by its (+)-enantiomer. Life Sci 30:1747–1755

Porsolt RD (1981) Behavioural despair. In: Enna SJ et al. (eds) Antidepressants: neurochemical, behavioural and clinical perspectives. Raven, New York, pp 121–139

Waldmeier PC, Baumann PA, Hauser K, Maitre L, Storni A (1982) Oxaprotiline, a noradrenaline uptake inhibitor with an active and an inactive enantiomer. Biochem Pharmacol 31:2163–2176

Wendt G, (in press) Levoprotiline-clinical antidepressive efficacy and tolerability. Neuropharmacology, Proceedings of the XVIth CINP Congress, Munich 1988

Evaluation of Clinical and Biological Parameters in Healthy Volunteers: More than Pharmacokinetics and Side Effects?

A. J. Puech, P. Danjou, D. Warot, G. Bensimon, and L. Lacomblez [1]

1 Introduction

For ethical, scientific and economic reasons, new drugs must be studied carefully before their first clinical evaluation in patients. The amount of data from animals and humans available before administration to patients has increased in recent years. Presently, most data available in healthy volunteers concern pharmacokinetics and side effects.

Assessment of dose-effect relationships for new drugs is usually poorly documented in patient populations. This step of development seems important when a pharmacological effect observed in animals is examined in humans in order initially to determine the pharmacologically active dose. These preliminary data may help clinicians to choose the range of doses to be evaluated in patients. Among the various biological and behavioural effects of drugs, some may thus be assessed in healthy volunteers.

2 Biological Effects

At the receptor level some binding sites which exist in the CNS and are implicated in therapeutic activity are present on peripheral cells (Hamilton and Reid 1986; Poirier et al. 1987). Drug-receptor interaction can be assessed by means of in vivo studies using blood cells (Garcia-Sevilla 1981). Such determinations may be of interest, but it may also be hazardous to predict the centrally active dose from such results. In the near future, positron-emission tomography using specific ligands may be adapted for this purpose (Samson et al. 1987; Farde et al. 1988; Pappata et al. 1988; Smith et al. 1988).

Some biochemical effects of psychoactive drugs can be evaluated in humans: (a) serotonin and dopamine uptake inhibition, evaluated ex vivo in platelets; (b) norepinephrine uptake inhibition in vivo, by studying the antagonism of tyramine-induced mydriasis or pressive effect (Freyschuss et al. 1970; Ghose and Turner 1975; Jackson et al. 1983); (c) MAO inhibition using the tyramine pressor test (Schultz and Bieck 1987). As is the case with peripheral binding studies, one must be careful in extrapolating information

[1] Departement de pharmacologie clinique, Groupe Hospitalier Pitié-Salpetrière, 47, Bd de l'Hôpital, 75651 Paris Cedex 13, France

Clinical Pharmacology in Psychiatry
Editors: S. G. Dahl and L. F. Gram
(Psychopharmacology Series 7)
© Springer-Verlag Berlin Heidelberg 1989

from biochemically active doses from such studies to the CNS. Since centrally active drugs may modify monoamine metabolism, it is possible to evaluate some consequences of these changes by measurement of amine metabolites in CSF, blood and urine (Charney et al. 1986; Struthers et al. 1986; Zametkin and Hamburger 1988). Despite some criticism, these changes at least reflect the penetration of the drugs into the CNS, when the CNS metabolite can be distinguished from the peripheral origin for instance with 3-methoxy-4-hydroxyphenylglycol (MHPG) sulphate.

As regards neuroendocrine responses, the neurotransmitter control of pituitary secretions, for example, prolactin and growth hormone, have been extensively studied in recent years (Lal et al. 1977; McCance et al. 1987; Lal 1988). Alteration of the levels of these hormones or of receptor sensitivities by specific drugs reflects the agonistic or the antagonistic effects of the drug. However, this approach has been disappointing for dopaminergic antagonists in term of the prediction of therapeutic doses, although such extrapolation may be possible for other drugs.

Psychoactive drugs modify EEG results, and increasingly sophisticated methods allow the EEG classification of drugs. However, the main difficulty is determining whether the modifications observed are related to the main pharmacological activity of the drug or to lateral effects (Fink 1980; Ott et al. 1982). Moreover, peripheral effects, as those induced by hydrophilic β-blockers, may induce changes in CNS and EEG modifications (Betts and Alford 1983). The qualitative relationship between EEG and therapeutic classification is still questionable; at the most, dose-effect relationships can be observed within a pharmacological class.

3 Behavioural Effects

Various tests have been described which evaluate CNS arousal and psychomotor performances in humans (e.g. critical frequency fusion or choice reaction time). These tests are sensitive to sleep deprivation and to the sedative effects of benzodiazepines, neuroleptics and antidepressants (Smith and Misiak 1976; Hindmarch 1980; Johnson and Chernik 1982). The sedative doses in healthy volunteers and in patients seem to resemble one another closely. Sedation, which is frequently considered a side effect, is a positive feature in hypnotics and may not be devoid of interest in the case of anxiolytics, antidepressants and antipsychotics. Conversely, the impairment of psychomotor functions induced by sleep deprivation is very sensitive to stimulant drugs. The evaluation of effects of psychoactive drugs on vigilance in normal volunteers (Table 1) seems useful for predicting the active sedative or stimulant doses in patients.

The amnesic effect of benzodiazepines and other psychoactive drugs after acute administration is now well documented in healthy volunteers (Table 1; Subhan 1984; Lister 1985; Curran 1986). The evaluation of promnesic drugs

Table 1. Comparative effects of sleep deprivation and psychoactive drugs on critical frequency fusion (CFF) and memory tests in healthy volunteers: means ($\pm$ SD)

	CFF (Hz)		Paired-Associate words (max. score, 7)		Free recall (number of pictures out of 12 or 20)	
Sleep deprivation ($n = 12$)						
(Bensimon 1988, unpublished data)						
12 h	28.9	(2.5)	6.5	(0.7)	16.8	(2.3)
24 h	27.2[a]	(2.1)	6.5	(0.8)	15.5	(3)
48 h	27.4[a]	(2.2)	5.4[a]	(1.3)	13.6[a]	(4.8)
Levomepromazine ($n = 12$)						
(Warot et al. 1988)						
0 mg	26.7	(1.7)	6.7	(0.4)	10.7	(1.1)
3 mg	26.1	(2.5)	6.4	(0.6)	10.2	(1.4)
6 mg	25.1[a]	(2.7)	6.2	(1.1)	9	(1.5)
12 mg	24.7[a]	(2.5)	6.2	(0.9)	8.4[a]	(2.8)
Maprotiline ($n = 12$)						
(Warot, 1989a)						
0 mg	28.9	(2.4)	5.9	(0.7)	9.3	(1.1)
25 mg	27.4	(2.3)	5.9	(0.8)	10.4	(1.1)
50 mg	29.1	(1.8)	6.3	(0.6)	8.9	(1.2)
75 mg	24.9[a]	(1.9)	6	(0.8)	9	(1.6)
Trimipramine ($n = 12$)						
(Warot 1989b)						
0 mg	27.2	(1.8)	6	(1.1)	9.9	(1.9)
25 mg	25.7[a]	(2.1)	6.3	(0.7)	9	(2.7)
50 mg	25.1[a]	(2.0)	6.4	(0.9)	9	(2.4)
100 mg	24[a]	(1.8)	5.6	(1.4)	8	(3.1)
Triazolam ($n = 12$)						
(Warot et al. 1987)						
0 mg	27.0	(2.3)	6.3	(0.75)	9.8	(2.4)
0,25 mg	25.4[a]	(2.4)	4.5[a]	(1.6)	3.3[a]	(3.4)
Alprazolam ($n = 10$)						
(Danjou et al. 1988)						
0 mg	27	(2.6)	5.3	(1.3)	7.7	(1.2)
0,50 mg	25.9[a]	(2.4)	5.3	(1)	4.8[a]	(2.1)
Flunitrazepam ($n = 12$)						
(Bensimon et al. 1986)						
0 mg	26	(2.6)	6.7	(0.5)	10	(1.2)
2 mg	24.9[a]	(2.7)	5.8[a]	(0.78)	6.5[a]	(2.4)
Zopiclone ($n = 12$)						
(Warot et al. 1987)						
0 mg	27.0	(2.3)	6.3	(0.75)	9.8	(2.4)
7,5 mg	25.0[a]	(2.4)	3.4[a]	(1.5)	2.5[a]	(2.3)

[a] $p < 0.05$.

in healthy volunteers, on the other hand, is currently a challenge for the clinical psychopharmacologist. Because so many new drugs seem able to antagonize scopolamine- or benzodiazepine-induced amnesia in animals, it seems reasonable to propose the same models in humans. It remains to be determined whether these drugs are effective in memory impairment in patients, and whether the active dose in drug-induced amnesia is predictive of the therapeutic dose or not.

Drug-induced anxiety has been described, but it is not a realistic model for studies of new drugs (Lader and Bruce 1986). The biological or clinical modifications induced by stress situations (stroop color-word test or delayed auditory feedback, etc.) are sensitive to anxiolytics (Taeuber et al. 1979; Kilminster et al. 1988). Although in these tests the active doses of anxiolytic are lower than the sedative doses, the drug-related changes are neither clearly linked to the anxiolytic effect nor predictive of the therapeutic dosage in patients. These models are presently not sufficiently validated, and it is difficult to determine their real value. According to some psychodynamic theories of anxiety, inhibition seems to be an important behavioural abnormality in anxious patients. Moreover, studies of behavioural pharmacology in rats suggest that inhibition is an important behavioural target for anxiolytics. In animals, the behavioural disinhibition is evaluated by the waiting capacity, which is decreased by benzodiazepines. Since it is difficult to evaluate anxiolytic activity in healthy subjects from these hypotheses, it may be easier to evaluate the disinhibitory effects of drugs by study the subject's waiting capacity and drug-induced changes in this parameter. We are presently using different experimental situations to evaluate anxiety, where the task of the subjects is to answer either very quickly with high reward and low probability or more slowly with lower reward but higher probability.

Learned helplessness is considered a reliable animal model in evaluating behavioural effects of antidepressants (Overmier and Seligman 1967). It is unethical to induce depression in the healthy subject; the induction of a short an reversible state of learned helplessness in humans would be preferable, using controllable or uncontrollable stimuli. Subjective ratings and biological parameters (ACTH, cortisol, noradrenaline are modified in different ways according to the controllable or uncontrollable stress (Gatchel and Proctor 1976; Breier et al. 1987). However, no data using this situation to evaluate antidepressants in healthy subjects are available in the literature, at least to our knowledge. Further development of these types of models might help us to understand the behavioural changes induced by antidepressants in humans and perhaps to predict active doses.

Some psychoactive drugs might exert their action by increasing serotonin transmission. In humans an intense drop in plasma total and free tryptophan, peaking at 80%, is observed after oral intake of tryptophan-free L-amino acid mixtures (Young et al. 1985; Moja et al. 1988). As serotonin synthesis is not rate limited by tryptophan hydroxylase but depends on only CNS uptake, serotonin levels can theoretically be modulated by altering plasma free tryptophan levels (Tagliamonte et al. 1973). In man, only indirect clues such as the decrease of prolactin levels can be used. Healthy volunteers have been shown to be more easily disturbed during a proof-reading task while listening to a tape with themes of hopelessness than with those of neutral content (Young et al. 1985; Smith et al. 1987). This deficit may be used to study the effects of serotonin uptake inhibitors in a behavioural model in humans.

Healthy subjects represent an inadequate population to study the effects of antidopaminergic drugs. In animals models, some effects of apomorphine (e.g. yawning), related to a specific localization of subclasses of dopamine receptors, are induced by very small doses. In healthy volunteers, apomorphine induces yawning at a very low dose (0.1 mg; Blin et al. 1988). This effect of apomorphine, in relation to the stimulation of the dopamine autoreceptor, could be useful in evaluating the dose of neuroleptics blocking the dopamine autoreceptors.

4 Conclusions

Very few central biological effects of psychoactive drugs can be assessed in humans. Presently, changes in monoamine metabolites and neurohormones seem the most predictive of a centrally active dose. In the future positron-emission tomography probably will be very useful for this purpose. The effects of drugs on CNS arousal and psychomotor performances have been the most widely studied. The study of mnemonic effects of psychoactive drugs in normal subjects represents an interesting challenge for the psychopharmacologist. Further data are required in order to validate the different models which have been described here.

References

Bensimon G, Warot D, Foret J, Thiercelin JF, Barthelet G, Simon P (1986) Lack of daytime sleepiness following an oral dose of the new non-benzodiazepine hypnotic, zolpidem administered at bedtime. 3rd Conference on Clinical Pharmacology and Therapeutics, July 27–August 1, Stockholm

Betts TA, Alford C (1983) Beta-blocking drugs and sleep (a controlled trial). Drugs 25:268–272

Blin O, Danjou P, Warot D, Fondarai J, Puech AJ (1988) Induction of yawning by low doses of apomorphine (0.1, 0.2 and 0.4 mg) in healthy volunteers. Psychiatr Psychobiol 3:195–199

Breier A, Albus M, Pickar D, Zahn TP, Wolkowitz OM, Paul SM (1987) Controllable and uncontrollable stress in humans: alterations in mood and neuroendocrine and psychophysiological function. Am J Psychiatry 144:1419–1425

Charney DS, Breier A, Jatlow PI, Heninger GR (1986) Behavioral, biochemical, and blood pressure responses to alprazolam in healthy subjects: interaction with yohimbine. Psychopharmacology (Berlin) 88:133–140

Curran HV (1986) Tranquillising memories: a review of the effects of benzodiazepines on human memory. Biol Psychol 23:179–213

Danjou P, Warot D, Puech AJ (1988) Effets de l'alprazolam sur la vigilance, la mémoire et le stress induit chez le volontaire sain. Therapie 43:93–96

Farde L, Pauli S, Hall H, Eriksson L, Halldin C, Hogberg T, Nilsson L, Sjogren I (1988) Stereoselective binding of 11C-raclopride in living human brain – a search for extrastriatal central D2-dopamine receptors by PET. Psychopharmacology (Berlin) 94:471–478

Fink M (1980) An objective classification of psychoactive drugs. Prog Neuropsychopharmacol 4:495–502

Freyschuss U, Sjøqvist F, Tuck D (1970) Tyramine pressor effects in man before and during treatment with nortriptyline or ECT: correlation between plasma level and effect of nortriptyline. Pharmacol Clin 2:72–78

Garcia-Sevilla JA, Zis AP, Hollingsworth PJ, Greden JF, Smith CB (1981) Platelet alpha-2-adrenergic receptors in major depressive disorder. Binding of tritiated clonidine before and after tricyclic antidepressant drug treatment. Arch Gen Psychiatry 38:1327–1331

Gatchel RJ, Proctor JD (1976) Physiological correlates of learned helplessness in man. J Abnorm Psychol 85(1):27–34

Ghose K, Turner P (1975) Intravenous tyramine pressor response in depression. Lancet 1:1317–1318

Hamilton CA, Reid JL (1986) Platelet alpha-adrenoceptors – a valid model for brain or vascular adrenoceptors? Br J Clin Pharmacol 22:623–626

Hindmarch I (1980) Psychomotor function and psychoactive drugs. Br J Clin Pharmacol 10:189–209

Jackson SHD, Turner P, Ehsanullah RSB (1983) A comparison of diclofensine and desmethylimipramine using tyramine pressor tests in normal subjects. Br J Clin Pharmacol 16:427–429

Johnson LC, Chernik DA (1982) Sedative-hypnotics and human performance. Psychopharmacology (Berlin) 76:101–113

Kilminster SG, Lewis MJ, Jones DM (1988) Anxiolytic effects of acebutolol and atenolol in healthy volunteers with induced anxiety. Psychopharmacology (Berlin) 95:245–249

Lader M, Bruce M (1986) States of anxiety and their induction by drugs. Br J Clin Pharmacol 22:251–261

Lal S (1988) Apomorphine in the evaluation of dopaminergic function in man. Prog Neuropsychopharmacol Biol Psychiatry 12:117–164

Lal S, Guyda H, Bikadoroff S (1977) Effect of methysergide and pimozide on apomorphine-induced growth hormone secretion in men. J Clin Endocrinol Metab 44:766–769

Lister RG (1985) The amnesic action of benzodiazepines in man. Neurosci Biobehav Rev 9:87–94

McCance SL, Cowen PJ, Waller H, Grahame-Smith DG (1987) The effect of metergoline on endocrine responses to L-tryptophan. J Psychopharmacol 2:90–94

Moja EA, Stoff DM, Gessa GL, Castoldi D, Assereto R, Tofanetti O (1988) Decrease in plasma tryptophan after tryptophan-free amino acid mixtures in man. Life Sci 42:1551–1556

Ott H, McDonald RJ, Fichte K, Herrmann WM (1982) Interpretation of correlations between EEG-power-spectra and psychological performance variables within the concepts of "subvigilance", "attention" and "psychomotoric impulsion". In: Herrmann WM (ed) EEG in drug research. Fischer, Stuttgart, pp 227–247

Overmier JB, Seligman MEP (1967) Effects of inescapable shock upon subsequent escape and avoidance responding. J Comp Physiol Psychol 63:28–33

Pappata S, Samson Y, Chavoix C, Prenant C, Mazière M, Baron JC (1988) Regional specific binding of 11C-RO 15 1788 to central type benzodiazepine receptors in human brain: quantitative evaluation by PET. J Cereb Blood Flow Metab 8(3):304–314

Poirier MF, Galzin AM, Loo H, Pimoule C, Segonzac A, Benkelfat C, Sechter D, et al. (1987) Changes in (3H)-5-HT uptake and (3H) imipramine binding in platelets after chlorimipramine in healthy volunteers. Comparison with maprotiline and amineptine. Biol Psychiatry 22:287–302

Samson Y, Pappata S, Hantraye P, Mazière M, Baron JC (1987) Récepteurs centraux aux benzodiazépines: études chez l'homme en tomographie d'émission de positons. Circ Metab Cerveau 4:1255–1266

Schultz R, Bieck PR (1987) Oral tyramine pressor test and the safety of MAO inhibitor drugs. Psychopharmacology (Berlin) 91:515–516

Smith JM, Misiak H (1976) Critical flicker frequency (CFF) and psychotropic drugs in normal human subjects. A review. Psychopharmacology (Berlin) 47:175–182

Smith M, Worf AP, Brodie JD, Arnett CD, Barouche F, Shiue CY, Fowler JS, et al. (1988) Serial (18F)N-methylspiroperidol PET studies to measure changes in antipsychotic drug D-2 receptor occupancy in schizophrenic patients. Biol Psychiatry 23:653–663

Smith SE, Pihl RO, Young SN, Ervin FR (1987) A possible cognitive and environmental influences on the mood lowering effect of tryptophan depletion in normal males. Psychopharmacology (Berlin) 91:451–457

Struthers AD, Burrin JM, Brown MJ (1986) Exercise-induced increases in plasma catecholamines and growth hormone are augmented by selective alpha-2-adrenoceptor blockade in man. Neuroendocrinology 44:22–28

Subhan Z (1984) The effects of benzodiazepines on short-term memory and information processing. Psychopharmacology (Berlin) [Suppl] 1:173–181

Taeuber K, Appel F, Badian M, Palm D, Rupp W, Schofer J, Sitting W (1979) Effects of betablockers and benzodiazepines on stress induced by delayed auditory feed back (DAF) (Abstr). NCDEU Annual Meeting, May 2–24, Key Biscayne

Tagliamonte A, Biggion G, Viargiu L, Gessa LG (1973) Free tryptophan in serum controls brain tryptophan level and serotonin synthesis. Life Sci 12:277–287

Warot D, Bensimon G, Danjou P, Puech AJ (1987) Comparative effects of zopiclone, triazolam and placebo on memory and psychomotor performance in healthy volunteers. Fundam Clin Pharmacol 1:145–152

Warot D, Krebs MO, Bensimon G, Payan C, Danjou P, Lacomblez L, Puech AJ (1988) Dose-effect study of levomepromazine on psychomotor and memory tasks in healthy volunteers. Hum Psychopharmacol 3:127–132

Warot D, Danjou P, Lacomblez L, Diquet B, Puech AJ (1989b) Effects de trois doses de maprotiline (25, 50 et 75 mg) sur la vigilance et la memoire chez le volontaire sain. Therapie (in press)

Warot D, Molinier P, Lacomblez L, Payan C, Danjon P, Puech AJ (1989a). Dose related effects of trimipramine on psychomotor junction memory and autonomic nervous septem activity in healthy volunteers. Hum Psychopharmacol (in press)

Young SN, Smith SE, Pihl RO, Ervin FR (1985) Tryptophan of depletion causes rapid lowering mood in normal males. Psychopharmacology (Berlin) 87:173–177

Zametkin AJ, Hamburger SD (1988) The effect of methylphenidate on urinary catecholamine excretion in hyperactivity: a partial replication. Biol Psychiatry 23:350–456

Dose Finding and Serum Concentrations of Neuroleptics in the Treatment of Schizophrenic Patients *

F.-A. WIESEL, G. ALFREDSSON, and E. JÖNSSON [1]

1 Introduction

The efficacy of neuroleptics in reducing psychotic symptoms has been demonstrated beyond doubt in a number of controlled studies. Nevertheless, the basis for dosage in the treatment of schizophrenic patients is not very well documented. In a survey of the best maintenance doses of neuroleptics in schizophrenics, Baldessarini and Davis (1980) did not find a dose-effect relationship among dose equivalents of about 100–2500 mg chlorpromazine per day.

Results from behavioural animal studies have been the major basis for titrating clinical dosage. Especially the potency of neuroleptics to induce cataleptic effects in animals has been used in this regard, since a high positive correlation between catalepsy and antipsychotic effects in man has been demonstrated (Stille and Hippius 1971). This fact may partly explain both the use of high doses in the treatment of schizophrenic patients and the wide range of doses used, which all seem to be equally effective. The efficacy has been ascertained for high doses, but the lower part of the dose–clinical-effect curve has not been documented (Jain et al. 1988). There is a pronounced dissimilarity in dosage for high-potency and low-potency neuroleptics. Baldessarini et al. (1984), for example, found that the mean chlorpromazine-equivalent daily dose of high-potency neuroleptic agents was 3.5 times as high as that of low-potency drugs. Clinical studies do not substantiate such a difference in dosage between high- and low-potency neuroleptics (Dahl 1986; Jain et al. 1988).

During the 1970s specific and sensitive methods were developed for the determination of drug concentrations in human body fluids. A number of studies have been performed to investigate relationships between drug concentrations and clinical effects in schizophrenic patients. No clear-cut evidence of a linear relationship between symptom reduction and drug concentrations has been obtained (Dahl 1986). At best, therapeutic plasma concentration ranges can be given for some antipsychotic drugs.

* This study was supported by grants from the Swedish Medical Research Council (07027, 07958, 08318) and the Karolinska Institute.
[1] Department of Psychiatry and Psychology, Karolinska Hospital, 10401 Stockholm, Sweden

Clinical Pharmacology in Psychiatry
Editors: S. G. Dahl and L. F. Gram
(Psychopharmacology Series 7)

Neuroleptic drugs are a heterogeneous group regarding both their chemistry and their pharmacokinetics and pharmacodynamics, which probably contributes to the negative findings concerning relationships between drug concentrations and therapeutic effects. Experimental and clinical data give strong support to the opinion that the antipsychotic effect in man is mediated by a blockade of D_2 dopamine receptors (Peroutka and Snyder 1980; Farde et al. 1988). The use of a selective D_2 dopamine receptor antagonist would therefore be more optimal in studying relationships between clinical effects and drug concentrations. Sulpiride, a benzamide, is a selective D_2 dopamine receptor antagonist (Jenner and Marsden 1981) and an effective antipsychotic drug (Härnryd et al. 1984). Sulpiride is used in a wide range of doses (800–3200 mg; Munk-Andersen et al. 1984) as an antipsychotic drug, but the basis for the dosage is poor. The results from a previous study by our group indicated that 800 mg sulpiride per day was an effective dose in the treatment of schizophrenic patients (Härnryd et al. 1984). Determination of sulpiride concentrations indicated that patients with a serum level below 1.5 µmol/l had a better clinical outcome than patients above that level (Alfredsson et al. 1984b, 1985). To further explore dose- and concentration-effect relationships of sulpiride in the treatment of schizophrenic patients a dose-response study was performed. Besides being a selective D_2 dopamine antagonist, sulpiride also has the advantages of not forming active metabolites (see Wiesel et al. 1980) and not being bound to proteins to a greater extent (40%, i.e. individual differences in protein binding do not produce major changes in the free serum concentrations of sulpiride; Alfredsson et al. 1984a).

2 Methods

The protocol of the study was approved by the ethics committee of the Karolinska Hospital, Stockholm, Sweden. Patients with an acute psychosis of the schizophrenic type were selected for the study. The research diagnostic criteria (RDC) and DSM-III-R for schizophrenia had to be fulfilled for inclusion in the study. Patients with organic brain disorder, somatic disease, or alcohol or drug abuse were excluded. No patient had taken oral neuroleptics for at least 2 weeks before the study was started. Depot neuroleptics had not been given during the last 6 months. A total of 26 patients were recruited to the study. However, two patients were excluded when it was found that they did not fulfil the inclusion criteria. Of the remaining patients 14 were men and 10 were women. The age range was 18–42 years. Physical examinations and routine blood and urine tests indicated that all the patients were physically healthy.

Sulpiride (200 mg; Dogmatil, Essex, UK; Läkemedel, Sweden) was administered to the 24 patients according to a double-blind procedure (the double-dummy technique) for 6 weeks. During the first 3 weeks a daily dose of

400 mg ($n=8$), 800 mg ($n=9$) or 1200 mg ($n=7$) was given. After 3 weeks of treatment the daily dose was increased from 400 to 800 mg ($n=8$) and from 800 to 1200 mg ($n=4$) or decreased from 800 to 400 mg ($n=5$) and from 1200 to 800 mg ($n=7$). Sulpiride was administered in two equal doses at 8 a.m. and 8 p.m.

Psychiatric morbidity of the patients was rated with the Comprehensive Psychopathological Rating Scale (CPRS). In the evaluation of the patients global morbidity scores (range, 0–3) and a subscale (CPRSΣ10) was used, consisting of the following 10 CPRS items: inattention, indecision, concentration difficulties, reduced sleep, feeling controlled, disrupted thoughts, ideas of persecution, commenting voices, lack of appropriate emotion, incoherent speech (Härnryd et al. 1984). Each item had a range of 0–3. Ratings were made before treatment and after 1, 3, 4 and 6 weeks of treatment. Ratings of observed extrapyramidal side effects and reported side effects were performed directly after the CPRS ratings (Härnryd et al. 1984).

The sulpiride concentrations in serum were analysed by high-performance liquid chromatography (Alfredsson et al. 1979). All patients had been fasting for 12 h before blood sampling, which was made at 8 a.m. before the morning dose. The serum fractions were stored below $-70\,°C$ pending the analysis. Blood sampling was made before and once per week during treatment.

Analysis of variance (ANOVA) for repeated measurements was used for comparison of differences among the four treatment groups. Student's t test was used for analysis of differences within groups (dependent data) and between groups (independent data). Two-tailed tests were used. The product-moment correlation coefficient was calculated to study relationships between clinical ratings and sulpiride concentrations.

3 Results

The different doses of sulpiride resulted in a wide range of serum concentrations (Fig. 1). The dose change after 3 weeks of treatment resulted in the expected changes of sulpiride concentrations, i.e. a dose elevation was related to an increase of sulpiride concentrations and a dose reduction with a decrease of sulpiride concentrations (Fig. 2).

Clinical morbidity scores, their changes from pretreatment scores or the occurrence of side effects were not dose dependent (ANOVA repeated measurements). The rating scores of psychotic symptoms (CPRSΣ10) were significantly decreased after 3 weeks of treatment in all groups (Fig. 3). After 6 weeks of treatment only the group with a decrease of the dose from 800 to 400 mg per day did not demonstrate a significant reduction in morbidity scores. Morbidity scores for autistic symptoms were significantly reduced only in the group who started the treatment with the highest dose 1200 mg per day. The reduction in scores was significant both after 3 weeks and after 6 weeks of treatment. Global morbidity was changed in a similar way as the scores of the CPRSΣ10.

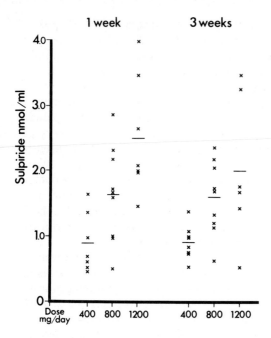

Fig. 1. Concentrations of sulpiride in serum from schizophrenic patients treated with different doses

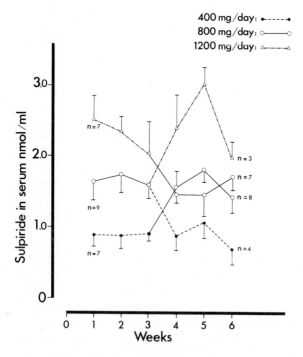

Fig. 2. Concentrations of sulpiride in serum from schizophrenic patients treated with sulpiride in three different dosages. After 3 weeks of treatment the dose was increased or decreased. In the 800 mg/day group, four patients were changed to 1200 mg/day and 5 patients to 400 mg/day. Differences in patient numbers are due to loss(es) of blood sample(s) at a particular day. Mean values ± SE

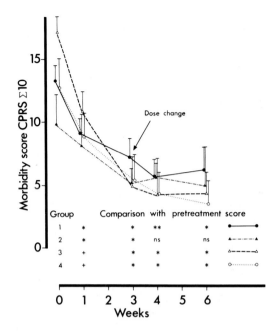

Fig. 3. The sum of morbidity scores from ten items in the CPRS. After 3 weeks of treatment the doses were changes: group 1, from 400 to 800 mg/day ($n=8$); group 2, from 800 to 400 mg/day ($n=5$); group 3, from 800 to 1200 mg/day ($n=4$); group 4, from 1200 to 800 mg/day ($n=7$). Mean values $\pm$ SE

Relationships between clinical effects and sulpiride concentrations were investigated by correlating all sulpiride and clinical measurements at each point in time. No significant correlations between sulpiride concentrations and morbidity scores or their changes from pretreatment levels were found, except a single negative correlation between the change in global scores and sulpiride concentrations after 1 week ($r = -0.45$, $p < 0.05$). Neither were there any significant correlations between sulpiride concentrations and side effects at any point in time.

To further analyse relationships between clinical morbidity and sulpiride concentrations patients were divided into three groups: (a) a low-concentration group ($n=4$; 0.48–0.71 µmol/l), i.e. patients below the median concentration level in the low-dose group (400 mg); (b) a high-concentration group ($n=4$; 2.36–3.44 µmol/l), i.e. patients above the median concentration in the high-dose group (1200 mg); and (c) a medium-concentration group consisting of the remaining patients ($n=16$). The division into the groups was made on the basis of each patient's average concentration of sulpiride calculated from the levels after 1, 2 and 3 weeks of treatment. Rating scores after 6 weeks of treatment were compared with the pretreatment scores within each group. Rating scores between groups were compared at each point in time. Scores on the CPRSΣ10 were significantly lower in the high-concentration group than in the medium-concentration group after 3, 4 and 6 weeks of treatment (Fig. 4). The autistic symptoms demonstrated similar significant changes as did the scores on the CPRSΣ10. Global morbidity was significantly reduced in all groups after 6 weeks of treatment. However, the high-concentration group had significantly lower scores than both the low- and medium-concentration groups.

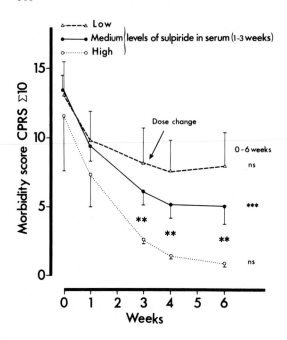

Fig. 4. Scores on the CPRSΣ10 in schizophrenic patients in relation to sulpiride concentrations in serum. Patients were divided into a low-concentration group (0.48–0.71 μmol/l; $n=4$), a high-concentration group (2.36–3.44 μmol/l; $n=4$), and a medium-concentration group (remaining patients, $n=16$). Mean values $\pm$ SE. $\star\star$, $p<0.01$; $\star\star\star$, $p<0.001$

4 Discussion

In a previous study we obtained indications of a therapeutic concentration level (<1.5 μmol/l) of sulpiride in the treatment of schizophrenic patients (Alfredsson et al. 1984b, 1985). The design of this study was made to investigate the hypothesis of a therapeutic concentration interval of sulpiride. However, we could not demonstrate a correlation between clinical improvement and the sulpiride dose or its serum concentration. This was also the case for side effects. Changes in dosage or drug concentrations during treatment did not seem to influence the clinical outcome.

A wide range of sulpiride concentrations was obtained, and indications of a lower limit of the concentration for the therapeutic response was found. This level was 0.6–0.7 μmol/l. It seemed as if the patients with this low concentration during the early phase of treatment had a worse outcome than the other patients after 6 weeks of treatment despite an increase of their drug concentrations during the final 3 weeks of treatment. From a clinical point of view the results indicate that a moderate dose (800–1200 mg) of sulpiride, resulting in drug concentrations above 0.7 μmol/l, should be used in the early phase of treatment. The utility of prompt dose changes should be carefully considered since there is obviously a delay in the clinical effect. It may be speculated that this delay corresponds to the kinetics of the D_2 dopamine receptor blockade (Farde et al. 1988).

The use of a selective D_2 dopamine receptor antagonist gave similar negative results as did the classical neuroleptics in the study of relationships between clinical response and drug concentrations (Dahl 1986). The negative findings may indicate that a diagnosis of schizophrenia includes too heterogenous a patient group to allow a demonstration of such a relationship. It is also possible that regardless of their mode of action, the pharmacodynamic effects of neuroleptics are not at all linearly related to their clinical effects. In fact, some studies have obtained results supporting a curvilinear relationship (Smith et al. 1984; Garver et al. 1984; Hansen et al. 1982). Such a relationship is in accordance with findings suggesting that the blockade of central D_2 dopamine receptors in the living human brain follows a hyperbolic function (Farde et al. 1988). In fact, in a sulpiride-treated patient a curvilinear relationship was demonstrated between central D_2 dopamine receptor occupancy and serum drug concentrations.

Acknowledgements. The assistance of Ms. B. Berthelsson and Ms. K. Lind is gratefully acknowledged as well as that of Ms. M. Youssefi for preparing the manuscript.

References

Alfredsson G, Sedvall G, Wiesel F-A (1979) Quantitative analysis of sulpiride in body fluids by high performance liquid chromatography with fluorescence detection. J Chromatogr 164:187–193

Alfredsson G, Bjerkenstedt L, Edman G, Härnryd C, Oxenstierna G, Sedvall G, Wiesel F-A (1984a) Relationships between drug concentrations in serum and CSF, clinical effects and monoaminergic variables in schizophrenic patients treated with sulpiride or chlorpromazine. Acta Psychiatr Scand [Suppl 311] 69:49–74

Alfredsson G, Härnryd C, Wiesel F-A (1984b) Effects of sulpiride and chlorpromazine on depressive symptoms in schizophrenic patients – relationship to drug concentrations. Psychopharmacology (Berlin) 84:237–241

Alfredsson G, Härnryd C, Wiesel F-A (1985) Effects of sulpiride and chlorpromazine on autistic and positive psychotic symptoms in schizophrenic patients – relationship to drug concentrations. Psychopharmacology (Berlin) 85:8–13

Baldessarini RJ, Davis JM (1980) What is the best maintenance dose of neuroleptics in schizophrenia? Psychiatry Res 3:115–122

Baldessarini RJ, Katz BK, Cotton P (1984) Dissimilar dosing with high-potency and low-potency neuroleptics. Am J Psychiatry 141:748–752

Dahl SG (1986) Plasma level monitoring of antipsychotic drugs. Clinical utility. Clin Pharmacokinet 11:36–61

Farde L, Wiesel F-A, Halldin C, Sedvall G (1988) Central D_2-dopamine receptor occupancy in schizophrenic patients treated with antipsychotic drugs. Arch Gen Psychiatry 45:71–76

Garver DL, Hirschowitz J, Glicksteen GA, Kanter DR, Mavroidis ML (1984) Haloperidol plasma and red blood cell levels and clinical antipsychotic response. J Clin Psychopharmacol 4:133–137

Härnryd C, Bjerkenstedt L, Björk K, Gullberg B, Oxenstierna G, Sedvall G, Wiesel F-A et al. (1984) Clinical evaluation of sulpiride in schizophrenic patients – a double-blind comparison with chlorpromazine. Acta Psychiatr Scand [Suppl 311] 69:7–30

Hansen LB, Larsen N-E, Gulmann N (1982) Dose-response relationships of perphenazine in the treatment of acute psychoses. Psychopharmacology (Berlin) 78:112–115

Jain AK, Kelwala S, Gershon S (1988) Antipsychotic drugs in schizophrenia: current issues. Int Clin Psychopharmacol 3:1–30

Jenner P, Marsden DD (1981) Substituted benzamide drugs as selective neuroleptic agents. Neuropharmacology 20:1285–1293

Munk-Andersen E, Behnke K, Heltberg J, Nielsen H, Gerlach J (1984) Sulpiride versus haloperidol, a clinical trial in schizophrenia. A preliminary report. Acta Psychiatr Scand [Suppl 311] 69:31–41

Peroutka SJ, Snyder SH (1980) Relationship of neuroleptic drug effects at brain dopamine, serotonin, α-adrenergic, and histamine receptors to clinical potency. Am J Psychiatry 137:1518–1522

Smith RC, Baumgartner R, Misra CH, Mauldin M, Shvartsburd A et al. (1984) Plasma levels and prolactin response as predictors of clinical improvement in schizophrenia: chemical v radioreceptor plasma level assays. Arch Gen Psychiatry 41:1044–1049

Stille G, Hippius H (1971) Kritische Stellungnahme zum Begriff der Neuroleptika (anhand von pharmakologischen und klinischen Befunden mit Clozapin). Pharmacopsychiatry 4:182–191

Wiesel F-A, Alfredsson G, Ehrnebo M, Sedvall G (1980) The pharmacokinetics of intravenous and oral sulpiride in healthy human subjects. Eur J Clin Pharmacol 17:385–391

Post-Marketing Surveillance of Psychotropic Drugs

R. BRINKMANN [1]

1 Introduction

At the end of a highly sophisticated scientific programme, the author has the honour as well as the difficulty to consider more generally the field of post-marketing surveillance of psychotropic drugs. Although post-marketing surveillance has gained considerable attention in recent years, little has been published about post-marketing surveillance of psychotropic drugs in general. In their introduction to *Post-marketing Surveillance of Psychotherapeutic Drugs,* Hollister and Balter (1987) do not touch upon any aspect of post-marketing surveillance that may be specific to patients and/or physicians dealing with psychoactive compounds as opposed to other compounds. This may be only partly explained by the fact that Hollister and Balter (1987) use the term post-marketing surveillance synonymously with phase IV studies, which usually include a minimum number of 10 000 patients and follow documented study protocols and statistical evaluation procedures. But post-marketing surveillance techniques refer to more than phase IV studies. Post-marketing surveillance is defined as *all methods to understand more precisely the benefits and risks of drugs under normal prescribing conditions.* For practical reasons, post-marketing surveillance can be divided into single-patient surveillance and population-oriented surveillance.

In this presentation some of the basic problems that are pertinent to both types of post-marketing surveillance techniques will be outlined. In addition, only the risk assessment part of post-marketing surveillance, i.e. the detection of adverse drug reactions, is elaborated further.

Pre-marketing clinical trials often fail to discover what are subsequently known to be rare but important adverse drug reactions (Hemminki 1980; Skegg 1979) simply because the number of patients involved in the usual three phases of new drug development may vary between 500 and 3000. This is also true for the development of psychotropic drugs.

Psychotropic drugs are not as clearly defined as one might wish. Certainly, they involve drugs for the treatment of mental disorders – psychotherapeutic drugs – but drugs for therapy of CNS-controlled functions such as pain, sleep and pleasure (and placebo drugs) may also be regarded as psychotropic drugs.

---

[1] F. Hoffmann-La Roche AG, Pharma Communications, Grenzacherstr. 124, 4002 Basel, Switzerland

Clinical Pharmacology in Psychiatry
Editors: S. G. Dahl and L. F. Gram
(Psychopharmacology Series 7)
© Springer-Verlag Berlin Heidelberg 1989

For the purpose of this presentation any drug which interferes with the regulation of brain functions and which modifies mental processes is regarded as a psychotropic drug.

2 Detection of Adverse Drug Reactions

Before any of the specificities of post-marketing surveillance of psychotropic drugs can be addressed, a basic model of the generation of adverse drug reactions must be presented. The model shown in Fig. 1 is not very elaborate but is sufficiently complex for our purposes. With regard to terminology, the term "adverse drug reaction" is used throughout this presentation although this actually implies that there is some kind of a causal relationship between the suspected drug and the observed adverse experience of the patient. This is why some prefer the term "adverse event" in order not to prejudge causal relationships, because all adverse drug reactions are adverse events, but not all adverse events are adverse drug reactions.

Included in the darkened area of Fig. 1 are the minimum requirements for an adverse drug reaction generation: exposure to a drug (drug 2), the exposed patient (organism), and the adverse drug reaction (R3) which is then *interpreted* as the adverse drug reaction. This is why all primary reactions (R1, R2, R3) are surrounded by a striped area indicating that this important part of objectivity will always reach the recipient of an adverse drug reaction report in an interpreted form. Hence, it must be borne in mind that other reactions of the organism (R1 and R2) will be interpreted as "normal" or "disease-related" behaviour/reaction. Other factors that might have influenced the adverse drug reaction are also shown in Fig. 1: the physico-chemical environment of the organism, the socio-cultural environment of the patient, and the co-medications, drug 1 and drug 3, which are interpreted as being apparently irrelevant to the adverse drug reaction in question.

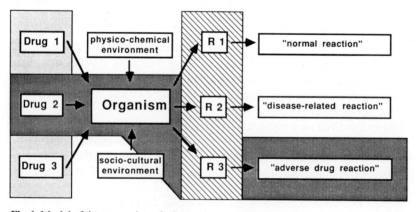

Fig. 1. Model of the generation of adverse drug reactions

When this general model of the generation of adverse drug reactions is applied to the realities of post-marketing surveillance, we must observe that usually nothing is known about all "normal" reactions; neither do we know anything about the physico-chemical environment of the organism. We also know little or nothing about the socio-cultural environment, and we usually have very little information on the organism, i.e. laboratory values, medical history, and other examinations and assessments. Most of the time we even know very little about concomitant medications as well as the pattern of reactions that were interpreted as being disease related.

The reality of adverse drug reaction generation is, again, substantially different from this adverse drug reaction model. First of all, only about 5%–10% of all adverse drug reactions are reported once a drug is on the market (Stephens 1985), and even this figure is true only for some of the highly industrialized Western countries. This high degree of underreporting is even more important when it is realized that at least 100 000 adverse drug reactions in hospitals alone delay recovery or threaten life each year (Imman 1985).

Within this framework of post-marketing surveillance we must now concentrate on aspects that are specific to patients and/or physicians dealing with psychotropic drugs. Specificity may be related to (a) the pharmacology of psychotropic drugs, (b) the kind of adverse drug reactions to be expected, or (c) the sources of information underlying the adverse drug reaction generation.

Adverse drug reactions due to psychotropic drugs affect predominantly the CNS, but all other organ systems may be involved. For further information the reader is referred to standard textbooks (Ammon 1986; Davies 1985; Gilman et al. 1985; Kuemmerle and Goosens 1984; Martindale 1982). The classification of adverse drug reactions proposed by Rawlins and Thompson (1985) is now widely accepted. According to them, adverse drug reactions can be separated into those which are an exaggerated, but otherwise normal, pharmacological action of a drug given in the usual therapeutic doses (type A reactions) and those which are totally aberrant effects that are not to be expected from known pharmacological actions of a drug when given in the usual therapeutic doses (type B reactions).

The sources of information are typically patients, lay observers or reports in lay media, pharmacists, medical doctors, the professional media, post-marketing surveillance studies, and surveillance institutions of public health authorities (Table 1). These sources provide a great variety of information on adverse drug reactions. With regard to psychotropic drugs, it is obvious that psychiatric patients differ in a number of aspects that are relevant to adverse drug reaction generation when compared to other patient groups, and the same is true for psychiatrists when compared to other medical doctors, although in a different sense, of course.

Table 1. Information sources in post-marketing surveillance

Single-patient surveillance
Spontaneous case reports
Literature case reports, letter-to-the-editor reports
Intensive monitoring
Semi-official ADR institutions
National ADR centres, public health authorities
Population-oriented surveillance
Intensive hospital monitoring
Prescription event monitoring (UK)
Record linkage (USA)
Case-control studies, cohort studies

3 Surveillance of Psychotropic Drugs

With regard to the fundamental question of this presentation, i.e. "What makes post-marketing surveillance of psychotropic drugs different from that of any other drug?", the author firmly believes that the specific distortions of the general adverse drug reaction model by patients and/or physicians dealing with psychotropic drugs are the main reason for any specificity in this field of post-marketing surveillance.

Three levels in the generation of adverse drug reactions must be looked at more closely: perception, cognition, or comprehension, and expression. Perception may be a problem if the sensory organs of the patient externally or internally, are not able to detect the adverse drug reaction, as in the case of haemolytic anaemia, liver dysfunction, or agranulocytosis, to mention only some sources of adverse drug reactions that led finally to withdrawal or heavy restrictions of some well-known psychotropic drugs (nomifensine, clozapine). On the other hand, psychiatric patients in particular may have a distorted perception per se. The physician or, as in our case, the psychiatrist, may not be equipped with appropriate devices for the detection of adverse drug reactions which do not fall into the realm of his standard diagnostic apparatus, as in the case of agranulocytosis due to clozapine.

With regard to cognition and comprehension, the psychiatric patient may be highly susceptible to internal or external influences because of hypochondria or because of a weak personality or low threshold for critical thinking. Psychiatric patients sometimes attribute causality on the basis of irrational conceptions: an example for this has been reported from the United States, where a patient claimed to have lost his ability to think after having had a computed-tomography scan of the head. The physician, on the other hand, may be somewhat careless or inconsiderate according to his socio-cultural background, and although this may sound like a rather harsh criticism, we must acknowledge that there are certainly differences among physicians with respect to their basic attitude towards adverse drug reaction detection. Even pharmaco-epidemiological studies may be misleading because of a lack of reliable and valid methodology, and this is particularly true for any distinction between disease-related reactions or behaviour and drug-related reactions or behaviour.

Finally, we must look at the way in which an adverse drug reaction is *expressed* by a psychiatric patient. In fact, patients may not be able to give an appropriate account because of age, underlying disease, or basic intelligence impairment. Also, Physicians other than psychiatrists may use misleading terminology. It is our experience that substantial confusion exists, for instance, about the use of terms such as addiction, dependence, misuse, abuse and overuse by physicians who have had no psychiatric training. On the other hand, a psychiatrist may also use inappropriate terminology for the description of dermatological reactions or other organic diseases that he heard of only during medical school.

Another problem is created by the fact that a physician may tend to give a distorted description of an adverse drug reaction in order to prevent criticism or prosecution for malpractice. An example of this is the inappropriate use of a sedative for conscious sedation in diagnostic procedures which leads to excessive sedation and life-threatening conditions for the patient. Finally, studies may apply inappropriate statistical evaluation methods and report "significant" results when in fact the wrong statistical method was chosen.

In conclusion, the author hopes to have contributed to a better understanding of adverse drug reactions as being one of the fundamentals of post-marketing surveillance. In addition, the basic role of perception, cognition, and expression with particular reference to patients and physicians dealing with psychotropic drugs has been pointed to as one of the main aspects that makes post-marketing surveillance of psychotropic drugs different from that of any other drug.

References

Ammon HPT (ed) (1986) Arzneimittelneben- und -wechselwirkungen, 2nd edn. Wissenschaftliche Verlagsgesellschaft, Stuttgart

Davies DM (ed) (1985) Textbook of adverse drug reactions, 3rd edn. Oxford University Press, Oxford

Gilman AG, Goodman LS, Rall TW, Murad F (eds) (1985) Goodman and Gilman's the pharmacological basis of therapeutics, 7th edn. Macmillan, New York

Hemminki L (1980) Study of information submitted by drug companies to licensing authorities. Br Med J 1:836

Hollister LE, Balter MB (1987) Postmarketing surveillance of psychotropic drugs. Psychopharmacol Bull 23:387–388

Inman WHW (1985) Detection and investigation of adverse drug reactions. In: Davies DM (ed) Textbook of adverse drug reactions, 3rd edn. Oxford University Press, Oxford, pp 49–62

Kuemmerle HP, Goosens N (1984) Klinik und Therapie der Nebenwirkungen, 3rd edn. Thieme, Stuttgart

Martindale (1982) The extra pharmacopoeia, 28th edn. Pharmaceutical Press, London

Rawlins MD, Thompson JW (1985) Mechanisms of adverse drug reactions. In: Davies DM (ed) Textbook of adverse drug reactions, 3rd edn. Oxford University Press, Oxford

Skegg DCG (1979) Adverse reaction monitoring in the future. In: Macleod N (ed) Pharmaceutical medicine. Livingstone, Edinburgh, p 144

Stephens MDB (1985) The detection of adverse drug reactions. Stockton, New York

List of Participants

AARBAKKE, JARLE, Dr.
Institute of Medical Biology
University of Tromsø
P.O.Box 977
N-9001 Tromsø
Norway

ÅGREN, HANS, Dr.
Department of Psychiatry
University Hospital
S-751 85 Uppsala
Sweden

ALTAMURA, A.C., Dr.
Department of Psychiatry
University of Milan
Via F. Sforza 35
I-20122 Milan
Italy

ARESVIK, STÅLE, Dr.
Janssen Pharma, Postboks 113
N-1415 Oppegård
Norway

BACCINO, ERIC, Dr.
Service Sébileau
Hôpital Augustin Morvan
5 avenue Foch
F-29 285 Brest Cedex
France

BALANT, LUC P., Dr.
Département de Psychiatrie
Case postale 79
CH-1211 Geneva 8
Switzerland

BALANT-GORGIA, A.E., Dr.
Unité Monitoring Thérapeutique
Département de Psychiatrie
Centre Médical Universitaire
CH-1211 Geneva 4
Switzerland

BARON, J.C., Dr.
INSERM Unit 320
CYCERON
Bôite Postale 5027
F-14021 Caen Cedex
France

BAUMANN, PIERRE, Dr.
Hopital de Cery
Clinique Psychiatrique
Universitaire
Canton de Vaud
CH-1008 Prilly
Switzerland

BECH, PER, Dr.
Frederiksborg General Hospital
Department of Psychiatry
Dyrehavevej 48
DK-3400 Hillerød
Denmark

BENITEZ, JULIO, Dr.
Department of Pharmacology
School of Medicine
University of Extremadura
E-06071 Badajoz
Spain

BERGMAN, THORVALD, Mr.
Essex Läkemedel AB
P.O. Box 27 190
S-102 52 Stockholm
Sweden

BERTILSSON, LEIF, Dr.
Department of Clinical
Pharmacology
Huddinge University Hospital
S-141 86 Huddinge
Sweden

BJERKE, CARSTEN, Dr.
Psychogeriatric Department
9010 Åsgård Psychiatric Hospital
N-9001 Tromsø
Norway

BJERKENSTEDT, LARS, Dr.
Department of Psychiatry
Danderyd Hospital
S-182 88 Danderyd
Sweden

BJÖRK, ANDERS, Dr.
AB Ferrosan
P.O. Box 839
S-201 80 Malmö
Sweden

BOLWIG, TOM G., Dr.
Psychiatric Department O
Rigshospitalet
Blegdamsvej 9
DK-2100 Copenhagen Ø
Denmark

BOURIN, MICHEL, Dr.
Pharmacologie Clinique
C.H.U. de Nantes
1, Rue Gaston Veil
F-44035 Nantes Cedex
France

BRÆSTRUP, CLAUS, Dr.
Pharmaceuticals R & D
NOVO Industri A/S
DK-2880 Bagsverd
Denmark

BRATLID, TROND, Dr.
9010 Åsgård Psychiatric Hospital
N-9001 Tromsø
Norway

BREKKE-NILSEN, BJØRN, Dr.
9010 Åsgård Psychiatric Hospital
N-9001 Tromsø
Norway

BRINKMANN, RUDIGER, Dr.
Pharma Communications
F. Hoffmann-La Roche
Grenzacherstr. 124
CH-4002 Basel
Switzerland

BRØSEN, KIM, Dr.
Dept. Clin. Pharmacology
Odense University
J.B. Winsløws vej 19
DK-5000 Odense C
Denmark

CALIL, HELENA M., Dr.
Depto. de Psicobiologia
Escola Paulista de Medicina
Rua Botucatu, 862 – 1° andar
04034 Sao Paulo
Brazil

CAMERON, ANNE, Dr.
Roche Norge A/S
P.O. Box 41, Haugenstua
N-0915 Oslo 9
Norway

CASEY, DANIEL E., Dr.
Psychiatric Service (116A)
V.A. Medical Center
P.O. Box 1034
Portland, OR 97207
USA

CHOPIN, PHILIP, Dr.
17 Avenue Jean Molin
Centre de Recherche Pierre Fabre
F-8100 Castres
France

CHRISTENSEN, ANNE V., Dr.
Sct. Hans Hospital
Department E
DK-4000 Roskilde
Denmark

DAHL, SVEIN G., Dr.
Instute of Medical Biology
University of Tromsø
P.O. Box 977
N-9001 Tromsø
Norway

DAHL-PUUSTINEN, M.-L., Dr.
Department of
Clinical Pharmacology
Huddinge University Hospital
S-141 86 Huddinge
Sweden

DELINI-STULA, ALEXANDRA, Dr.
Ciba-Geigy Ltd.
PH 2.19
Ch-4002 Basel
Switzerland

DENCKER, SVEN J., Dr.
Klinik II
Lillhagen's Hospital
Box 3005
S-422 03 Hisings Backa
Sweden

DOROW, RAINER, Dr.
Schering AG Pharm. Research
Postfach 650 311
D-1000 Berlin (West) 65
FRG

DOSE, MATHIAS, Dr.
Max-Planck-Institut für Psychiatrie
Kraepelinstrasse 10
D–8000 München 40
FRG

DREYFUS, J.-F., Dr.
Jouveinal Laboratoires
1, rue des Moissons
Sofilic 423
F-94 263 Fresnes Cedex
France

EBERHARD, GÖRAN, Dr.
Department of Psychiatry
Malmö General Hospital
S-214 01 Malmö
Sweden

EKDAL, PER, Dr.
9012 Åsgård Psychiatric Hospital
N-9001 Tromsø
Norway

EMRICH, H.M., Dr.
Max-Planck-Institut für Psychiatrie
Kraepelinstrasse 10
D-8000 München 40
FRG

FARDE, LARS, Dr.
Department of Psychiatry
Karolinska Hospital
S-10401 Stockholm
Sweden

FOG, RASMUS, Dr.
Sct. Hans Hospital
Department E
DK-4000 Roskilde
Denmark

GAILLOT, JEAN, Dr.
Département de Biodynamique
Institut de Biopharmacie
Rhône-Poulenc Santé
20 Avenue Raymond Aron
F-92160 Antony
France

GARVER, DAVID L., Dr.
Department of Psychiatry
231 Bethesda Avenue (ML 559)
Cincinnati, OH 45267
USA

GENTIL, VALENTIM, Dr.
Universidade De Sao Paulo
Rua Oscar Freire, 587
01426 Sao Paulo
Brazil

GEREBTZOFF, ALEXANDER, Dr.
Ciba-Geigy Ltd.
PH 2.19
CH-4002 Basel
Switzerland

GHANY, IGBAL M., Dr.
St. Ann's Hospital
110 Frederick Street
Port-of-Spain
Trinidad W.I.
Spain

GRAM, LARS F., Dr.
Dept. Clin. Pharmacology
Odense University
J.B. Winsløws vej 19
DK-5000 Odense C
Denmark

GREENWOOD, DAVID, Dr.
Medical Research Dept.
ICI Pharmaceuticals Div.
Mereside Alderly Park
Macclesfield
Cheshire SK10 4TG
United Kingdom

HAFFNER, FRODE, Dr.
Lier Psychiatric Hospital
N-1340 Lier
Norway

HALL, HÅKAN, Dr.
Astra Research Centre Södertälje,
CNS Research and Development,
Neuropharmacology, CNS 2,
S-151 85 Södertälje
Sweden

HALS, PETTER-ARNT, Dr.
Department of Pharmacology
Nycomed AS
P.O. Box 4220 Torshov
N-0401 Oslo 4
Norway

HEFFNER, THOMAS G., Dr.
Department of Pharmacology
Parke-Davis
Pharmaceutical Research
2800 Plymouth Road
Ann Arbor, MI 48105
USA

HENINGER, GEORGE R., Dr.
Abraham Ribicoff
Research Facilities
Yale University
34 Park Street
New Haven, CT 06508
USA

HENNING, MATTS, Dr.
Ciba-Geigy
P.O. Box 605
S-421 26 Västra Frölunda
Sweden

HYTTEL, JOHN, Dr.
H. Lundbeck A/S
Ottiliavej 7–9
DK-2500 Valby
Denmark

JOHNSEN, HELGE, Dr.
Norwegian Defence Research
Establishment
Div. for Environmental
Toxicology
P.O. Box 25
N-7002 Kjeller
Norway

KALOW, WERNER, Dr.
Department of Pharmacology
Medical Sciences Building
University of Toronto
Toronto
Canada M5S 1A8

KLEIN, MARCEL, Dr.
Institut Roussel Uclaf
102,111, Route de Noisy – B.P. 9
F-93 230 Romainville
France

KNORRING, LARS VON, Dr.
Departments of Psychiatry
University of Umeå
S-90 185 Umeå
Sweden

KNORRING, ANNE-LIS VON, Dr.
Department of Child and Youth
Psychiatry
University of Umeå
S-90 185 Umeå
Sweden

KOSSMANN, LOUIS, Dr.
Laboratoires Delagrange
1, avenue Pierre Brossolette
F-91380 Chilly-Mazarin
France

LAVOISY, J., Dr.
Laboratoires ICI-Pharma
1, rue des Chauffours
B.P. 127
F-95022 Cergy Cedex
France

LECRUBIER, YVES, Dr.
Hôpital de la Salpêtrière
Chargé de Recherche INSERM
47, Bd de L'Hôpital
F-Paris 75651 Cedex 13
France

LIDÉN, ANDERS, Dr.
Dept. Psychiatry
and Neurochemistry
University of Lund
P.O. Box 638
S-220 06 Lund
Sweden

LINDBERGET, JOSTEIN, Dr.
Organon A/S
P.O. Box 325
N-1372 Asker
Norway

LINGJÆRDE, ODD, Dr.
Gaustad Psychiatric Hospital
P.O. Box 24 Gaustad
N-0320 Oslo 3
Norway

LINK, C.G.G., Dr.
Beecham Pharmaceuticals
Medicinal Research Centre
Coldharbour Road
The Pinnacles
Harlow, Essex CM19 5AD
United Kingdom

LOVENBERG, WALTER, Dr.
Merrell Dow Research Institute
Strasbourg Research Center
16, rue d'Ankara
F-67084 Strasbourg Cedex
France

LUND, JØRGEN, Dr.
Ferrosan Group
Sydmarken 5
DK-2860 Søborg
Denmark

MELTZER, HERBERT Y., Dr.
Department of Psychiatry
Case Western Reserve University
School of Medicine
2040 Abington Road
Cleveland, OH 44106
USA

MARDER, STEVEN R., Dr.
West L.A. VA Medical Center
Brentwood Division
11301 Wilshire Blvd.
Los Angeles, CA 90073
USA

MESTIKAWY, S. EL, Dr.
INSERM U 288
91 Boulevard de l' Hôpital
F-75 634 Paris Cedex 13
France

MEYER, URS, Dr.
Department of Pharmacology
Biocenter
University of Basel
CH-4056 Basel
Switzerland

MONTGOMERY, STUART A., Dr.
Academic Dept. of Psychiatry
St. Mary's Hospital
Praed Street
London W2 1NY
United Kingdom

MUSCH, BRUNO, Dr.
CNS Clinical Research
Rhône-Poulenc Santé
20, Avenue Raymond Cedex
F-92165 Antony Cedex
France

MÅRTENSSON, ERIK, Dr.
Psychiatric Department III
Lillhagen's Hospital
S-42203 Hisings Backa 3
Sweden

NELSON, J. CRAIG, Dr.
Department of Psychiatry
Yale Univ. School of Medicine
333 Cedar Street
New Haven, CT 06504
USA

NILSEN, CLAES, Dr.
Eli-Lilly
Tømmerup Stationsvej 10
DK-2770 Kastrup
Denmark

NILSSON, HEIMO L., Dr.
Ciba-Geigy
Box 605
S-421 26 Västra Frölunda
Sweden

NYBERG, GÖSTA, Dr.
Department III
Lillhagen Hospital
S-422 03 Hisings Backa
Sweden

POLLOCK, BRUCE G., Dr.
Department of Psychiatry
University of Pittsburgh
School of Medicine
Western Psychiatric
Institute and Clinic
3811 O'Hara Street
Pittsburgh, PA 15213
USA

POTTER, WILLIAM Z., Dr.
Clinical Psychobiology Branch
NIMH, Building 10 Room 2D46
9000 Rockville Pike
Bethesda, MD 20892
USA

POURRIAS, B., Dr.
Centre de Recherche Delalande
10, rue des Carriers
F-92 500 Rueil-Malmaison
France

PRESKORN, SHELDON H., Dr.
Department of Psychiatry 452/116
University of Kansas
School of Medicine-Wichita
1010 N. Kansas
Wichita, KS 67214
USA

PUECH, ALAIN, Dr.
Département de
Pharmacologie Clinique
Groupe Hospitalier Pitié-Salpêtrière
47, Boulevard de l'Hôpital
F-75651 Paris Cédex 13
France

REISBY, NILS. Dr.
Århus Psychiatric Hospital
DK-8240 Risskov
Denmark

REITEN, ÅSLAUG, Dr.
Upjohn Informasjon
Postboks 6749 St. Olavs plass
N-0130 Oslo 1
Norway

RUTZ, WOLFGANG, Dr.
Norrahansegatan 4
S-621 00 Visby
Sweden

SAGER, GEORG, Dr.
Institute of Medical Biology
University of Tromsø
P.O. Box 977
N-9001 Tromsø
Norway

SCHUSTER, MARTIN, Dr.
9010 Åsgård Psychiatric Hospital
N-9001 Tromsø
Norway

SCHWARTZ, J.C., Dr.
Unité de Neurobiologie
Centre Paul Broca de l' INSERM
2 ter, Rue d' Alesia
F-75014 Paris
France

SIEGHART, WERNER, Dr.
Psychiatrische Universitätsklinik
Währinger Gürtel 18–20
A-1090 Wien
Austria

SIMON, PIERRE, Dr.
Societé Sanofi Recherche
37 Avenue Pierre 1er de Serbie
F-75008 Paris
France

SITSEN, J.M.A., Dr.
Scientific Development Group
Organon International BV
P.O. Box 20
NL-5340 BH Oss
The Netherlands

SJÖQVIST, FOLKE, Dr.
Department of Clinical
Pharmacology
Huddinge University Hospital
S-141 86 Huddinge
Sweden

SPINA, EDOARDO, Dr.
Institute of Pharmacology
University of Messina
Piazza XX Settembre, 4
I-98100 Messina
Italy

TEIGEN, LISE, Dr.
Sentipharm AG
Aslakveien 14
N-0753 Oslo 7
Norway

THIEKÖTTER, THOMAS, Dr.
Springer-Verlag
Postfach 10 52 80
D-6900 Heidelberg 1
FRG

VESTERGAARD, PER, Dr.
Århus Psychiatric Hospital
DK-8240 Risskov
Denmark

VON BAHR, CHRISTER, Dr.
Department of Clinical
Pharmacology
Astra Research Centre
S-151 85 Södertälje
Sweden

WAHLÉN, ANITA, Dr.
Astra Alab AB
S-151 85 Södertälje
Sweden

WAKELIN, J.S., Dr.
Duphar
Clinical Research Department
P.O. Box 900
NL-1380 DA Weesp
The Netherlands

WIESEL, FRITS-AXEL, Dr.
Department of
Psychiatry and Psychology
Karolinska Hospital
S-10401 Stockholm
Sweden

WIK, GUSTAV, Dr.
9012 Åsgård Psychiatric Hospital
N-9001 Tromsø
Norway

WILLIAMS, D. CLIVE, Dr.
Dept. of Biochemistry
Trinity College
Dublin 2
Ireland

Subject Index

Page numbers given are the first pages of chapters in which the subject listed is discussed